KU-659-218

indian head massage

4th edition

Helen McGuinness

HODDER EDUCATION
AN HACHETTE UK COMPANY

Although every effort has been made to ensure that website addresses are correct at time of going to press, Hodder Education cannot be held responsible for the content of any website mentioned in this book. It is sometimes possible to find a relocated web page by typing in the address of the home page for a website in the URL window of your browser.

Hachette UK's policy is to use papers that are natural, renewable and recyclable products and made from wood grown in sustainable forests. The logging and manufacturing processes are expected to conform to the environmental regulations of the country of origin.

Orders: please contact Bookpoint Ltd, 130 Milton Park, Abingdon, Oxon OX14 4SB. Telephone: +44 (0)1235 827827. Fax: +44 (0)1235 400401. Lines are open from 9.00a.m. to 5.00p.m., Monday to Saturday, with a 24-hour message-answering service. Visit our website at www.hoddereducation.co.uk

© Helen McGuinness 2012

First edition published 2000
Second edition published 2004
Third edition published 2007
This edition published 2012

Hodder Education
An Hachette UK Company
338 Euston Road
London NW1 3BH

Impression number	10	9	8	7	6	5	4	3	2	1
Year	2017	2016	2015	2014	2013	2012				

All rights reserved. Apart from any use permitted under UK copyright law, no part of this publication may be reproduced or transmitted in any form or by any means, electronic or mechanical, including photocopying and recording, or held within any information storage and retrieval system, without permission in writing from the publisher or under licence from the Copyright Licensing Agency Limited. Further details of such licences (for reprographic reproduction) may be obtained from the Copyright Licensing Agency Limited, Saffron House, 6–10 Kirby Street, London EC1N 8TS.

Cover photo © Andrew Callaghan

Illustrations by Cactus

Typeset by Integra

Printed in Italy

A catalogue record for this title is available from the British Library

ISBN: 978 1444 16822 8

Contents

Acknowledgements

I would like to acknowledge and thank the following people for their support in the development of the 4th edition of this book:

My husband Mark, for his considerable help and contributions (especially with updating Chapter 9, Health, safety, security and employment standards, and for updating the resource section for this edition), for his constant love and support, and for inspiring and encouraging me to write this book originally; to our beautiful daughter Grace for being so patient while I was writing and for providing lots of love and laughter; my dear friend (and surrogate Mum) Dee Chase, for her constant support, love and much needed encouragement throughout the writing of this book; Dr Nathan Moss for his invaluable advice for Chapter 3, Conditions affecting the head, neck and shoulders; the Maharishi Ayurvedic Centre in Lancashire, for their kind permission to use references and information on the ingredients of their hair oils; and finally, all the Indian head massage students who have encouraged me to write, and develop my writing in this edition of the book.

This edition is dedicated to my Mum Valerie, who always believed in me and encouraged me to write.

The publishers would like to thank the following for permission to reproduce copyright material:

Figure 1.1 © Floris Leeuwenberg/The Cover Story/Corbis; Figure 1.4 © Around the World in a Viewfinder/Alamy; Figure 1.5 ©Vikram Raghuvanshi/iStockphoto.com; Figure 1.6 Dragan Trifunovic/iStockphoto.com; Figure 2.6 DR P. MARAZZI/SCIENCE PHOTO LIBRARY; Figure 2.7 DR P. MARAZZI/SCIENCE PHOTO LIBRARY; Figure 2.8 DR H.C.ROBINSON/SCIENCE PHOTO LIBRARY; Figure 2.9 DR. CHRIS HALE/SCIENCE PHOTO LIBRARY; Figure 2.10 Wellcome Images; Figure 2.11 DR P. MARAZZI/SCIENCE PHOTO LIBRARY; Figure 2.12 DR P. MARAZZI/SCIENCE PHOTO LIBRARY; Figure 2.13 BIOPHOTO ASSOCIATES/SCIENCE PHOTO LIBRARY; Figure 2.14 JOHN HADFIELD/SCIENCE PHOTO LIBRARY; Figure 2.15 Wellcome Images; Figure 2.16 SCIENCE PHOTO LIBRARY; Figure 2.17 TOM MYERS/SCIENCE PHOTO LIBRARY; Figure 2.18 DR P. MARAZZI/SCIENCE PHOTO LIBRARY; Figure 2.19 Wellcome Images; Figure 2.20 CUSTOM MEDICAL STOCK PHOTO/SCIENCE PHOTO LIBRARY; Figure 2.21 JAMES STEVENSON/SCIENCE PHOTO LIBRARY; Figure 2.22 DR P. MARAZZI/SCIENCE PHOTO LIBRARY; Figure 2.23 DR P. MARAZZI/SCIENCE PHOTO LIBRARY; Figure 6.10 nito – Fotolia; Figure 6.11 eyewave – Fotolia; Figure 6.12 photocrew – Fotolia; Figure 6.13 volff – Fotolia; Figure 6.14 jeff gynane – Fotolia; Figure 6.15 Swapan – Fotolia; Figure 6.16 Unclesam – Fotolia; Figure 6.17 Aarti S. Khale; Figure 7.2 © Veena Kumbargadde/iStockphoto.com; p. 143 © Imagestate Media (John Foxx)/Yoga V3033; p. 145 absolut – Fotolia; p. 147 © Design Pics Inc./Alamy.

Commissioned photos © Andrew Callaghan.

With thanks to our wonderful models Annabelle Tripp, Paige Harding and Charis Read from Basingstoke College of Technology.

Every effort has been made to trace and acknowledge all copyright holders, but if any have been inadvertently overlooked the Publishers will be pleased to make the necessary arrangements at the first opportunity.

Preface

Originally existing as a family tradition in its country of origin, Indian head massage has developed from being a technique mainly practised on the head by family members to a comprehensive holistic therapy skill that addresses the widespread problems of stress in the western world.

This book has been written for those undertaking a professional qualification in Indian head massage, and addresses all the skills and knowledge required for commercial practice and competency in the workplace.

I am delighted to see the growth in popularity of Indian head massage since the late 1990s. It has become an integral part of the Beauty Therapy and Hairdressing standards at Level 3, and has become a skill much in demand, in salons and spas both in the UK and abroad.

This fully updated 4th edition meets the requirements of the following awarding bodies offering Level 3 Diploma qualifications in Indian Head Massage:

- Edexcel (BTEC)
- City & Guilds
- Confederation of International Beauty Therapy and Cosmetology (CIBTAC)
- International Therapy Examination Council (ITEC)
- Vocational Training Charitable Trust (VTCT)

This 4th edition also benefits from a unique accompanying free digital website that provides a number of resources (see below) to help make learning fun and stimulating. The resources will also help students to generate sufficient evidence to reach a competent level for commercial practice.

Guide to lecturers and students

Dear colleague,

This edition of *Indian Head Massage* has been completely revised to include new interactive features that can be accessed online at **www.hodderplus.co.uk/indianhead.**

The range of digital resources available online includes video clips of massage routines, interactive examples of the multiple-choice questions provided at the end of each chapter, drag-and-drop labelling activities, answers to the knowledge checks and multiple-choice questions, crosswords and other worksheets and resources.

Wherever you see this box in the text you will be able to scan the QR code using your mobile phone or webcam to take you directly to associated digital resources. Alternatively you can access the resources at **www.hodderplus.co.uk/indianhead**. See page vi for more details on how to access the online resources.

I sincerely hope you enjoy your studies, and find the resources helpful in stimulating your development in Indian head massage.

Helen McGuinness

Accessing the online resources

Using the QR codes

Videos of massage routines, answers to knowledge check activities and multiple-choice self-assessment questions, and other useful worksheets and resources are available online. You will see a QR code in the margin of the text where this content is provided.

To use the QR codes you will need a QR code reader for your smartphone/tablet. There are many free QR code readers available dependent on the smartphone/tablet you are using. We have supplied some suggestions below of well-known QR readers, but this is not an exhaustive list and you should only download software compatible with your device and operating system. We do not endorse any of the third-party products listed below and downloading them is at your own risk:

iphone/ipad – Qrafter – **http://itunes.apple.com/app/qrafter-qr-code-reader-generator/id416098700**

Android – QR Droid – **https://market.android.com/details?id=la.droid.qr&hl=en**

Blackberry – QR Scanner Pro – **http://appworld.blackberry.com/webstore/content/13962**

Windows/Symbian – Upcode – **http://www.upc.fi/en/upcode/download/**

Once you have downloaded a QR code reader, simply open the reader app and use it to take a photo of the code. The resource will then load on your smartphone/tablet.

Answers to knowledge check activities and multiple-choice questions are supplied as PDF files. PDF files are best read on your mobile device using Adobe® Reader® X. Visit www.adobe.com to download for your mobile device.

Via the website

If you do not have a smartphone/tablet, you can view any of these resources online, along with interactive versions of the multiple-choice questions at the end of each chapter and drag-and-drop labelling activities, by visiting the website http://www.hodderplus.co.uk/indianhead. The resources are listed by chapter.

We are interested in your feedback on the QR codes included with this title. If you have any comments, please send them to zelah.pengilley@hoddereducation.co.uk.

1 Introduction to Indian head massage

Introduction

Massage has always been an important feature of Indian family life.

Indian head massage is a treatment that has evolved from traditional techniques that have been practised in India as part of a family ritual for thousands of years.

Learning objectives

By the end of this chapter you will be able to relate the following to your work as a holistic therapist:

- The basic principles of Ayurveda
- The history and development of Indian head massage as a holistic therapy
- The benefits and effects of Indian head massage.

The history and development of Indian head massage

The traditional art of Indian head massage is based on the ancient system of medicine known as Ayurveda, which has been practised in India for thousands of years.

Ayurveda

Ayurveda is recorded as India's oldest healing system. The word 'Ayurveda' comes from Sanskrit and means the 'science of life and longevity'. The Ayurvedic approach to health is the balance of body, mind and spirit, and the promotion of long life; it recommends the use of massage together with diet, herbs, cleansing, yoga, meditation and exercise.

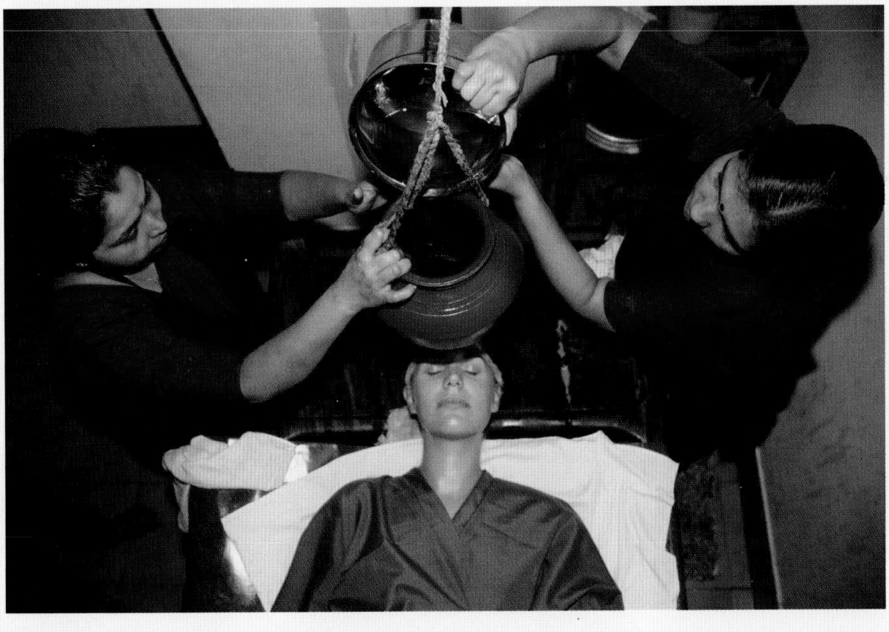

Figure 1.1 Ayurvedic treatment

The ancient texts say that the human lifespan should be around 100 years, and that all those years should be lived in total health, physically and emotionally. The whole aim of Ayurveda is in illness prevention and in the promotion of positive health, beauty and long life.

The early Ayurvedic texts, dating back nearly 4,000 years, feature massage and the principles of holistic treatment, in that health results from harmony within one's self. The Ayur-Veda, a sacred book among Hindus, written around 1800 BC, included massage among its Ayurvedic principles. The Hindus used techniques preserved in the Sanskrit texts 2,500 years ago, which detail the underlying principles of Ayurveda in maintaining balance in the body.

Key fact

The word 'Ayurveda' comes from Sanskrit and means the 'science of life and longevity'.

Ayurvedic principles

The Ayurvedic view of health is in physical, emotional and spiritual well-being. The purpose of Ayurveda is to nourish the 'root of life' in order to help keep ourselves healthy and happy.

The Ayurvedic principle identifies three main roots of life, or three main principles in nature itself. These three principles, or doshas, are known in Ayurveda as **vata**, **pitta** and **kapha**. Everyone has a unique natural balance of these three principles, and if that balance is maintained in our everyday lives we will be healthy and happy. If the balance is disturbed then problems may develop.

Ayurveda and the five elements

Ayurveda is also based on the principles of the five elements.
The five elements are:

- ether
- air
- fire
- water
- earth.

The elements are responsible for the structure of the universe, and are the building blocks of the material world. Everything in the universe, both animate and inanimate, is made up of the five elements. Each object and being in the universe contains a varying degree and combination of the five elements providing its unique features.

The density of the five elements increases from ether to air, to fire, to water, to earth.

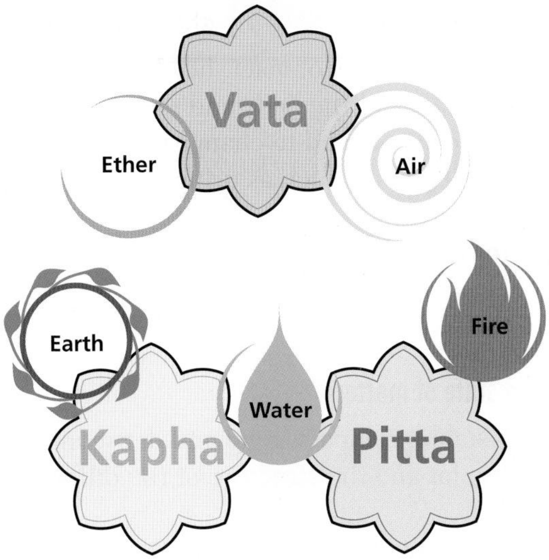

▲ Figure 1.2 The five elements

The theory of the five elements

Ether represents space and expansion

- Ether is the space in which everything exists and acts, and is always present.
- It is fine, subtle, soft, light, porous and smooth in quality.
- In the body ether is found where there is empty space such as in blood and lymph vessels, openings, pores and the intestinal tract.
- Ether also contributes the sounds of the heart, lungs, intestines and swallowing.
- Ether represents space; all sound is transmitted through space and is related to the sense of hearing and sound.

Air represents movement and direction

- Air is the gaseous form and matter.
- It is mobile, dynamic, light, cold, rough, fine, subtle, dry and exists without form.
- All empty spaces are filled with air.
- Air flows freely throughout the body, controls breathing, feeds the cells with oxygen and helps to give movement to biological functions.
- Air relates to the sense of touch and the skin.

Fire represents heat and transformation

- Fire is energy and is hot, sharp, subtle, fine, light, slightly sticky and radiant in quality.
- Fire is found in the heat and energy of the body.
- Fire exists in all metabolic processes and chemical reactions.
- Fire relates to vision because of its qualities of heat, light and colour.

Water represents cohesion and balance

- Water is liquid, sticky, cold, soft, compact, heavy and moist in quality.
- Water constitutes the liquids of the body and represents the force of cohesion, as well as the abilities to attract and to change that are associated with water.
- Water provides the bodily fluids, such as urine, plasma and lymph, and makes up most of our bodily weight.
- Water is necessary for nutrition and to maintain the water/electrolyte balance in the body.
- Water is related to the sense of taste.

Earth represents the solid state of matter

- Earth is heavy, hard, stable, compact, rigid and dense in quality.
- Bones, teeth, muscles, fat and the structure of the different organs are derived from the earth element.
- Earth is related to the sense of smell.

The five elements in relation to the body and cell structure

The five elements can be explained with the example of an atom:

- **Ether** represents the **space** that the protons and neutrons occupy, as well as the space in which the electrons revolve.
- **Air** represents the force of **movement** of the electrons around the nucleus.
- **Fire** represents the **energy** in an atom, as well as the released energy when an atom is broken down.
- **Water** gives the force of **cohesion** that allows the protons, neutrons and electrons to remain attracted towards each other.
- **Earth** contributes the solid portion of the atom – that is, the electrons, protons and neutrons.

If you consider a single cell:

- The cellular vacuoles represent the element ether or space.
- The metabolic processes and movement in the cell represent the element air.
- Nucleic acid and all chemical components of the cell represent the element fire.
- The cytoplasm represents the element water.
- The cell membrane represents the element earth.

The Ayurvedic principles and the five elements

The Ayurvedic principle shows how the five subtle elements are projected through the five senses.

- Through the sense of **hearing** the element **space** is generated.
- Through **touch** the **air** element arises.
- The **fire** element is projected by the sense of **sight**.
- **Water** arises from the sense of **taste**.
- **Earth** arises from the sense of **smell**.

The five elements make up the basic elements of life, and they form the building blocks of the universe.

Element	Sanskrit name	Its role in existence	Sense	Sense organ
Ether	*Aakash*	Space	Hearing	Ears
Air	*Vayu*	Movement	Touch	Skin
Fire	*Agni*	Heat	Sight	Eyes
Water	*Jala*	Cohesion	Taste	Tongue
Earth	*Prithvi*	Solid state of matter	Smell	Nose

▲ Table 1.1 Summary of the five elements

How the five elements apply to health

In Ayurveda, a person is seen as a unique individual made up of five primary elements: **ether** (space), **air, fire, water** and **earth**. When any of these elements is imbalanced in the environment, it will have an influence on how an individual feels. The foods we eat and the weather are just two of the influences on these elements.

The human body is made up of the five elements and so is everything we consume. Because natural substances such as foods, herbs, minerals, sunlight, air and water are of the same composition as our structure, our bodies are able to utilise them in a harmonious way. The Ayurvedic concept can be applied to maintain health and promote healing.

In a healthy body the five elements are maintained in a particular proportion. When the state of the body is not in its natural harmony, the body will try to maintain its equilibrium by eliminating excess elements and taking in others. All disorders of the body are manifested because of a disturbance in this balance of the body's components.

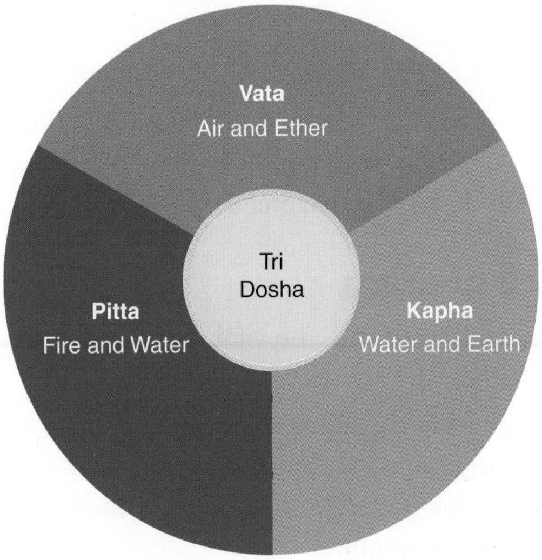

▲ Figure 1.3 Tridosha

Principles of the five elements and the dosha

While each individual is a composite of the five primary elements, certain elements are seen to have an ability to create various physiological functions.

The elements with ether and air in dominance combine to form **vata**, which governs the principle of movement and therefore can be seen as the force which directs nerve impulses, circulation, respiration and elimination.

The elements with fire and water in dominance combine to form **pitta**, which is responsible for the process of transformation or metabolism. The transformation of foods into nutrition is an example of pitta function.

It is predominantly the elements of water and earth that combine to form **kapha**, which is responsible for growth. It also offers protection – for example, in the form of cerebrospinal fluid, which protects the brain and spinal column. The mucosal lining of the stomach is another example of the kapha dosha protecting the tissues.

Knowledge check 1

1. Ayurveda is based on the principles of the five elements. Name the five elements.
2. For each of the five elements, state the significance of each element in existence.
3. How do the five elements relate to health?

To see the answers to this knowledge check, scan the QR code below or visit www.hodderplus.co.uk/indianhead/chapter-1.

The Ayurvedic perspective

In the Ayurvedic philosophy, the most fundamental aspect of life is in one's inner self, which operates through the five senses to create the five subtle elements that make up the life-giving doshas.

The Ayurvedic view of health is in physical, emotional and spiritual well-being, and that health is maintained by the balance of the three subtle life-giving forces or doshas: vata, pitta and kapha.

Each of the three doshas has a role to play in the body and each dosha possesses individual qualities.

- **Vata** is the driving force, and relates mainly to the nervous system and the body's energy centre.
- **Pitta** is fire and relates to metabolism, digestion, enzymes, acid and bile.
- **Kapha** is related to water in the mucous membranes, phlegm, moisture, fat and lymphatics.

The sub-doshas

Each of the three doshas has a subdivision of five aspects, known as sub-doshas, each one controlling a function or system of the body. These are useful to know, as they can indicate which dosha is unbalanced.

The importance of prana

The secret of Ayurveda lies in **prana**, the vital force (pra = before, ana = breath). In Ayurveda, strong prana is the source of good health.

There are five major pranas in the human body to support all movement and bodily functions. The five pranas are normally called vayus. The descriptions of the pranas outlined below are not definitive, as they interrelate to each other and are very complex in their movements.

Prana vayu

This is the 'inward-moving' air that is located in the head and the heart. It controls thinking, inhalation, emotions, sensory functioning, memory and receiving the cosmic prana from the sun (hot or solar prana). It provides the basic energy that moves us in life.

Apana vayu

This is the 'downward-moving' air seated in the colon. It controls all the processes of elimination, including urine, sweat, menstruation, orgasm and defecation. The apana receives cosmic prana from the earth and moon (cool or lunar prana). It also rules the elimination of negative emotions and provides mental stability. It is the basis of our immune system and when disturbed is the cause of most diseases.

Udana vayu

This is the 'upward-moving' air located in the throat. It controls speech, connects us to the solar and lunar forces (sky and earth; masculine and feminine) and is responsible for spiritual development. Udana controls psychic powers and creative expression.

Samana vayu

This is known as the 'equalising or balancing air'. It is seated in the navel and controls the digestive system and harmonises the prana and apana vayus. Samana also governs the digestion of air, emotions and feeling. It is hot and solar in nature.

Vyana vayu

This is called the 'pervading' or 'outward-moving' air. It is seated in the heart, yet pervades the whole body. It unites the other pranas and the tissues and controls nerve and muscle action. It holds the body together and is responsible for all circulation in the body: food, blood and emotions. Vyana provides strength and stability to the body.

Profile of the dosha vata

Vata is a combination of the elements air and ether. Vata is the driving force, and relates mainly to the nervous system and the body's energy centre. It is responsible for all movements of the body, mind and senses, and the process of elimination. Vata may be dry, light, cold, mobile, active, clear, astringent and dispersing. Due to the dry quality, a person with excess vata will tend to have dry hair, dry skin, a dry colon and a tendency towards constipation.

Key fact

A unique characteristic of vata is dryness.

- Due to the light quality (opposite of heavy), the vata person will tend to have a light body frame, light muscles, light fat and be thin and/or underweight.
- Due to the cold quality, the vata person will have cold hands, cold feet and poor circulation.
- Due to the mobile quality, vata people are very active. They like jogging and jumping and do not like sitting in one place for very long.

Key fact

Restoring balance to the dosha vata

When vata is balanced, mind and body are integrated and all movements flow with ease. When out of balance, thoughts can become disturbed by fear, anxiety and panic; inspiration disappears and forgetfulness may set in. Body aches/pains and constipation may also occur.

Vata sub-dosha profile

In general, vata controls all movement in the body and mind, and is related directly to the nervous system. Vata creates dryness in the body when too high, and sluggishness when too low. Together with pitta, it controls the hormonal function. The other two doshas are inert without vata.

The five subdivisions that control various aspects of vata are as follows:

1. **Prana vayu** controls inhalation, the other four vayus, the five senses, thinking, health and proper growth.

   Indications of imbalance: loss of senses, anxiety and worry, insomnia, dryness, emaciation, disease in general.
2. **Apana vayu** controls elimination, sexual function, menstruation, downwards movements in the body and disease.

   Indications of imbalance: constipation, menstrual problems, dryness, urinary problems; generally all diseases are involved.
3. **Samana vayu** controls movement of the digestive system, the solar plexus and balances the prana and apana vayus.

   Indications of imbalance: upset digestion, indigestion, diarrhoea and malabsorption of nutrients, dryness.
4. **Udana vayu** controls exhalation, speech and the upward movements in the body, growth as a child.

   Indications of imbalance: problems with speech and the throat, weakness of will, general fatigue, lack of enthusiasm.
5. **Vyana vayu** pervades the whole body as the nervous system, yet it controls heart function and circulation of blood.

   Indications of imbalance: arthritis, nervousness, poor circulation, poor motor reflexes, problems with the joints, bone disorders, nervous disorders.

Study tip

To balance vata it is best to get plenty of rest, eat nourishing foods, slow down, keep warm and have an Indian head massage with an oil that has properties to help balance vata.

Profile of the dosha pitta

Pitta is a combination of the elements fire and water. Pitta is fire and relates to metabolism, digestion, enzymes, acid and bile. It is responsible for heat, metabolism and energy production and digestive functions of the body. The unique characteristics of pitta are heat, sharp, light, liquid, sour, oily and spreading qualities.

> **Key fact**
>
> A unique characteristic of pitta is heat.

Due to the heat characteristic, the pitta person will tend to have a strong appetite and warm skin. The body temperature is a little higher than that of the vata person. Due to the oily characteristics, a pitta person can have oily skin, but also be sensitive. They have warm, soft skin. Because pitta is light, pitta people are moderate in body frame.

> **Key fact**
>
> Restoring balance to the dosha pitta
>
> When pitta is balanced, you will feel content, cheerful, warm-hearted and have great physical energy. Imbalance of pitta may cause feelings of anger, resentment, jealousy, aggression or obsession, and can lead to physical ailments such as heartburn, cystitis, diarrhoea, skin rashes and fever, as well as excess hunger and thirst.

Pitta sub-dosha profile

In general, pitta is responsible for all metabolic processes. Pitta enables us to digest thoughts, feelings or food. Pitta controls all the heat disorders and relates to the fiery organs in the body and the blood. Together with vata it controls the hormonal function.

Low pitta will cause the whole metabolism to slow down and usually goes with high kapha. Excess pitta causes all kinds of heat-related disorders and inflammations.

The five subdivisions that control various aspects of pitta are:

1. **Alochaka pitta** controls the ability to see and the digestion of what we see.

   Indications of imbalance: eye problems and difficulties in digesting what we see.
2. **Sadaka pitta** controls functions of the heart and the digestion of thoughts and emotions.

   Indications of imbalance: heart failure, repressed emotions and feelings, excessive anger or unprocessed feelings.
3. **Pachaka pitta** controls stomach digestion.

   Indications of imbalance: ulcers, heartburn, cravings, indigestion.
4. **Ranjaka pitta** controls liver/gall bladder digestion.

   Indications of imbalance: anger, irritability, hostility, excessive bile, liver disorders, skin problems, toxic blood, anaemia.

5. **Bhrajaka pitta** controls metabolism of the skin.

   Indications of imbalance: all skin problems, acne, inflammation of the skin.

> **Study tip**
>
> To help balance pitta, it is best to avoid pressure, eat foods of a cooling nature, schedule rest to avoid overworking (and overheating), and have an Indian head massage with an oil that has properties to help balance pitta.

Profile of the dosha kapha

Kapha is a combination of the elements earth and water. Kapha is related to water in the mucous membranes, phlegm, moisture, fat and lymphatics. It is responsible for physical stability, proper body structure and fluid balance.

> **Key fact**
>
> A unique characteristic of kapha is heaviness.

The characteristics of kapha are heaviness, slowness, cool, oily, dense, thick, static and cloudy qualities. Kapha is sweet and salty. Due to the heavy quality, kapha people have a slower metabolism and digestion, and have a tendency to put on weight. Because kapha is cool, kapha people have a cool, clammy skin.

> **Key fact**
>
> Restoring balance to the dosha kapha
>
> When kapha is balanced, you will feel strong, even-tempered, kind, compassionate, slow to anger and unflappable. Imbalance of kapha may cause sluggishness, lethargy, depression. Physical complaints such as colds, coughs, allergies, asthma and sinusitis may also occur.

Kapha sub-dosha profile

In general, kapha is responsible for the stability of the body and mind. It is the principal cohesion of mind and body. Flexibility and growth are controlled by kapha; moisture and fluid retention are maintained by kapha.

When kapha is too high it restricts vata and subdues pitta, thereby creating congestion on all levels. When kapha is too low it results in dryness and ungrounded thoughts and actions.

1. **Tarpaka kapha** controls fluids in the head, the sinuses and cerebral fluids.

   Indications of imbalance: sinus problems, headaches, loss of smell.

2. **Bodhaka kapha** controls taste and the cravings of taste, digestion and saliva.

   Indications of imbalance: overeating and cravings for sweets, loss of taste, congestion in the throat and mouth areas.

3. **Avalambaka kapha** controls lubrication and the fluids around the heart, lungs and upper back.

   Indications of imbalance: congestion in the lungs or heart, stiffness in the back and upper spine, lethargy.

4. **Kledaka kapha:** controls the lubrication of the digestive processes, maintains a balance with the pitta's bile, provides mental lubrication.

Indications of imbalance: bloated stomach, slow or congested digestion, excess mucus.

5. **Slesaka kapha** controls the lubrication of the joints in the body and aids in all movements.

   Indications of imbalance: swollen joints, stiff joints, painful movements.

Study tip

To help balance kapha, it is best to eat lightly, exercise more and have an Indian head massage with an oil that has properties to help balance kapha.

Dosha	Elements	Main characteristics	Represents	Signs of imbalance
Vata	Air and ether	Dry, light, cold, mobile, active	Movement of the body, mind and senses	Body pains/constipation Thoughts of fear, anxiety and panic
Pitta	Fire and water	Heat, sharp, light, liquid, oily	Heat, metabolism and energy production	Heartburn, cystitis, skin rashes, diarrhoea Feelings of anger, resentment, aggression
Kapha	Earth and water	Heavy, slow, cool, oily, thick	Physical stability and fluid balance	Cold, coughs, allergies, asthma, sinusitis Feelings of depression, lethargy

▲ Table 1.2 Summary of the dosha profiles

Balance and harmony of the three doshas

When the three doshas are well harmonised and balanced, good health and well-being will result. However, when there is imbalance or disharmony in the elements it can lead to various types of ailments.

The Ayurvedic concept of physical health revolves around the three doshas, and the primary purpose is to maintain them in a balanced state to prevent disease and disharmony. This theory is not unique to Indian medicine; the yin and yang theory in Chinese medicine and the Hippocratic theory in Greek medicine are very similar.

Each individual is made up of unique proportions of vata, pitta and kapha. The ratio of the doshas varies for each individual, and Ayurveda sees each person as a special combination, which accounts for our diversity. Each individual's constitution is determined by the state of their parents' doshas at the time of conception: at birth, a person has the balance of the three doshas that is right for them. Life and all its forces and influences can cause the doshas to become unbalanced, which can lead to ill health.

Ayurveda offers a model for seeing each person with a unique make-up of the three doshas, and designs a treatment protocol to specifically address an individual's health challenges.

When any of the doshas becomes accumulated, Ayurveda will suggest specific lifestyle and nutritional guidelines to assist the individual in reducing the dosha that has become excessive. Also herbal medicines will be suggested to cure the imbalance and diseases.

Key fact

The Ayurvedic principle of life shows us how to identify our own natural balance of doshas, and then how to keep them in balance.

To see the answers to this knowledge check, scan the QR code below or visit www.hodderplus.co.uk/indianhead/chapter-1.

Understanding the main principle of Ayurveda offers an explanation as to why people respond differently to a treatment or diet, and why individuals with the same disease may require different treatments and medication.

Knowledge check 2

The Ayurvedic view of health is that health is maintained by the balance of the three subtle life-giving forces.

1. What is the name given to the life-giving forces?
2. Name the individual life-giving forces and what they represent.
3. State a unique characteristic of each of the life-giving forces.

Study tip

Go to www.whatsyourdosha.com for a free questionnaire to help establish your own dosha profile and those of your clients.

Massage in Indian family life

Traditionally, massage has been an important feature of family life across the generations. In Indian traditions, it is believed that massage preserves the body's life force and energy, and is the most powerful way of relaxing and rejuvenating the body.

In India, it is customary for babies to be massaged every day from birth, and to be massaged continually until they are three years old. This encourages the bonding process, keeps baby healthy and happy, and helps to create a secure family environment. From the age of six, children are taught to show love and respect by sharing a massage with family members.

It is considered compulsory for a bride and groom to receive a massage with chemicals and oils before marriage. This ceremonial massage is believed to help relax the bride and groom, give them stamina and psychic strength, as well as promote health and fertility.

It is also tradition to massage expectant mothers to help them cope with the physical and emotional demands of labour; massage is applied daily for a minimum of 40 days after the birth. Weekly massage is a family event in India, and for the majority continues throughout life to old age.

The Indian head massage techniques practised today have evolved from traditional rituals of Indian family grooming. Over generations, Indian women have been taught by their mothers to massage different oils, such as coconut, sesame, olive, almond, herbal oils, buttermilk, mustard oil and henna, into their scalp in order to maintain their hair in beautiful condition.

Barbers have developed a more stimulating and invigorating head massage, known as 'champi', to incorporate into their daily treatments, which leaves their clients feeling revitalised and alert. In India their particular techniques are passed down through the generations from barber father to barber son.

The tradition of Indian head massage has therefore been passed down through the family generations, as Indian women have been taught the tradition of hair massage and grooming from their mothers, and barbers' sons have learnt techniques from their fathers. Head massage forms an integral part of family life and is often a ritual that is not only carried out at home within families, but is commonly seen being performed on street corners, beaches and marketplaces.

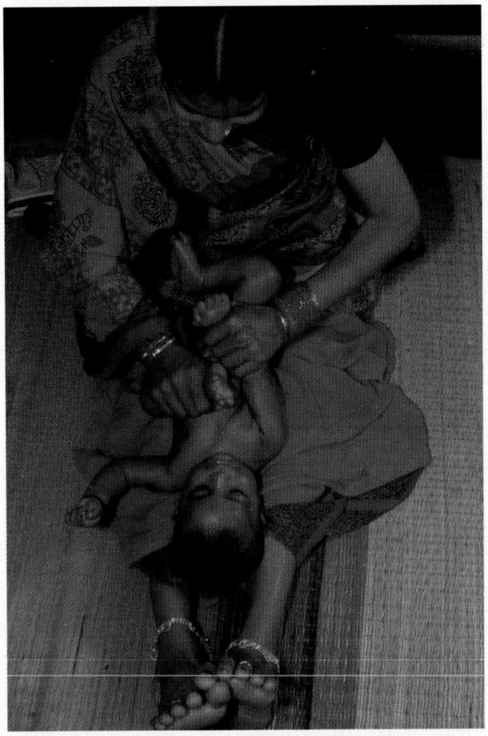

▲ Figure 1.4 Massage in Indian family life

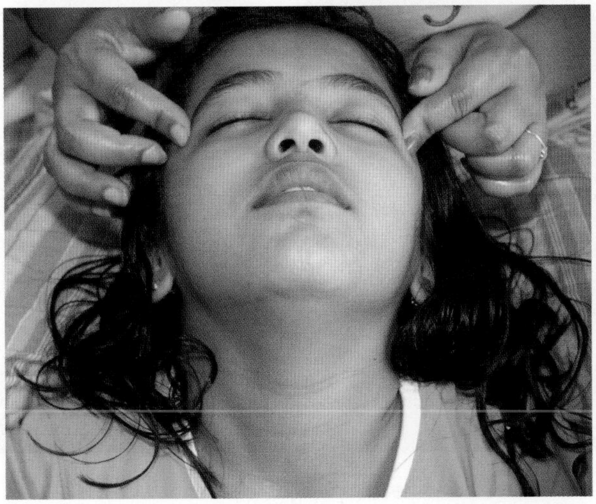

▲ Figure 1.5 Indian mother giving head massage to her daughter

Indian head massage in the western world

Despite its existence on the Indian subcontinent for thousands of years, Indian head massage has only recently started to gain popularity in the West. Though Indian head massage was originally designed for use on the head only, today it has been westernised to include other parts of the body vulnerable to stress, such as the shoulders, upper arms and neck.

It is important to realise that there is a relationship between the head, neck, shoulders and upper arms, and by incorporating these parts the treatment becomes more of a stress management treatment than a treatment designed to stimulate the head and improve the hair growth and condition.

Although the techniques are applied to the upper part of the body only (shoulders, upper arms, neck and head), collectively they represent a de-stressing programme for the whole body. Indian head massage has therefore become a primary form of stress management treatment in the western world.

Clients seeking relief from stress and tension often find Indian head massage a convenient form of treatment to receive in that:

- there is no need to undress
- it is quick and effective in terms of results
- it may be performed anywhere, due to its portable nature.

Therapists find Indian head massage a convenient form of treatment to offer in that:

- no special resources are needed
- the techniques used are quick and effective
- clients with special needs (a heavily pregnant client or a client in a wheelchair) may receive treatment with minimum fuss.

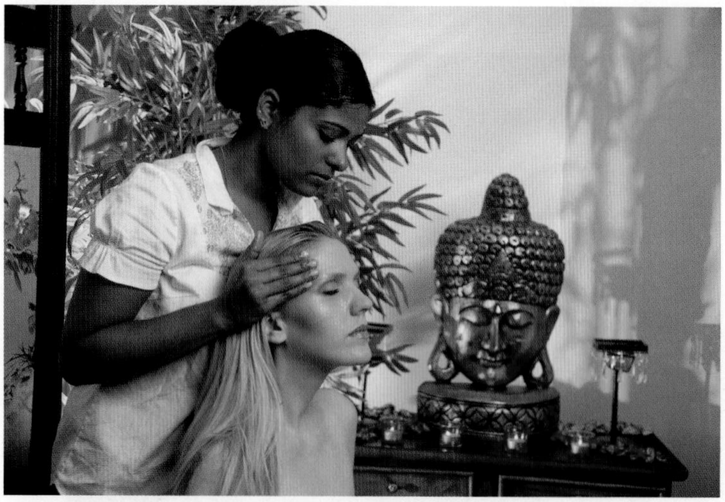

▲ Figure 1.6 An Indian head massage treatment

The future of Indian head massage

Today Indian head massage is one of the fastest-growing holistic therapies. In 1996, in response to market demand for the skill, Indian head massage was first formalised into a Diploma qualification by the Vocational Training

Charitable Trust (VTCT). Other awarding bodies, such as the International Therapy Education Council (ITEC), the Confederation of International Beauty Therapy and Cosmetology (CIBTAC), and City & Guilds have also developed qualifications in this field.

Indian head massage has now been incorporated into the National Occupational Standards for both **Hairdressing and Beauty Therapy at Level 3**. This is a significant development, in that what was previously a variable form of treatment passed down through Indian families has become a professional qualification, with national and international standards in the health and beauty industry.

Indian head massage is now available in hairdressing and beauty salons, spas, health farms, health clinics, in the workplace, at airports, on airlines, at conferences and exhibitions, on cruise liners and in private practice.

The diversity of practice of Indian head massage is due to both its versatility and its accessibility. Despite its diversity of development, there is still significant potential for the practice of Indian head massage to be widened in the market. Being a portable skill and the perfect antidote to stress and tension, Indian head massage is beneficial to all members of the community (from young to elderly).

A relatively untapped area of potential is the corporate market. The treatment can be tailored to be performed within a lunch break, and marketed as a stress management tool and preventative health care therapy. As at September 2011, the latest information from the Labour Force Survey from the Health and Safety Executive shows that stress, depression or anxiety and musculoskeletal disorders accounted for the majority of days lost due to work-related ill health, 10.8 and 7.6 million days respectively; the average days lost per case for stress, depression or anxiety (27 days) was higher than for musculoskeletal disorders (15 days) (www.hse.gov.uk/statistics/dayslost.htm). The development of Indian head massage in the workplace can help to reduce the harmful effects of stress in the workplace, while energising and motivating the workforce.

Although the techniques involved in Indian head massage involve only the upper part of the body, the potential benefits are widespread. It can be said that Indian head massage is a truly holistic therapy, in that it has many physiological and psychological benefits; many clients comment on the fact that they feel as if their whole body is balanced after the treatment.

The effects and benefits of Indian head massage

There are many benefits of Indian head massage in that it helps to treat the symptoms of stress-related conditions. It is particularly effective for helping in the relief of:

- muscular tension caused by occupational stress (long periods sitting at a computer)
- emotional stress (feelings of anxiety and depression)
- headaches caused by stress and tension
- poor sleep patterns resulting from the effects of stress on the mind and body.

Effects	Benefits
Increase in blood flow to the head, neck and shoulders	❍ Nourishes the tissues and encourages healing ❍ Improves the circulation; the delivery of oxygen and nutrients is improved via the arterial circulation and the removal of waste is hastened via the venous flow ❍ Dilates the blood vessels, helping them to work more efficiently ❍ Helps to temporarily decrease blood pressure, due to the dilation of capillaries
Increased lymphatic flow to the head, neck and shoulders	❍ Aids the elimination of accumulated toxins and waste products ❍ Reduces oedema ❍ Stimulates immunity, due to an increase in white blood cells
Relaxes the muscle and nerve fibres of the head, neck and shoulders	❍ Relieves muscular tension, soreness and fatigue ❍ Increases flexibility ❍ Improves muscle tone, balance and posture ❍ Can help to relieve tension headaches and aches and pains
Reduces spasms, restrictions and adhesions in the muscle fibres	❍ Relieves pain and discomfort ❍ Improves joint mobility
Decreases inflammation in the tissues, reducing any thickening of the connective tissue	❍ Pain relief ❍ Reduces stress placed on bones and joints
Decreases stimulation of the sympathetic nervous system	❍ Slows down and deepens breathing ❍ Slows down the heart and pulse rate ❍ Helps reduce blood pressure ❍ Reduces stress and anxiety
Stimulates the parasympathetic nervous system	❍ Helps promote rest, relaxation and sleep ❍ Reduction of stress
Stimulates the release of endorphins from the brain	❍ Helps relieve pain ❍ Helps relieve emotional stress and repressed feelings ❍ Elevates the mood ❍ Helps relieve anxiety and depression
Deepens external respiration and increases rate of internal respiration	❍ Improves lung capacity ❍ Relaxes tightness in the respiratory muscles ❍ Increased blood and lymphatic flow helps eliminate toxins more efficiently
Improves circulation and nutrition to the skin and the hair	❍ Encourages cell regeneration ❍ Increases desquamation (shedding of dead skin cells) ❍ Improved elasticity of the skin
Increases sebum production	❍ Helps to increase the skin's suppleness and resistance to infection
Promotes vasodilation of the surface capillaries in the skin	❍ Helps improve the skin's colour

▲ Table 1.3 Effects and benefits of Indian head massage

Effects	Benefits
Increases circulation to the scalp	❍ Promotes healthy hair growth ❍ Increases desquamation (shedding of dead skin cells) ❍ Helps improve the condition of the hair
Increases the supply of oxygen to the brain	❍ Helps relieve mental fatigue ❍ Promotes clearer thinking ❍ Improves concentration ❍ Helps increase productivity
Relaxes and soothes tense eye muscles	❍ Helps relieve tired eyes and eye strain ❍ Brightens the eyes
Encourages the release of stagnant energy	❍ Creates a feeling of balance and calm and restores the energy flow to the body

▲ Table 1.3 *Continued*

Knowledge check 3

1. How long has Indian head massage been practised in India?
2. Give a brief description of what an Indian head massage treatment involves.
3. State six physical effects of Indian head massage.

To see the answers to this knowledge check, scan the QR code opposite or visit www.hodderplus.co.uk/indianhead/chapter-1.

Multiple-choice self-assessment questions

1. **Indian head massage has evolved from**
   a Sanskrit texts dating from 2,500 years ago
   b the sacred book of Ayur-Veda dating from 1800 BC
   c an Indian family tradition
   d the ancient system of Indian medicine, Ayurveda.

2. **The Ayurvedic principle is that health is maintained by**
   a having a regular Indian head massage
   b balancing of the three doshas
   c eating the correct diet
   d using special oils on the hair.

3. **In Ayurveda the five elements that make up an individual are**
   a ether, air, food, water and earth
   b ether, air, fire, water and earth
   c earth, water, fire, wind and space
   d earth, cells, fire, water and space.

4. **In Ayurveda, which of the following is a unique characteristic of the dosha kapha?**
   a Dry
   b Light
   c Rough
   d Heavy

5. **One of the unique characteristics of the dosha pitta is**
   a cold
   b heat
   c dry
   d soft.

6. **Which of the following statements is *true* in relation to the dosha vata?**
   a Vata is a combination of the elements fire and water.
   b Vata is responsible for physical stability and fluid balance.
   c Vata is the driving force and is responsible for all movements of the mind, body, senses and the process of elimination.
   d Excess vata causes heat-related disorders.

7. **Which of the following statements is *incorrect*?**
   a Imbalances in the doshas can lead to ill health.
   b Each individual is made of the same proportions of vata, pitta and kapha.
   c Life and all its forces and influences can cause the doshas to become unbalanced.
   d Each individual's constitution is determined by the state of their parents' doshas at the time of conception.

8. **Which of the following statements is *incorrect*?**
   a Indian head massage helps reduce stress and anxiety.
   b Indian head massage decreases the release of endorphins from the brain.
   c Indian head massage increases the blood flow to the head, neck and shoulders.
   d Indian head massage helps relieve tired eyes and eye strain.

9. **Increased lymphatic flow to the head, neck and shoulders from an Indian head massage can**
   a increase blood pressure
   b increase oedema
   c aid the elimination of accumulated toxins
   d deepen breathing.

10. **Indian head massage has the following effect on the skin:**
   a increases desquamation
   b increases sweat
   c increases vasoconstriction of blood vessels
   d increases skin density.

To see the answers, scan the QR code opposite or visit www.hodderplus.co.uk/indianhead/chapter-1.
To access an interactive version of these multiple-choice self-assessment questions visit www.hodderplus.co.uk/indianhead.

To access an interactive crossword for this chapter visit www.hodderplus.co.uk/indianhead/chapter-1.

2 Essential anatomy and physiology for Indian head massage

Introduction

It is important for a holistic therapist to have a good knowledge of essential anatomy and physiology in order to carry out treatments safely and effectively, and to be able to understand the physiological effects of Indian head massage on the body. This chapter is devoted to the anatomy and physiology relevant to Indian head massage.

Learning objectives

By the end of this chapter you will be able to relate the following knowledge to your practice in Indian head massage:

- the structure and functions of the skin and hair
- diseases and disorders in relation to skin and hair
- the structure of bone
- the bones of the head, neck, shoulders, thorax and upper limbs
- the structure and function of muscle
- muscles of the head, neck, upper back, shoulders and upper limbs
- the blood flow relating to the head and neck
- the lymphatic drainage of the head and neck
- the outline of the nervous system
- the mechanism of respiration
- the outline of the endocrine system.

The skin

The skin is the largest organ of the body and provides the therapeutic foundation for treatment. Providing more than just an external covering, the skin is a highly sensitive boundary between our bodies and the environment. A thorough knowledge of the structure and functions of the skin will help the therapist to treat clients more effectively.

Functions of the skin

The skin has several important functions.

Sensation

The skin is like an extension of the nervous system in that it receives stimuli such as pressure, pain and temperature from the external environment and brings this information to the central nervous system.

Study tip

It is helpful to think of the acronym SHAPES V to help you remember the functions of the skin.

Heat regulation

The skin helps to regulate the body's temperature at 37 degrees Celsius.

- When the body is losing too much heat, the blood capillaries near the skin's surface constrict to keep warmth in and closer to major organs.
- When the body is too warm, the blood capillaries dilate to allow more blood to flow near the surface in order to cool the body.
- The sweat glands help to cool the body down through the production of sweat.

Absorption

The skin has limited absorption properties. Fat-soluble substances, such as oxygen, carbon dioxide, fat-soluble vitamins and steroids, can be absorbed by the epidermis, as can small amounts of water.

Protection

- The skin acts as a physical barrier, protecting the underlying tissues from abrasion. Keratin, a protein found in the skin, provides protection by waterproofing the skin's surface, helping to keep water in and out.
- The skin also provides limited protection from ultraviolet radiation through specialised cells called melanocytes found in the basal cell layer of the epidermis.
- The skin's acidic secretions (sweat and sebum), known as the acid mantle, act as a barrier against foreign agents such as bacteria and viruses.
- Fat cells in the subcutaneous layer of the skin help protect bones and major organs from injury.

Excretion

The skin functions as a minor excretory system, eliminating waste through perspiration. The eccrine glands produce sweat, which helps to remove waste materials such as urea, uric acid, ammonia and lactic acid from the skin.

Secretion

The specialised glands in the skin called the sebaceous glands secrete the oily substance sebum, which lubricates the skin's surface, keeping it soft and pliable.

Storage

The skin acts as a storage depot for fat and water. About 15 per cent of the body's fluids are stored in the subcutaneous layer.

Vitamin D production

Located in the skin are molecules that are converted by the ultraviolet rays in sunlight to vitamin D. The vitamin D produced is then absorbed into the blood vessels and used by the body for the maintenance of bones and the absorption of calcium and phosphorus in the diet.

Study tip

Each person's skin varies in its colour, texture and condition. A client's skin can reflect their physiological as well as psychological state, and it is through touch that therapists can help to evaluate this information. Physiological signs of the skin may be shown by the client's colour and circulation, whereas psychological status may be reflected by muscular tightness.

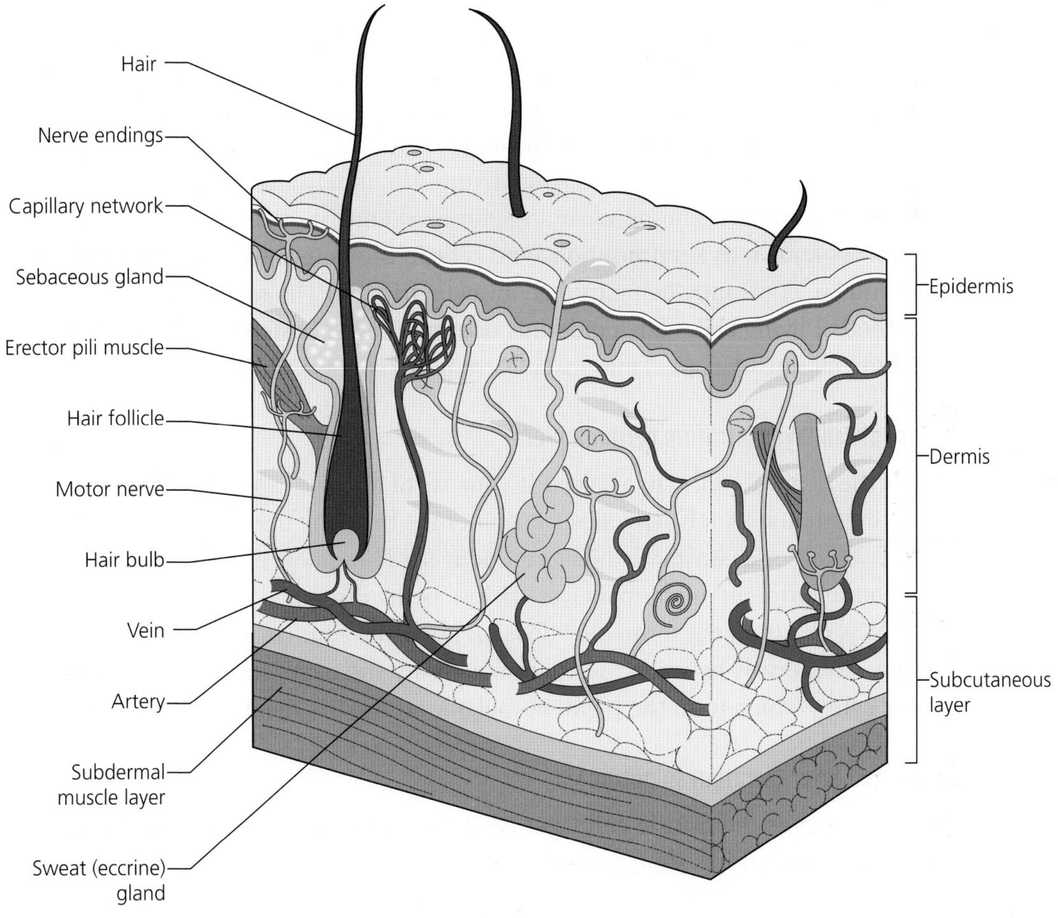

▲ Figure 2.1 Cross section of the skin

Structure of the skin

There are two main layers of the skin:

- the **epidermis**, which is the outer, thinner layer
- the **dermis**, which is the inner, thicker layer.

Below the dermis is the **subcutaneous layer**, which attaches to organs and tissues.

To access a drag and drop labelling exercise for the skin visit www.hodderplus.co.uk/indianhead/chapter-2.

The epidermis

The epidermis is the most superficial layer of the skin and consists of five layers of cells:

- the horny layer (stratum corneum, the outermost layer)
- the clear layer (stratum lucidum)
- the granular layer (stratum granulosum)
- the prickle cell layer (stratum spinosum)
- the basal cell layer (stratum germinativum, the innermost layer).

The three outer layers (horny, clear and granular) consist of dead cells as a result of the process known as keratinisation. The cells in the outermost layer are dead and scaly, and are constantly being rubbed away by friction. The inner two layers are composed of living cells. The epidermis does not have a system of blood vessels; therefore, all nutrients pass into its cells from blood vessels in the deeper dermis.

The basal cell layer (stratum germinativum)

This is the deepest of the five layers. It consists of a single layer of column cells on a base membrane which separates the epidermis from the dermis. In this layer, new epidermal cells are constantly being reproduced. These new cells move upwards through the different epidermal layers before being discarded into the horny layer. New column cells formed by division push adjacent cells towards the skin's surface. At intervals between the column cells are the large, star-shaped cells called melanocytes, which form the pigment melanin, the skin's main colouring agent.

Prickle cell layer (stratum spinosum)

This is known as the prickle cell layer because each of the rounded cells contained within it has short projections that make contact with the neighbouring cells and give them a prickly appearance. The living cells of this layer are capable of dividing by the process known as mitosis.

Granular layer (stratum granulosum)

This layer consists of flattened cells containing a number of granules that are involved in the hardening of cells through **keratinisation**. Keratinisation is the process that cells undergo when they change from living cells with a nucleus to dead cells without a nucleus. This layer links the living cells of the epidermis to the dead cells above.

Clear layer (stratum lucidum)

This layer consists of transparent cells that permit light to pass through. It consists of three or four rows of flat, dead cells that are completely filled with keratin; they have no nuclei as these have degenerated through the keratinisation process. The clear layer of the epidermis is thought to form a barrier zone that controls the movement of water through the skin. This layer is very shallow in facial skin, but thick on the soles of the feet and the palms of the hands, and is generally absent in hairy skin.

Horny layer (stratum corneum)

This is the most superficial outer layer, consisting of dead, flattened, keratinised cells. The cells of the horny layer form a waterproof covering for the skin and help to prevent the penetration of bacteria. This outer layer of dead cells is continually being shed; this process is known as **desquamation**.

Cell regeneration of the epidermis

Cell regeneration occurs in the epidermis by the process mitosis (cell division). It takes approximately a month for a new cell to complete its journey from the basal cell layer where it is reproduced, through the granular layer where it becomes keratinised, to the horny layer where it is desquamated.

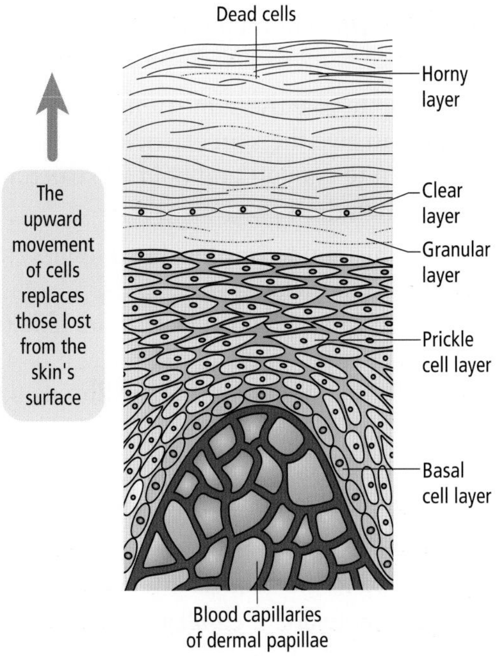

▲ Figure 2.2 Cell regeneration of the epidermis

The dermis

The **dermis** lies below the epidermis and is the deeper layer of the skin. Its key functions are to provide nourishment to the epidermis and to give a supporting framework to the tissues. The dermis has two layers: a superficial **papillary layer** and a deeper **reticular layer**.

Epidermal layer	Significance
Horny layer	Dead skin cells are subject to shedding (desquamation)
Clear layer	Important transitional stage in the development of the horny layer
Granular layer	Keratinocytes becomes less flexible, more granular in appearance and hardened, thereby completing the keratinisation process
Prickle cell layer	The cells of this layer are living and are therefore capable of dividing by the process mitosis
Basal cell layer	Concerned with cell regeneration; as new cells are formed by division, they push adjacent cells towards the skin's surface

▲ Table 2.1 Summary of the journey of cell regeneration through the epidermal layers

Study tip

Think of the dermis as the skin's scaffolding, as it gives support and holds all the layers.

The superficial papillary layer is made up of fatty connective tissue and is connected to the underside of the epidermis by cone-shaped projections called **dermal papillae**, which contain nerve endings and a network of blood and lymphatic capillaries.

The deeper reticular layer is formed of tough, fibrous, connective tissue, which contains the following:

- collagen fibres, which help to give the skin strength and resilience
- elastic fibres, which help to give the skin elasticity
- reticular fibres, which help to support and hold all structures in place.

Cells present in the dermis include:

- mast cells, which secrete histamine (involved in allergies), causing dilation of blood vessels to bring blood to the area
- phagocytic cells, which are white blood cells that are able to travel around the dermis, destroying foreign matter and bacteria
- fibroblasts, which are cells that help to form new fibrous tissue.

Blood supply

Unlike the epidermis, an abundant supply of blood vessels runs through the dermis and the subcutaneous layer.

Arteries carry oxygenated blood to the skin via arterioles; these enter the dermis from below and branch into a network of capillaries around active or growing structures. These capillary networks form in the dermal papillae to provide the basal cell layer of the epidermis with food and oxygen. They also surround the sweat glands and **erector pili muscles**, two appendages of the skin.

The capillary networks drain into venules, small veins which carry the deoxygenated blood away from the skin and remove waste products. The dermis is therefore well supplied with capillary blood vessels to bring nutrients and oxygen to the germinating cells in the basal cell layer of the epidermis and to remove waste products from them.

Lymphatic vessels

There are numerous lymphatic vessels in the dermis. They form a network in the dermis, facilitating the removal of waste from the skin's tissue. The lymphatic vessels in the skin generally follow the course of veins and are found around the dermal papillae, glands and hair follicles.

Nerves

There is a wide distribution of nerves throughout the dermis. Most nerves in the skin are sensory, which send signals to the brain and are sensitive to heat, cold, pain, pressure and touch. The dermis also has motor nerves, which relay impulses to the brain and are responsible for the dilation and constriction of blood vessels, the secretion of perspiration from the sweat glands and the contraction of the erector pili muscles attached to hair follicles.

The subcutaneous layer (hypodermis)

This is a thick layer of connective tissue found below the dermis. The type of tissue found in this layer (areolar and adipose) helps to support delicate structures such as blood vessels and nerve endings.

The subcutaneous layer contains the same collagen and elastin fibres as the dermis, and contains the major arteries and veins that supply the skin and form a network throughout the dermis. The fat cells contained within this layer help to insulate the body by reducing heat loss.

Below the subcutaneous layer lies the subdermal muscle layer.

Knowledge check 1

1. List seven functions of the skin.
2. List the five layers of the epidermis, from the bottom layer upwards.
3. In which layer/s of the epidermis are cells subject to
   i. regeneration?
   ii. keratinisation?
   iii. desquamation?
4. The dermis is the deeper layer of the skin. Name its two layers and their significance.
5. Where is the subcutaneous layer found in the skin?

To see the answers to this knowledge check, scan the QR code below or visit www.hodderplus.co.uk/indianhead/chapter-2.

Appendages of the skin

The appendages are accessory structures that lie in the dermis of the skin and project on to the surface through the epidermis. These include the hair, the erector pili muscle and the sweat and sebaceous glands.

Hair

Hair is an appendage of the skin that grows from a sac-like depression in the epidermis called a hair follicle. Hair grows all over the body, with the exception of the palms of the hands and the soles of the feet.

The function of hair

The primary function of a hair is in physical protection and insulation. For example, the hair on the scalp provides partial shading from the sun's rays, and the hairs in the nostrils, eyelashes and eyebrows provides protection from foreign particles.

The structure of hair

The hair is composed mainly of the protein keratin and therefore is a dead structure. Longitudinally, the hair is divided into three parts:

- **hair shaft** – the part of the hair lying above the surface of the skin
- **hair root** – the part found below the surface of the skin
- **hair bulb** – the enlarged part at the base of the hair root.

Internally, the hair has three layers, which all develop from the matrix (the active, growing part of the hair):

Hair layer	Location	Description	Function
Cuticle	Outer layer	Made up of transparent, protective scales, which overlap	Protects the cortex and gives the hair its elasticity
Cortex	Middle layer	Made up of tightly packed, keratinised cells containing the pigment melanin, which gives the hair its colour	Helps to give strength to the hair
Medulla	Inner layer	Made up of loosely connected, keratinised cells and tiny air spaces	Determines the sheen and colour of hair, due to the reflection of light through the air spaces

▲ Table 2.2 Layers of the hair

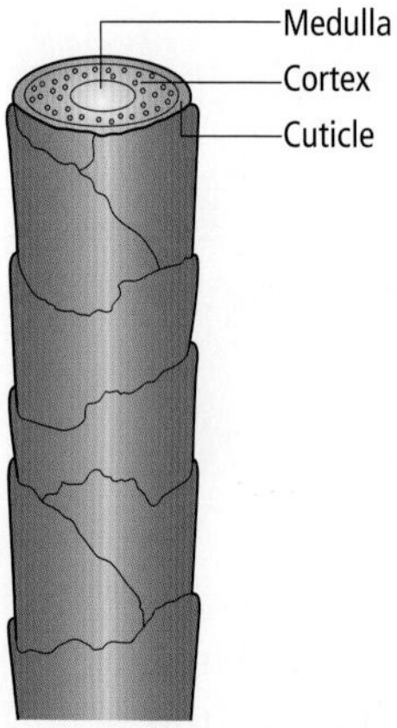

▲ Figure 2.3 Layers of the hair

To access a drag and drop labelling exercise for the layers of the hair visit www.hodderplus.co.uk/indianhead/chapter-2.

Types of hair

There are three main types of hair in the body: lanugo, vellus and terminal hair.

Type of hair	Description	Where found in body
Lanugo	Fine, soft hair, often unpigmented	On a foetus; grows from around the third to the fifth month of pregnancy and is eventually shed to be replaced by secondary vellus hairs, around the seventh to eighth month of pregnancy
Vellus	Soft, downy hair, often unpigmented and without a medulla or a well-developed bulb Lies close to the surface of the skin and therefore has a shallow follicle	All over the face and body, except for the palms of the hands, soles of the feet, eyelids and lips
Terminal	Longer, coarser hairs, most are pigmented Vary greatly in shape, diameter, length, colour and texture Deeply seated in the dermis, with well-defined bulbs	On the scalp, under the arms, eyebrows, pubic regions, arms and legs

▲ Table 2.3 Types of hair

The structure of a hair in its follicle

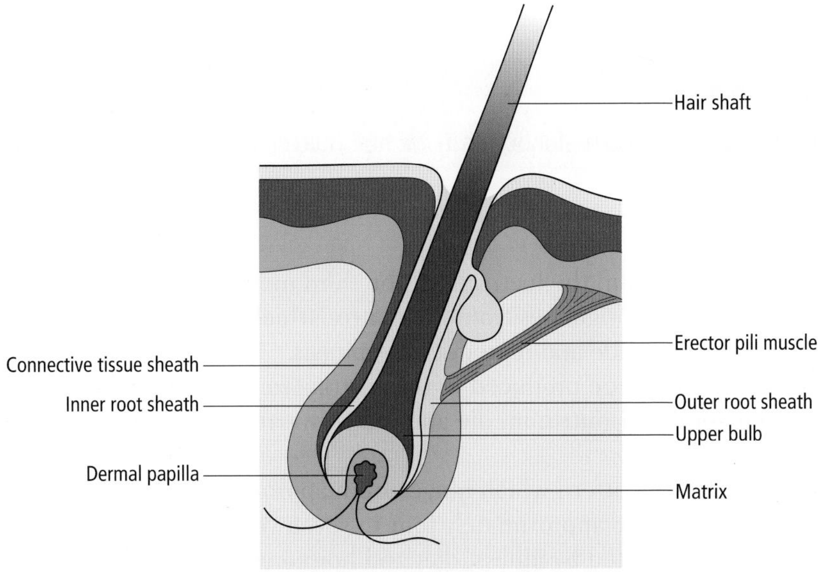

▲ Figure 2.4 A hair in its follicle

The individual parts of a hair's structure are as follows:

Structure	Location	Function
Connective tissue sheath	Surrounds hair follicle and sebaceous gland	Supplies follicle with nerves and blood Main source of sustenance for the follicle
Outer root sheath	Forms the follicle wall and is continuous with the basal cell layer of the epidermis	Provides a permanent source of growing cells (hair germ cells) to enable the follicle to grow and renew cells during its life cycle
Dermal papilla	Elevation at the base of the hair bulb, which contains a rich blood supply	Crucial source of nourishment for hair, providing the hair cells with food and oxygen
Inner root sheath	Originates from the dermal papilla at the base of the follicle and grows upwards with the hair (it ceases to grow when level with the sebaceous gland)	Shapes and contours the hair, helping to anchor it into the follicle
Hair bulb	Enlarged part at the base of the hair root	Area where the cells grow and divide by the process of mitosis
Matrix	Lower part of the hair bulb	Area of mitotic activity of the hair cells

▲ Table 2.4 Structure, location and function of hairs

Hair colour

Hair colour is due to the presence of melanin in the cortex and medulla of the hair shaft. In addition to the standard black colour, the melanocytes in the hair bulb produce two colour variations of melanin: brown and yellow. Blond, light-coloured and red hair has a high proportion of the yellow variant. Brown and black hair possesses more of the brown and black melanin.

Key fact

Hair turns grey when the melanocytes in the hair bulb stop producing melanin.

Facts about hair growth

- Hair begins to form in the foetus from the third month of pregnancy.
- The growth of hair originates from the matrix, which is the active growing area where cells divide and reproduce by mitosis.
- Living cells, which are produced in the matrix, are pushed upwards, away from their source of nutrition, die and are converted to keratin to produce a hair.
- Hair has a growth pattern which ranges from approximately four to five months for an eyelash hair to approximately four to seven years for a scalp hair.
- Hair growth is affected by illness, diet and hormonal influences.

The growth cycle of a hair

Each hair has its own growth cycle and undergoes three distinct stages of development: anagen, catagen and telogen.

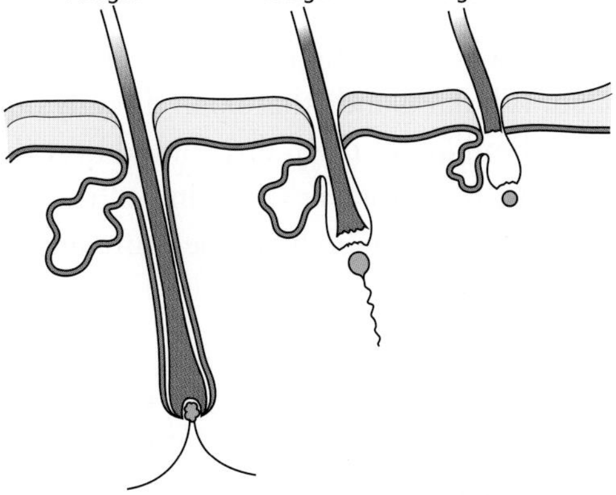

▲ Figure 2.5 The hair growth cycle

Study tip

It is helpful to think of the acronym ACT when thinking of the stages of hair growth.

Anagen is the active, growing stage:

- lasts from a few months to several years
- hair germ cells reproduce at matrix
- new follicle is produced which extends in depth and width
- the hair cells pass upwards to form hair bulb
- hair cells continue rising up the follicle, and as they pass through the bulb they differentiate to form individual structures of hair
- inner root sheath grows up with the hair, anchoring it into the follicle
- when cells reach the upper part of bulb they become keratinised
- two-thirds of its way up the follicle, the hair leaves an inner root sheath and emerges on to surface of skin.

Catagen is the transitional stage of growth from active to resting:

- lasts approximately two to four weeks
- hair separates from dermal papilla and moves slowly up the follicle
- follicle below retreating hair shrinks
- hair rises to just below level of sebaceous gland, where the inner root sheath dissolves and the hair can be brushed out.

Telogen is the short, resting stage:

- shortened follicle rests until stimulated once more
- hair is shed on to skin's surface
- new replacement hair begins to grow.

Erector pili muscle

This is a small, smooth muscle, attached at an angle to the base of a hair follicle, which serves to make the hair stand erect in response to cold, or when experiencing emotions such as fright and anxiety.

Sweat glands

There are two types of sweat glands. The majority are called eccrine glands, which are simple, coiled, tubular glands that open directly on to the surface of the skin. There are several million of them distributed over the surface of the skin, although they are most numerous in the palms of the hands and the soles of the feet. Their function is to regulate body temperature and help eliminate waste products. Their active secretion sweat is under the control of the sympathetic nervous system.

The other type of sweat glands are called apocrine glands; these are connected with hair follicles and are only found in the genital and underarm regions. They produce a fatty secretion; breakdown of this secretion by bacteria leads to body odour.

Sebaceous glands

These glands are found all over the body, except for the soles of the feet and the palms of the hands. They are more numerous on the scalp, face, chest and back.

Sebaceous glands commonly open into a hair follicle, but some open on to the skin's surface. They produce an oily substance called sebum, which contains fats, cholesterol and cellular debris. Sebum coats the surface of the skin and the hair shafts, where it prevents excess water loss, lubricates and softens the horny layer of the epidermis and softens the hair.

To see the answers to this knowledge check, scan the QR code below or visit www.hodderplus.co.uk/indianhead/chapter-2.

Knowledge check 2

1. List the three layers of the hair, stating their location.
2. Hair colour is due to the presence of melanin in which layers of the hair shaft?
3. What is the main function of hair?
4. Which area of the hair's structure does growth originate from?
5. State the three stages of hair growth and their significance.

Key fact

Indian head massage can help to bring about an improvement in a client's skin and hair condition over a period of time. The increased circulation to the skin can increase cell nutrition and regeneration, as well as increase elimination of waste from the skin's tissues. Dead keratinised cells that are blocking the pores of the skin can be loosened by massage, and the blood supply can flow more freely to feed the skin and hair with nutrients.

Indian head massage can also help to increase the production of sebum from the sebaceous glands, helping to lubricate the skin and hair and improve its condition.

Factors affecting the skin

There are many factors, both external and internal, which affect a person's skin.

Internal factors affecting the skin

Age

The natural process of ageing naturally affects the skin, as cell regeneration starts to decrease with age.

Free radicals

These also contribute to skin ageing. Free radicals are parts of molecules – for example, oxygen molecules – that are found in the body. As a result of external factors, like ultraviolet radiation, nicotine or unhealthy food, the free radicals become prone to react. This means they are constantly looking for other chemical substances to bond with. Hence they attack the collagen fibres, cellular membrane and lipid layer of the skin. Free radicals change the inherited properties stored in the cell nucleus, so that the quality of newly formed skin cells deteriorates.

Stress and lifestyle

When the body is subjected to regular stress and tension, it can cause sensitivity and allergies in the skin, as well as encourage the formation of lines around the eyes and the mouth.

Hormones

The natural glandular changes of the body have an effect on the condition of the skin throughout life. During puberty, the sex hormones stimulate the sebaceous glands, which may cause some imbalance in the skin.

At the onset of menstruation, the skin may erupt due to the adjustment of hormone levels at that time. During pregnancy, pigmentation changes may occur, but usually disappear at birth. During the menopause, the activity of the sebaceous glands is reduced and the skin becomes drier.

Smoking

The effects of smoking have been linked to premature ageing and wrinkling of the skin. Nicotine weakens the blood vessels that supply blood to the tissues; this deprives the tissues of essential oxygen, and therefore the skin may appear dull and grey in colour.

Smoking affects the skin's cells and destroys vitamins B and C, which are important for a healthy skin. Smoking dulls the skin by polluting the pores and increases the formation of lines around the eyes and the mouth.

Medication

Medication can affect the skin by causing dehydration, or sensitivity and/or allergies.

Diet

A healthy body is needed for a healthy skin. The skin can be thought of as a barometer of the body's general health.

- Vitamin A: helps repair the body's tissues and helps prevent dryness and ageing
- Vitamin B: helps improve the circulation and the skin's colour, and is essential to cellular oxidation
- Vitamin C: is essential for healing and to maintain levels of collagen in the skin
- Vitamin E: helps to heal damaged tissues and can help heal structural damage to the skin.

Water consumption

The skin is approximately 70 per cent water. Drinking an adequate amount of water (approximately six to eight glasses per day) aids the digestive system and helps to prevent a build-up of toxicity in the skin's tissues.

Alcohol

Alcohol has a dehydrating effect on the skin by drawing essential water from the tissues. Excess consumption causes the blood vessels in the skin to dilate, resulting in a flushed appearance.

Exercise

Regular exercise promotes good circulation, increased oxygen intake and blood flow to the skin.

Sleep

Sleep is essential to physical and emotional well-being and is one of the most effective regenerators for the skin.

External factors affecting the skin

Photoageing

Photoageing is the process by which the skin undergoes accelerated ageing after ultraviolet exposure. The sun and its ultraviolet rays are therefore one of the most dominant factors in how the skin ages.

As we age naturally, the collagen and elastin fibres in the dermis weaken. This natural occurrence is accelerated with frequent exposure to ultraviolet rays, as exposure to the rays weakens the skin's collagen and elastin fibres, which causes wrinkling and sagging of the tissues.

It is important to note that tanning machines/sunbeds can also cause accelerated ageing of the skin, due to the fact that they produce large quantities of long-wave ultraviolet light (UVA). Overexposure may lead to the same risks as with overexposure to natural sunlight – that is, sagging and wrinkling – and to an increased risk of some skin cancers.

Environmental exposure

Exposure to adverse weather conditions, pollutants or poor air quality can affect the condition of the skin, often resulting in dryness and dehydration.

Occupation

The client's occupation could be a factor involved in the cause of a client's skin condition. For instance, they could be working in a hot or humid environment, or in dusty and dirty conditions.

Poor care

Lack of or incorrect skin care can be a major affecting the skin. The use of products that are too aggressive can strip the skin and effectively damage the barrier function of the skin. The correct use of sunscreens can provide the best protection against premature ageing.

Factors affecting hair growth

The way our hair looks has a great impact on the way we feel. Shiny, lustrous hair is synonymous with good health and vitality. Factors such as diet, age and hormones directly determine its appearance.

Hormonal influences

The hair is often affected by hormonal changes occurring in the body, such as puberty, pregnancy and the menopause.

- Hair can become more greasy during menstruation.
- Hair may become dry due to a thyroid problem, or there may be temporary hair loss during pregnancy (especially after delivery).
- A drop in oestrogen during the menopause can have a profound effect on the hair, causing it to become dry, coarse and brittle.

Medication

Medication can affect the hair by drying the skin, which in turn blocks the follicles with dead, keratinised cells, blocking the circulation to the scalp.

Diet

Health of the hair comes from within and therefore a poor diet can affect the condition of the hair. For healthy hair, it is important to have a diet rich in protein, essential fatty acids, and essential vitamins and minerals.

- Vitamin B complex and vitamin C help provide nourishment for hair follicles.
- Minerals such as iron, sulphur and zinc can help the hair if the important mineral content of the hair is missing and the hair is dull in appearance.
- Vitamin B5 is important to help relieve stress in the hair.
- Vitamin A is useful for a dry and scaly scalp.

Allergies

Reaction to products used on the hair and scalp may cause sensitisation of the scalp, and this can affect the circulation of blood to the hair. Some clients may develop dandruff in response to sensitisation of hair products.

Illness

Prolonged illness and stress can cause both hair loss and greying, due to the fact that the body is starved of essential nutrients and cell metabolism is slowed down due to infection and/or disease.

Overprocessing

Straightening, perming and dyeing the hair can alter the shaft of the hair, often making it dry and brittle. Frequent use of shampoos full of detergents and chemicals can also dry out the scalp.

Stress and tension

Tension in the scalp can reduce the circulation of oxygen and starve the hair root of nutrients needed for healthy growth. Stress can also cause hair loss and premature greying.

Skin types and their characteristics

When talking of skin types, the classifications are predetermined from genetics and ethnicity.

DNA is carried in chromosomes and is the factor that programmes and influences skin characteristics, such as follicle size, skin thickness, circulation and nerve endings.

The primary factors in determining skin types are:

- level of lipid (fat) secretions that are produced between the skin cells (this determines how well the skin retains moisture)
- the amount of secretion produced by the sebaceous glands.

Skin types are generally broadly classified into five main types:

1. Normal
2. Dry
3. Oily
4. Combination
5. Sensitive

Skin type	Main recognition factors	Pore size	Elasticity
Normal	Soft, supple, smooth Free from blemishes	Fine	Good; firm
Dry	Papery, thin, flaky	Small and tight	Generally not good
Oily	Shiny, thick, coarse and uneven Sallow colouring Blocked pores, comedones, papules and pustules may be present	Enlarged	Good; firm
Combination	Dry on cheeks and neck, oily/blemished in T-zone	Variable; enlarged in T-zone and fine and small on cheeks	Poor in dry areas; good in oily areas
Sensitive	Warm to touch, thin, dry and flaky, high colouring, easily irritated	Variable; tend to be small and tight	May be poor in areas of sensitivity

▲ Table 2.5 Main skin types

Ethnic skin types

All ethnic skin types vary in the degree of melanin they produce. Although all ethnic skin types have the same number of melanocyte cells, black skins have melanocytes capable of making large amounts of melanin.

Ethnic skin type	Colouring	Characteristics
White skin (British, Scandinavian, East and West European, North American, South Australian, Canadian, New Zealand origin)	Generally a pale buff; some skins may appear pinkish, while others have a sallowish tone	Relatively small amounts of melanin present Melanin produced to varying degrees Ages faster than black skins
Oriental/light Asian skin (Chinese, Japanese, Middle Eastern origin)	Creamy colour, with a tendency to yellow and olive tones, with more melanin present	Rarely shows blemishes and defies normal signs of ageing Scars are more likely to occur and hyper-pigment, causing unevenness
Dark Asian skin (Pakistani, Indian, Sri Lankan, Malaysian origin)	Very dark skin colour, which is deeply pigmented with melanin	Smooth and supple, with minimal signs of ageing Sweat glands are larger and more numerous Has a sheen that is often mistaken for oiliness Deeply pigmented, it does not reveal the blood capillaries
Mediterranean skin (Italian, Spanish, Greek, Portuguese, Yugoslavian, South American, Central American origin)	Looks sallow, with some reddish pigment	Good degree of melanin present, which obscures the colour of the blood vessels Tends to be oily (more sebum) Tans easily and deeply without burning

▲ Table 2.6 Ethnic skin types

Ethnic skin type	Colouring	Characteristics
African Caribbean/black skin (West Indian/African origin)	Darker, with a higher degree of melanin	Open pores Oily, with higher degree of sebaceous glands Thick and tough Desquamates easily Forms keloid scars when damaged More likely to be affected by several different types of disfiguring bumps
Mixed skin	Usually a combination of characteristics of all of the above skin types	Shades of colour and characteristics will vary greatly depending on the mix

▲ Table 2.6 *Continued*

Skin conditions

Skin conditions develop over a period of time and can apply to all skin types.

Common examples of skin conditions that may be encountered during an Indian head massage treatment include comedones, blocked/enlarged pores, papules, pustules, dehydration, milia, wrinkles, signs of ageing, sun damage, sensitivity, dehydration, poor elasticity and pigmentation problems.

Causes of skin conditions may be internal or external.

Blocked pores

This is where sebum begins to build up in a pore. The pore will appear enlarged, and sebaceous matter inside will be evident. The excess sebum needs to be released to prevent further build-up within the pore.

Enlarged pores

Larger pores are due to excess oil and debris trapped in the follicles, or expansion due to loss of elasticity.

Comedone

A collection of sebum, keratinised cells and waste, which accumulates in the entrance of a hair follicle. It may be open or closed.

An open comedone is a 'blackhead' contained within the follicle, whereas a closed comedone is a small bump just beneath the skin's surface and is not open to the air.

As comedones are technically 'skin blockages', trapped by dead skin cells, they need to be exfoliated and extracted.

Dehydration

Water intake is necessary for the healthy functioning of the body and skin cells. Dehydration means that there is a lack of moisture in the intercellular system of the skin. Key indicators of dehydration are flakiness, visible fine lines and a feeling of tightness on the skin.

A dehydrated skin lacks moisture and can affect any skin type, even an oily skin.

If an oily skin is dehydrated, this usually results from using products that are too harsh and have left the skin stripped of its protective coating of sebum.

Many skin types can suffer from temporary dehydration, such as that caused through illness, medication, overexposure to the elements (cold, wind and heat), central heating and dehydrating drinks, such as caffeine and alcohol.

As well as a dehydrated skin presenting a parched, dry-looking, rough surface, it will also tend to soak up any product applied very quickly.

Dilated capillaries

The technical term for dilated capillaries is telangiectasia (often called couperose). This condition presents as diffused areas of redness on the cheeks, nose and neck.

It occurs primarily as a result of poor elasticity in the capillary wall.

It is caused by sun exposure, smoking, alcohol, poor health – in fact, any factor that puts stress on the capillaries.

Signs of skin maturity/lines and wrinkles

Once the underlying structure of the skin has become damaged and the skin starts to lose its elasticity, exaggerated lines and wrinkles start to form on the face and neck.

These may be formed as a result of the normal ageing process, but often are formed prematurely due to sun and environmental damage.

The fine lines around the eye area are known as crow's feet, which appear with age, are precipitated by squinting and exposure to ultraviolet light (not wearing adequate protection for the eyes), and may also be aggravated by rough handling of the skin when removing cosmetics.

Milia

These are white pearly lumps that appear under the skin (often called whiteheads). They are a combination of oil and dead skin cells, and because they are trapped in a blind duct, they must be lanced with a sterile probe to remove them.

Pigmentation problems

Pigmentation may be associated with a client's ethnic skin type, or may be caused by environmental or other factors.

Pigmentation problems may result from the uneven distribution of melanin over the skin surface, due to either an accumulation of pigment or uneven production by the melanocytes.

The melanocyte cells are located in the basal cell layer of the epidermis, and they surround a large number of regular skin cells (keratinocytes).

The melanocytes are responsible for producing melanin, the black-brown pigment that gives the skin its colour.

Melanin production varies from individual to individual, and is greater in those with darker skins. Melanin has a protective function in that it acts as a filter to help protect the skin against the harmful effects of the sun's radiation.

Any surface irritation of the skin (including exposure to the sun) is capable of increasing melanin production.

Hyperpigmentation

This is an excess of skin pigment, resulting in brown discolouration/darkening of the skin from the overproduction of melanin.

The overproduction of pigment results when the melanocytes produce a greater amount of melanin in a given area of the skin, and/or when the melanin is not properly absorbed by the keratinocytes.

Hyperpigmentation is usually caused by exposure to the sun or environmental damage, although a type of hyperpigmentation may occur during pregnancy (chloasma).

Hyperpigmentation may also result from injuries, rashes or chemical irritation, and is especially common in clients with darker skins.

Hypopigmentation

This condition presents as white, colourless areas resulting from less than the normal melanin production, or the absence of pigmentation. It may be due to long-term sun exposure or irritation, which causes a dysfunction in the melanocytes (cells that produce melanin).

Poor elasticity

Skin lacking elasticity will tend to feel soft and flaccid, rather than firm and tight, as in a well-toned skin.

To test for skin elasticity, gently lift the skin between the thumb and forefinger and then release. If the skin snaps back quickly it has good elasticity. If the skin takes any time to snap back it is lacking elasticity.

Poor elasticity, or elastosis, resulting in sagging or loose skin, is a sign of ageing (sometimes prematurely) or damage from the sun.

Sensitivity

Sensitivity is a condition that may affect any skin type, and should not be confused with genetically predisposed sensitive skin.

Sensitivity will usually manifest itself as redness, itching or burning.

Sensitivity reactions are very complex, and will depend on the client experiencing them. Because the chemical composition of each person's skin varies, one client may react sensitively to a particular ingredient, while another may not.

It is important to note that an ingredient may not be sensitising as a rule, but that a client's skin may be sensitive to that particular ingredient. An ingredient can only be deemed sensitising if most clients react to it with sensitivity.

Sensitivity and allergies may occur due to exposure to specific product ingredients, misuse of products, medication, diet or other internal or external factors (hot and cold weather, and the wind). Major ingredients that can cause sensitivity are those found in fragrances, preservatives and some chemical sunscreens.

Knowledge check 3

1. State three recognition factors of the following skin types:
   i. dry
   ii. oily
   iii. sensitive.
2. What are the key recognition factors of the following skin conditions?
   i. sensitivity
   ii. dehydration
   iii. skin maturity.
3. Which of the ethnic skin types have melanocytes capable of making large amounts of melanin?

To see the answers to this knowledge check, scan the QR code below or visit www.hodderplus.co.uk/indianhead/chapter-2.

Allergic reaction	A disorder in which the body becomes hypersensitive to a particular allergen. When irritated by an allergen, the body produces histamine in the skin as part of the body's defence or immune system. The effects of different allergens are diverse; they affect different tissues and organs. For instance, certain cosmetics and chemicals can cause rashes and irritation in the skin; certain allergens, such as pollen, fur, feathers, mould and dust, can cause asthma and hay fever. If severe, allergies may result in anaphylactic shock.
Comedone	A collection of sebum, keratinised cells and waste that accumulate in the entrance of a hair follicle. It may be open or closed. An open comedone is a 'blackhead' contained within the follicle, whereas a closed comedone is a 'whitehead', trapped underneath the skin's surface.
Cyst	An abnormal sac containing liquid or a semi-solid substance. Most cysts are harmless.
Erythema	Reddening of the skin due to the dilation of blood capillaries in the dermis, just below the epidermis.
Fissure	A crack in the epidermis exposing the dermis.
Keloid	An overgrowth of an existing scar that grows much larger than the original wound. The surface may be smooth, shiny or ridged. The onset is gradual and is due to an accumulation or increase in collagen in the immediate area. The colour varies from red, fading to pink and white.
Lesion	A zone of tissue with impaired function, as a result of damage by disease or wounding.
Macule	A small, flat patch of increased pigmentation or discolouration – for example, a freckle.
Milia	Sebum trapped in a blind duct with no surface opening, usually found around the eye area. They appear as pearly, white, hard nodules under the skin.
Mole	Moles are also known as a pigmented naevi. They appear as round, smooth lumps on the surface of the skin. They may be flat or raised and vary in size and colour, from pink to brown or black. They may have hairs growing out of them.
Naevus	A mass of dilated capillaries. May be pigmented, as in a birthmark.
Papule	Small, raised elevation on the skin, less than 1 cm in diameter, which may be red in colour. Often develops into a pustule.
Pustule	Small, raised elevation on the skin that contains pus.
Skin tag	Small growth of fibrous tissue, which stands up from the skin and is sometimes pigmented (black or brown).
Scar	A mark left on the skin after a wound has healed. Scars are formed from replacement tissue. Depending on the type and extent of damage, the scar may be raised (hypertrophic), rough and pitted (ice pick) or fibrous and lumpy (keloid). Scar tissue may appear smooth and shiny or form a depression in the surface.
Telangiecstasis	This is a term for dilated capillaries, where there is persistent vasodilation of capillaries in the skin. Usually caused by extremes of temperature and overstimulation of the tissues, although sensitive and fair skins are more susceptible to this condition.

▲ Table 2.7 Glossary of useful terms

Tumour	A tumour is formed by an overgrowth of cells and almost every type of cell in the epidermis and dermis is capable of benign or malignant overgrowth. Tumours are lumpy, and even when they cannot be seen, they can be felt underneath the surface of the skin.
Ulcer	A break or open sore in the skin, extending to all its layers.
Vesicles	Small, sac-like blisters. A bulla is a vesicle larger than 0.5 cm and is commonly called a blister.
Wart	Well-defined, benign tumour, which varies in size and shape. (See viral infections of the skin on page 44.)
Weal	A raised area of skin, containing fluid, which is white in the centre, with a red edge, commonly seen in the condition urticaria.
Xanthoma	Xanthoma is a skin condition in which certain fats build up under the surface of the skin. A xanthoma looks like a sore or bump under the skin. It is usually flat, soft to the touch and yellow in colour. It has sharp, distinct edges. It is particularly common among older adults and people with high blood lipids. A common type of xanthoma appears on the eyelids and may occur without any underlying medical condition.

▲ Table 2.7 *Continued*

To access a matching exercise for skin types and skin conditions visit www.hodderplus.co.uk/indianhead/chapter-2.

Disorders of the sebaceous gland

Acne vulgaris

A common inflammatory disorder of the sebaceous glands which leads to the over-production of sebum. It involves the face, back and chest and is characterised by the presence of comedones, papules, pustules and, in more severe cases, cysts and scars.

Acne vulgaris is primarily androgen-induced and appears most frequently at puberty and usually persists for a considerable period of time.

There are four different grades of acne, the grade being dependent on the severity of the disorder.

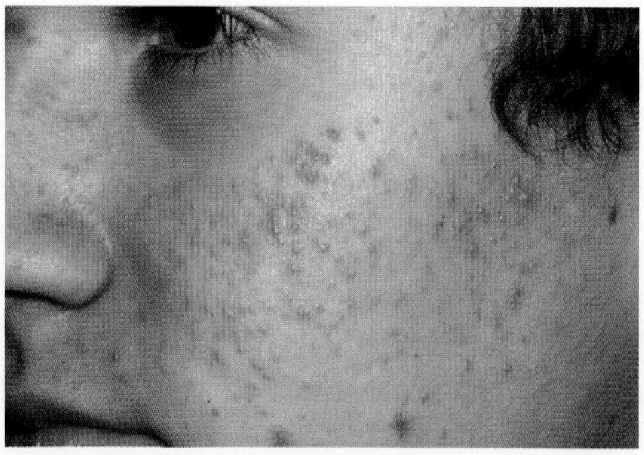

▲ Figure 2.6 Acne vulgaris

Grade I acne	Presence of a few papules and pustules, minor breakout. Mainly open comedones present, with some closed comedones. Typical in a teenager just beginning puberty.
Grade II acne	Greater incidence of papules and pustules, presence of many closed comedones and more open comedones.
Grade III acne	Skin appears very red and inflamed, with many papules and pustules present.
Grade IV acne	Cysts present, with comedones, papules, pustules. Skin appears inflamed.

▲ Table 2.8 Four grades of acne

Rosacea

A chronic inflammatory disease of the face in which the skin appears abnormally red. The condition is gradual and begins with flushing of the cheeks and nose; as the condition progresses it may become pustular. Aggravating factors include hot, spicy foods, hot drinks, alcohol, menopause, the elements and stress.

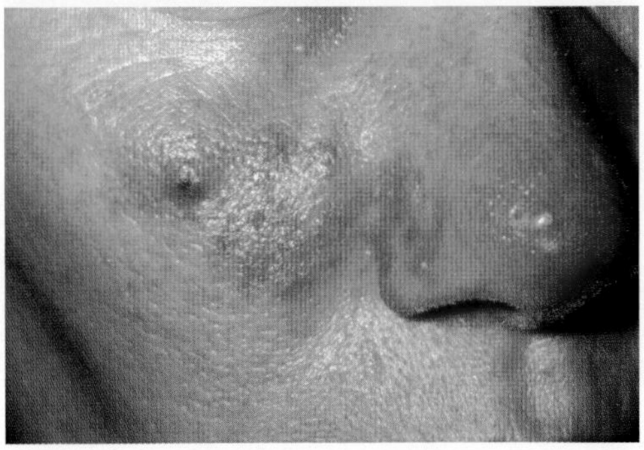

▲ Figure 2.7 Rosacea

Sebaceous cyst

A round, nodular lesion with a smooth, shiny surface, which develops from a sebaceous gland. They are usually found on the face, neck, scalp and back. They are situated in the dermis and vary in size from 5 to 50 mm. The cause is unknown.

Seborrhoea

This condition is defined as an excessive secretion of sebum by the sebaceous glands. The glands are enlarged and the skin appears greasy, especially on the nose and the centre zone of the face. The condition may develop into acne vulgaris and is common at puberty, lasting for a few years.

Disorders of the sweat glands

Hyperhidrosis

Excessive production of sweat affecting the hands, feet and underarms.

Bacterial infections

Boil

A boil begins as a small, inflamed nodule, which forms a pocket of bacteria around the base of a hair follicle or a break in the skin. Local injury or lowered constitutional resistance may encourage the development of boils.

Conjunctivitis

This is a bacterial infection following irritation of the conjunctiva of the eye. In this condition, the inner eyelid and eyeball appear red and sore and there may be a pus-like discharge from the eye. The infection spreads by contact with the secretions from the eye of the infected person.

Health and safety note

Clients who present with acne that is acutely inflamed (Grade III or IV) need to be referred to their GP and/or dermatologist, to ensure that the correct treatment is offered and that any infection that has impacted at the base of the follicle is treated.

Health and safety note

In the case of clients with rosacea, it is important to avoid products that are harsh, abrasive, fragranced or too heavy, and to avoid a very stimulating massage.

Health and safety note

A client who presents with what appears to be a sebaceous cyst should be referred to their GP, who may recommend it is removed surgically.

Health and safety note

In the case of an infectious skin disorder, no treatment can be carried out until all signs of infection have ceased. This is to prevent cross-infection and to avoid the condition spreading and/or worsening. Clients should also be referred to their GP to ensure that the proper treatment is carried out to help clear the condition.

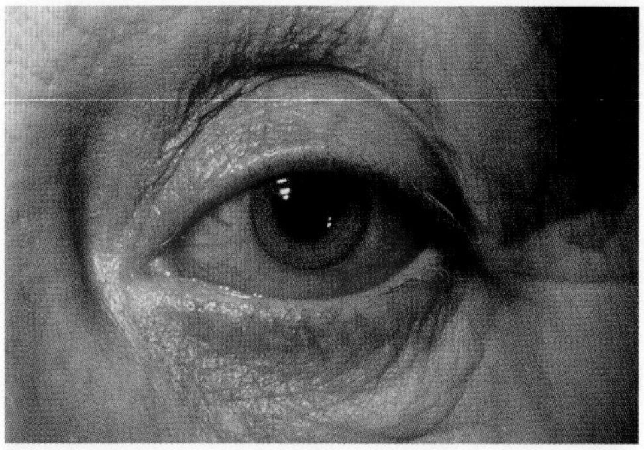

▲ Figure 2.8 Conjunctivitis

Blepharitis

This is a condition where the rims of the eyelids become inflamed (red and swollen), which can result in symptoms such as burning, soreness or stinging in the eyes, crusty eyelashes or itchy eyelids. There are three main types of blepharitis, all of which can cause symptons similar to those described above:

1. Staphylococcal blepharitis is caused by a bacterial infection.
2. Seborrhoeic blepharitis is closely associated with a skin condition called seborrhoeic dermatitis.
3. Meibomian blepharitis (the meibomian glands are tiny glands in the eyelids that lie just behind the eyelashes).

Folliculitis

This is a bacterial infection and appears as a small pustule at the base of a hair follicle. There is redness, swelling and pain around the hair follicle.

Pseudo-folliculitis is often referred to as razor bumps, and resembles folliculitis without the pus.

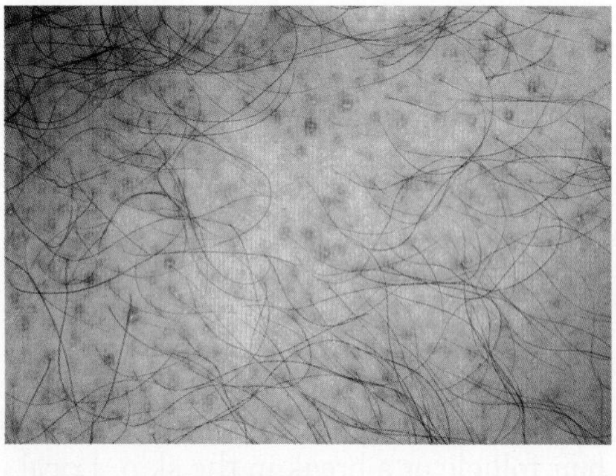

▲ Figure 2.9 Folliculitis

Sycosis barbae

Sycosis barbae is a chronic folliculitis in which there are pustules in the hair follicles and inflammation of the surrounding skin area. Folliculitis is characterised by burning and itching, with pain on manipulation of the hair.

Chronic, persistent infection results in spread to the surrounding skin, which becomes red and crusted, resembling eczema. The upper lip is particularly susceptible in patients who suffer from chronic nasal discharge from sinusitis or hay fever.

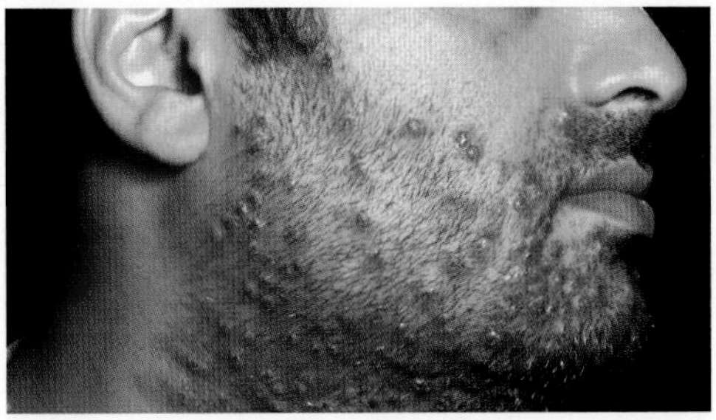

▲ Figure 2.10 Sycosis barbae

Impetigo

A superficial, contagious, inflammatory disease caused by streptococcal and staphylococcal bacteria. It is commonly seen on the face and around the ears, and features include weeping blisters which dry to form honey-coloured crusts. (The bacteria are easily transmitted by dirty fingernails and towels.)

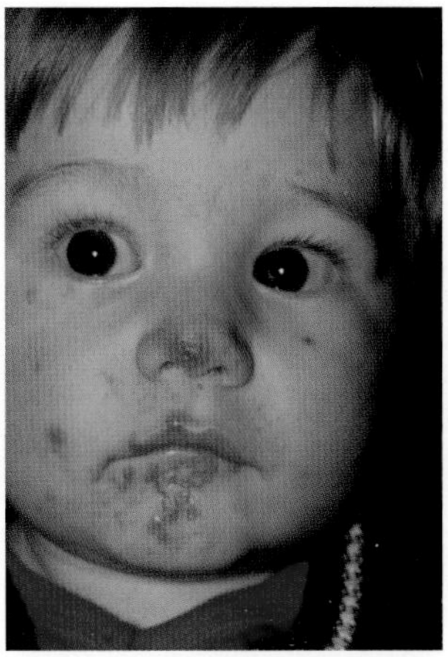

▲ Figure2.11 Impetigo

Stye

This acute inflammation of a gland at the base of an eyelash is caused by bacterial infection. The gland becomes hard and tender, and a pus-filled cyst develops at the centre.

Viral infections of the skin

Herpes simplex (cold sores)

Herpes simplex is normally found on the face and around the lips. It begins as an itching sensation, followed by erythema and a group of small blisters, which then weep and form crusts. This condition will generally persist for approximately two or three weeks. It will recur at times of stress, ill health or exposure to sunlight.

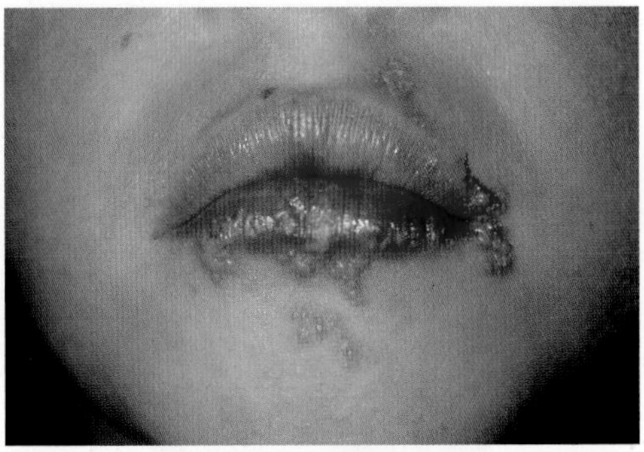

▲ Figure 2.12 Herpes simplex

Herpes zoster (shingles)

This is an infection along the sensory nerves due to the virus that causes chicken pox. Lesions resemble herpes simplex with erythema and blisters along the lines of the nerves. Areas affected are mostly on the back or upper chest wall. This condition is very painful due to acute inflammation of one or more of the peripheral nerves. Severe pain may persist at the site of shingles for months or even years after the apparent healing of the skin.

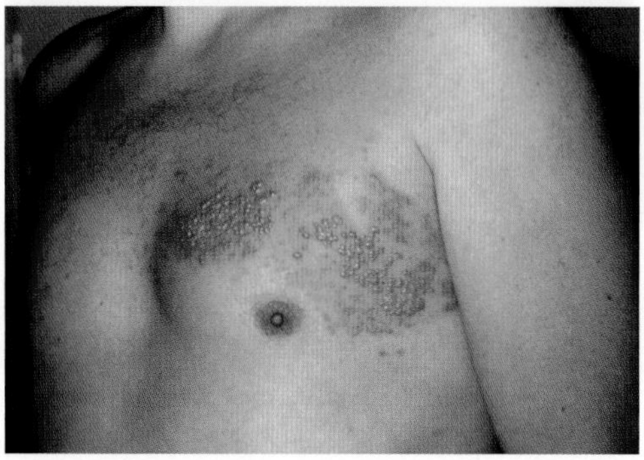

▲ Figure 2.13 Herpes zoster

Warts

A wart is a benign growth on the skin caused by infection with the human papilloma virus.

- Plane warts are smooth in texture, with a flat top, and are usually found on the face, forehead, the back of the hands and the front of the knees.
- Plantar warts or verrucae occur on the soles of the feet. These warts are often grey and the centre frequently has pinpoint black spots.

Fungal infections of the skin

Ringworm

This is a fungal infection of the skin, which begins as small, red papules that gradually increase in size to form a ring. Affected areas on the body vary in severity, from mild scaling to inflamed, itchy areas.

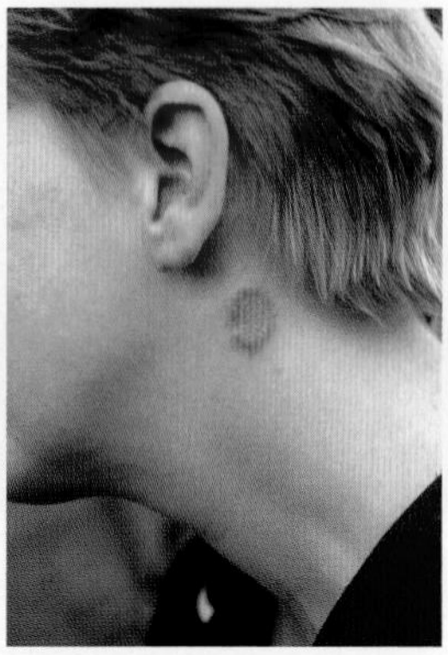

▲ Figure 2.14 Ringworm

Tinea barbae (ringworm of the beard)

Tinea barbae is the name used for fungal infection of the beard and moustache areas. It is less common than tinea capitis and generally affects only adult men. The skin is usually very inflamed, with red lumpy areas, pustules and crusting around the hairs. The hairs can be pulled out easily. Surprisingly, it is not excessively itchy or painful.

The cause of tinea barbae is most often an animal fungus, originating from cattle or horses. It most often affects farmers and is due to direct contact with an infected animal. It is rarely passed from one person to another.

Tinea capitis (ringworm of the scalp)

This appears as painless, round, hairless patches on the scalp. Itching may be present and the lesion may appear red and scaly.

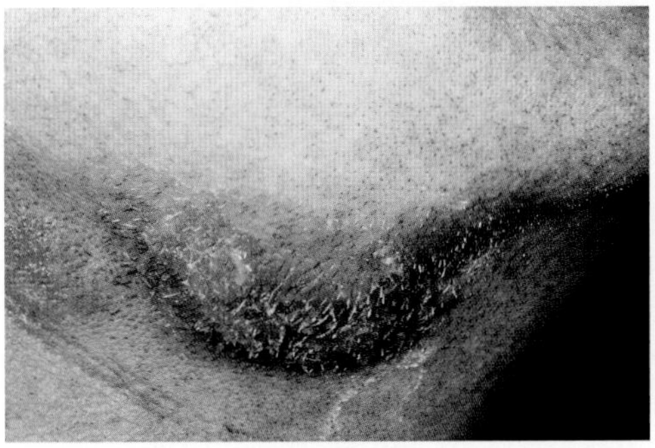

▲ Figure 2.15 Tinea barbae

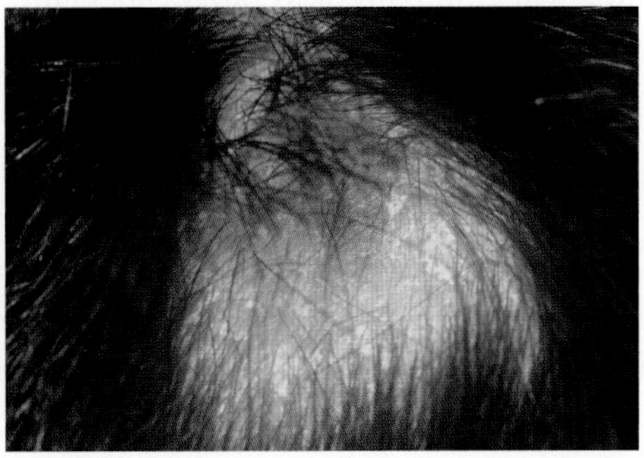

▲ Figure 2.16 Tinea capitis

Tinea pedis (athlete's foot)

This is a highly contagious condition that is easily transmitted in damp, moist conditions, such as swimming pools, saunas and showers. Athlete's foot appears as flaking skin between the toes, which becomes soft and soggy. The skin may also split and the soles of the feet may occasionally be affected.

Tinea corporis (ringworm of the body)

This fungal infection involves areas of the skin not covered by hair, and is characterised by a pink to red rash and is often considerably itchy. Tinea corporis is highly contagious.

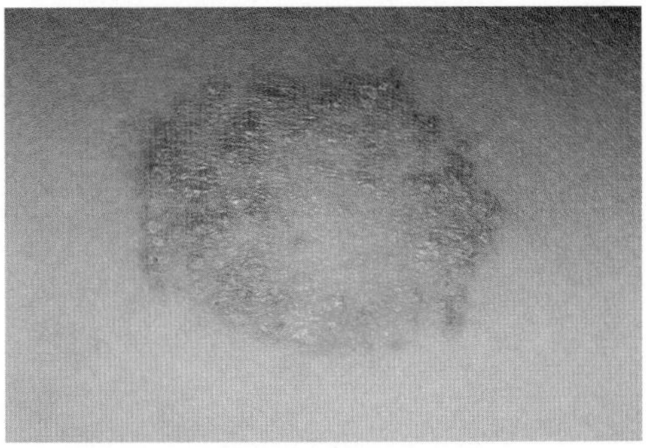

▲ Figure 2.17 Tinea corporis

Infestation disorders of the skin

Pediculosis (lice)

This condition is commonly known as lice and is a contagious parasitic infection, where the lice live off blood sucked from the skin. Head lice are frequently seen in young children and, if not dealt with quickly, may lead to a secondary infection as a result of scratching (impetigo). The eggs of head lice (nits) may be found in the hair; these are pale grey or brown, oval structures found on the hair shaft close to the scalp. The scalp may appear red and raw due to scratching.

Body lice are rarely seen. They will occur on an individual with poor personal hygiene; they live and reproduce in seams and fibres of clothing, feeding off the skin. Lesions may appear as papules, scabs and, in severe cases, pigmented, dry, scaly skin. Secondary bacterial infection is often present. A client affected by body lice will complain of itching, especially in the shoulder, back and buttock areas.

Scabies

A contagious, parasitic skin condition, caused by the female mite, which burrows into the horny layer of the skin where she lays her eggs. The first noticeable symptom of this condition is severe itching, which worsens at night; papules, pustules and crusted lesions may also develop.

Common sites for this infestation are the ulnar borders of the hand, the palms and between the fingers and toes. Other sites include the axillary folds, buttocks, the breasts in the female and the external genitalia in the male.

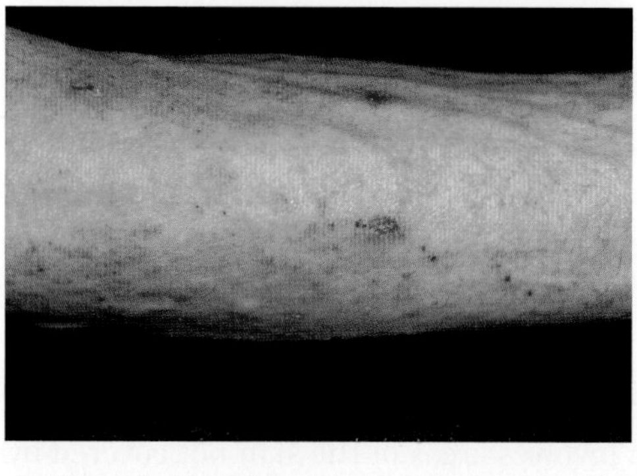

▲ Figure 2.18 Scabies

Pigmentation disorders

Albinism

A condition in which there is an inherited absence of pigmentation in the skin, hair and eyes, resulting in white hair, and pink skin and eyes. The pink colour is produced by underlying blood vessels that are normally masked by pigment. Other clinical signs of this condition include poor eyesight and sensitivity to light.

Chloasma

This is a pigmentation disorder that presents with irregular areas of increased pigmentation, usually on the face. It commonly occurs during pregnancy and sometimes when taking the contraceptive pill, due to stimulation of melanin by the female hormone oestrogen.

Dermatosis papulosa nigra

This is a unique, benign skin condition that is common among black skins. It is characterised by multiple, small, hyperpigmented, asymptomatic papules.

It appears as small, dark bumps and most commonly affects the face, neck, chest and back. The cause of dermatosis papulosa nigra is uncertain. There is a strong genetic basis for the disorder, and often the lesions can be seen in several members of the same family. Under the microscope, the lesions are a type of keratosis that is harmless.

Dermatosis papulosa nigra (DPN) is not a skin cancer, and it will not turn into a skin cancer. The condition is chronic, with new lesions appearing over time. No treatment is necessary other than for cosmetic concerns.

Health and safety note

In certain circumstances, if the lesions of DPN are symptomatic (painful, inflamed, itchy or catch on clothing), clients should be referred to their GP, as they can be treated via a minor surgical procedure.

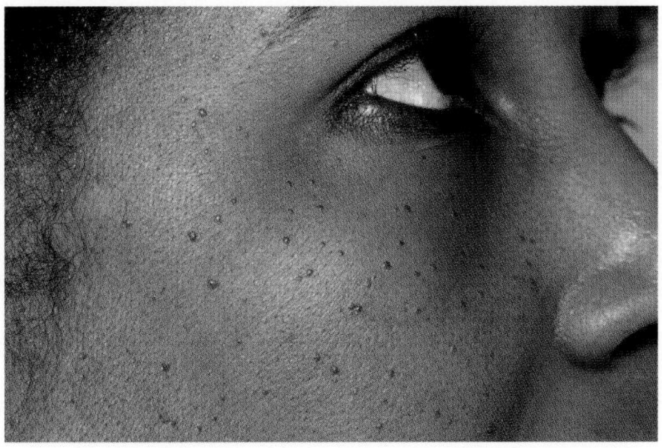

▲ Figure 2.19 Dermatosis papulosa nigra

Ephelides

This is another name for freckles. These are small, harmless, pigmented areas of skin. They appear where there is excessive production of the pigment melanin (after exposure to sunlight).

Lentigo

Also known as liver spots, these are flat, dark patches of pigmentation, which are found mainly in the elderly on skin exposed to light.

Papilloma

This is a wart-like growth on the skin or on a mucous membrane, derived from the epidermis and usually benign.

Vitiligo

This condition presents with areas of the skin that lack pigmentation, due to the basal cell layer of the epidermis no longer producing melanin. The cause of vitiligo is unknown.

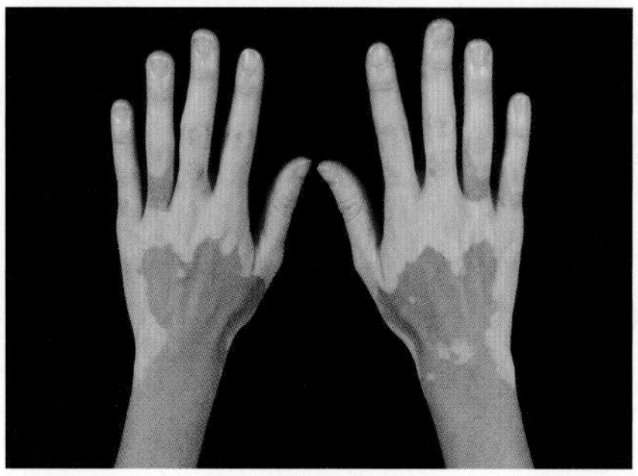

▲ Figure 2.20 Vitiligo

Naevi

Port wine stain

Also known as a deep capillary naevus, this is present at birth and may vary in colour from pale pink to deep purple. It has an irregular shape, but is not raised above the skin's surface. It is usually found on the face, but may also appear on other areas of the body.

Spider naevi

This is a collection of dilated capillaries which radiate from a central papule. They often appear during pregnancy or as the result of 'picking a spot'.

Strawberry mark

This usually develops before or shortly after a baby is born, but fades and disappears spontaneously before the child reaches the age of ten. It is raised above the skin's surface.

Hypertrophic disorders

Hyperkeratosis

Keratoses are generally defined as a build-up of cells.

Hyperkeratosis is a rare skin disorder in which there is a gross thickening of the skin due to a mass of keratinocytes that builds up to a horny overgrowth of skin cells.

Health and safety note

Care needs to be taken with hyperkeratosis to avoid harsh treatment or use of oils that are too stimulating, as this may cause irritation and sensitivity.

Malignant melanoma

A malignant melanoma is a deeply pigmented mole that is life-threatening if it is not recognised and treated promptly. Its main characteristic is a blue-black nodule, which increases in size, shape and colour and is most commonly found on the head, neck or trunk. Overexposure to strong sunlight is a major cause and its incidence is increased in young people with fair skins.

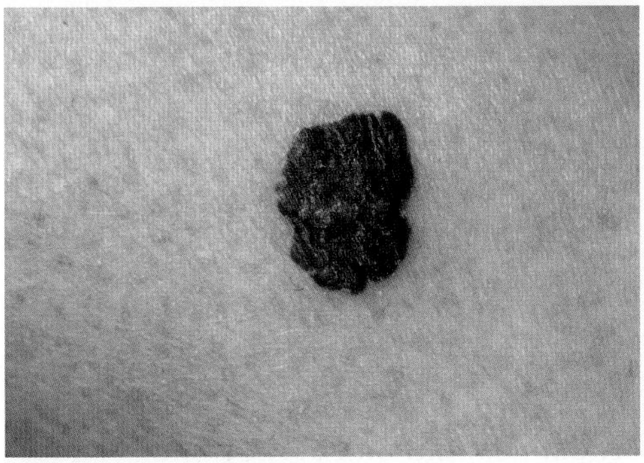

▲ Figure 2.21 Malignant melanoma

Health and safety note

Any client who presents with an abnormal growth or undiagnosed lump on the skin should be referred to their medical practitioner.

Rodent ulcer

This is a malignant tumour, which starts off as a slow-growing, pearly nodule, often at the site of a previous skin injury. As the nodule enlarges, the centre ulcerates and refuses to heal. The centre becomes depressed and the rolled edges become translucent, revealing many tiny blood vessels. Rodent ulcers do not disappear and, if left untreated, may invade the underlying bone. *This is the most common form of skin cancer*.

Squamous cell carcinoma

This is a malignant tumour that arises from the prickle cell layer of the epidermis. It is hard and warty and eventually develops a 'heaped-up, cauliflower appearance'. It is most frequently seen in elderly people.

Inflammatory/congenital skin conditions

Contact dermatitis

Dermatitis literally means 'inflammation of the skin'. Contact dermatitis is caused by a primary irritant that causes the skin to become red, dry and inflamed. Substances that are likely to cause this reaction include acids, alkalis, solvents, perfumes, lanolin, detergents and nickels. There may be skin infection as well.

Eczema

A mild to chronic inflammatory skin condition, characterised by itchiness, redness and the presence of small blisters that may be dry or may weep if the surface is scratched. It can cause scaly and thickened skin, mainly at flexures – for example, the cubital area of the elbows and the back of the knees.

Health and safety note

In the case of inflammatory skin disorders, care would be needed to avoid any form of stimulation (through product or treatment method) that may increase or worsen the inflammation.
If there is severe inflammation and the skin is broken, or if there are any signs of infection, treatment would need to be avoided and the client referred to their GP.

Eczema is not contagious; the cause may be genetic or due to internal and external influences.

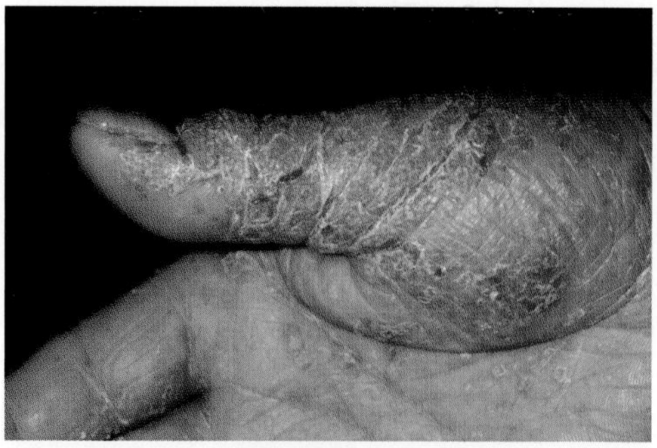

▲ Figure 2.22 Eczema

Psoriasis

A chronic inflammatory skin condition. Psoriasis may be recognised as the development of well-defined red plaques, varying in size and shape, covered by white or silvery scales. Any area of the body may be affected by psoriasis, but the most commonly affected sites are the face, elbows, knees, nails, chest and abdomen. It can also affect the scalp, joints and nails.

Psoriasis is aggravated by stress and trauma, but is improved by exposure to sunlight.

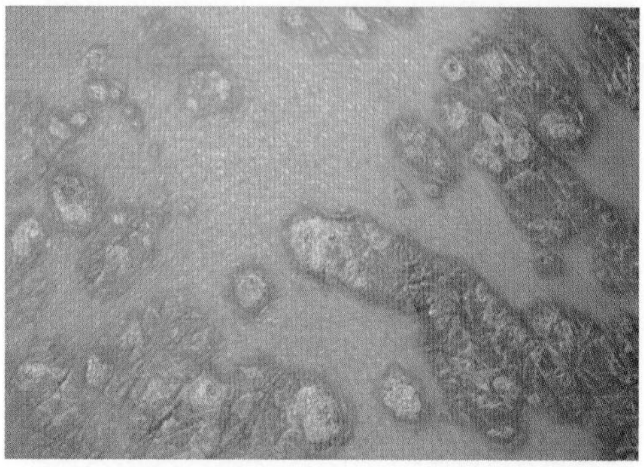

▲ Figure 2.23 Psoriasis

Seborrhoeic dermatitis

This is a mild to chronic inflammatory disease of those hairy areas that are well supplied with sebaceous glands. Common sites are the scalp, face, axilla and groin. The skin may appear to have a grey tinge or may be dirty yellow in colour. Clinical signs include slight redness, scaling and dandruff in the eyebrows.

Pityriasis simplex capitis (dandruff)

Dandruff is a popular collective name signifying a scaly, flaking scalp condition. Pityriasis simplex capitis is a non-inflammatory scalp condition that presents as exfoliation of the stratum corneum (outer layer of epidermal cells).

Health and safety note

In the case of a client with dandruff, place a towel across the client's upper back, to prevent dead skin cells from dropping on to clothes during treatment.

Urticaria

This is also known as hives. In this condition, lesions appear rapidly and disappear within minutes or gradually over a number of hours. The clinical signs are the development of red weals, which may later become white. The area becomes itchy or may sting.

There are a number of causes of urticaria, some of which are an allergic reaction – for example, to foods like strawberries or shellfish, or to penicillin, house dust or pet fur. Other causes include stress and sensitivity to light, heat or cold.

Knowledge check 4

1. Which skin disorder begins as an itching sensation, followed by erythema and a group of small blisters, which then weep and form crusts?
2. How would you recognise a malignant melanoma?
3. Which skin condition presents with areas of the skin that lack pigmentation?
4. How would you recognise tinea capitis?
5. What is a papule?
6. What action would you take in the event of a client with herpes zoster enquiring about having an Indian head massage?

To see the answers to this knowledge check, scan the QR code below or visit www.hodderplus.co.uk/indianhead/chapter-2.

Skin disease/disorder	Avoid contact	GP referral	Adapt
Boil	✓	✓	
Conjunctivitis	✓	✓	
Blepharitis	✓	✓	
Folliculitis	✓	✓	
Sycosis barbae	✓	✓	
Impetigo	✓	✓	
Stye	✓	✓	
Herpes simplex	✓	✓	
Herpes zoster	✓	✓	
Warts	✓	✓	
Ringworm	✓	✓	
Tinea capitis	✓	✓	
Tinea corporis	✓	✓	
Pediculosis	✓	✓	
Scabies	✓	✓	
Contact dermatitis	if severe		✓
Eczema	if severe		✓
Psoriasis	if severe		✓
Seborrhoeic dermatitis			✓

▲ Table 2.9 Summary of main skin diseases and disorders affecting Indian head massage

To access a sorting exercise for skin disorders visit www.hodderplus.co.uk/indianhead/chapter-2.

Skin disease/disorder	Avoid contact	GP referral	Adapt
Dandruff (pityriasis simplex capitis)			✔
Acne vulgaris		if severe	✔
Acne rosacea		if severe	✔
Sebaceous cyst		✔	✔
Dermatosis papulosa nigra			✔
Malignant melanoma		✔	
Rodent ulcer		✔	
Squamous cell carcinoma		✔	
Hyperkeratosis			✔

▲ Table 2.9 *Continued*

The skeleton

The skeleton is the structure and framework on which other body systems depend for support and protection; it is therefore the physical foundation of the body. The main functions of the skeleton are to provide a means of protection, support and attachment for muscles. The skeleton is very important to a therapist, as it provides landmarks for locating muscles.

Functions of the skeleton

Support

The skeleton bears the weight of all other tissues. Without it, we would be unable to stand up.

Shape

The bones of the skeleton give shape to structures such as the skull, thorax and limbs.

Protection of vital organs and delicate tissue

The skeleton surrounds vital organs and tissue with a tough and resilient covering, such as the ribcage protecting the heart and lungs, and the vertebral column protecting the spinal cord.

Attachments for muscles and tendons

Bones are like anchors that allow the muscle to function efficiently.

Movement

This happens as a result of the coordinated action of muscles on bones and joints. Bones are therefore levers for muscles.

Formation of blood cells

These develop in red bone marrow found in cancellous bone tissue.

Mineral reservoir

The skeleton acts as a storage depot for important minerals such as calcium, which can be released when needed for essential metabolic processes like muscle contraction and the conduction of nerve impulses.

The structure of bone

Bone is one of the hardest types of connective tissue in the body, and when fully developed is composed of water, calcium salts and organic matter. Bone tissue is living tissue made from special cells called osteoblasts. There are two main types of bone tissue: compact and cancellous. All bones have both types of tissue, the amount being dependent on the type of bone.

Compact (dense) bone

This is the hard portion of the bone that makes up the main shaft of the long bones and the outer layer of other bones. It protects spongy bone and provides a firm framework for the bone and the body.

Cancellous (spongy) bone

This is lighter in weight than compact bone. It has an open, sponge-like appearance, and is found at the ends of long bones or at the centre of other bones.

The development of bone

The process of bone development is called ossification. This process begins in the embryo near the end of the second month, and is not complete until about the twenty-fifth year of life.

Types of bone

Bones are classified according to their shape. The classifications are long bones, short bones, flat bones, irregular bones and sesamoid bones.

Bone type	Characteristics	Examples
Long	Weight-bearing bones, designed to provide structural support	Arms and legs
Short	Look like blocks, allow a wider range of movement than larger bones	Wrist and ankle bones
Flat	Plate-like structures with broad surfaces Designed for protection	Skull, scapula, ribs, sternum, pelvic bones
Irregular	Have a variety of shapes; usually have projections that muscles, tendons and ligaments can attach to	Vertebral column, some facial bones
Sesamoid	Small, rounded bone embedded in a tendon	Kneecap/patella

▲ Table 2.10 Different types of bone

Long bones

Long bones have a long shaft (a diaphysis) and one or more endings, or swellings (epiphysis). Smooth hyaline cartilage covers the articular surfaces of the shaft endings. Between the diaphysis and epiphysis of growing bone is a flat plate of hyaline cartilage called the epiphyseal cartilage or growth plate. This is the site of bone growth, and as fast as this cartilage grows it is turned into bone, allowing the bone to continue to grow in length.

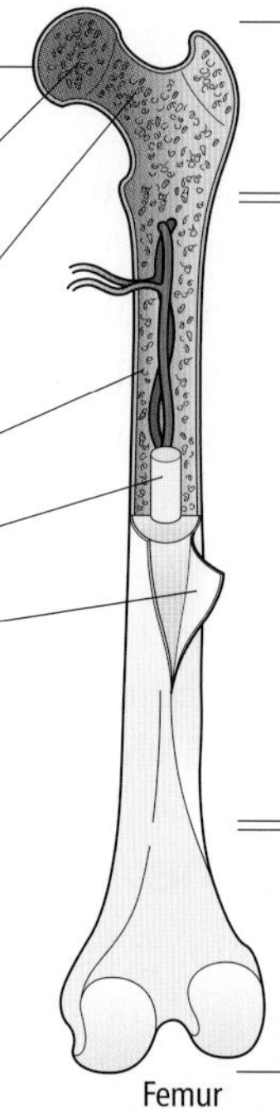

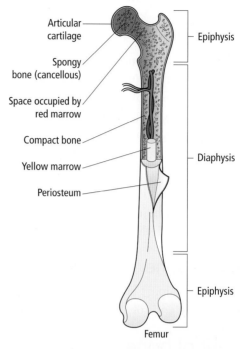

▲ Figure 2.24 Structure of a long bone

Key fact

Children's bones are more flexible than adults', as their bodies contain more cartilage and soft bone cells because complete calcification has not yet taken place. In older adults the opposite is true, as bone cells outnumber cartilage cells and the bone becomes more brittle, due to the fact that it contains more minerals and fewer blood vessels. This explains why elderly people's bones are more prone to fracture and slower to heal.

Vertebrae

The spine, which provides a central axis to the body, consists of 33 individual irregular bones called vertebrae. The spine is made up of the following:

- 7 cervical vertebrae – bones in the neck
- 12 thoracic vertebrae – bones of the mid-spine
- 5 lumbar vertebrae – bones of the lower back
- 5 sacral vertebrae – fused to form sacrum
- 4 coccygeal vertebrae – fused to form coccyx or tail bone.

Vertebrae of the neck

The neck comprises seven bones known as the cervical vertebrae. Although they are the smallest vertebrae in the spine, their bone tissue is denser than those in any other region of the vertebral column.

The top two cervical vertebrae are named C1 and C2.

- C1 is called the atlas and is the bone that sits at the top of the vertebral column, embedded in the base of the skull. The atlas supports and balances the head. Sliding joints on either side of the atlas allow the head to move up and down.
- C2 is called the axis and has a peg-like hook that fits into a notch in the atlas. The ring-and-peg structure of the atlas and axis allows for movement of the head from side to side.

The transverse processes of the cervical vertebrae are distinctive in that they have transverse foramina (or holes), which serve as passageways for arteries leading to the brain.

The spinous processes of the second through to the fifth cervical vertebrae are uniquely forked to provide attachment for the elaborate lattice of muscles of the neck. The spinous process of the seventh cervical vertebrae is longer and can be felt through the skin as it protrudes beyond the other cervical spines.

Vertebrae of the mid-spine

There are 12 thoracic vertebrae of the mid-spine and these lie in the thorax, where they articulate with the ribs. These vertebrae lie flatter and downwards to allow for muscular attachment of the large muscle groups of the back.

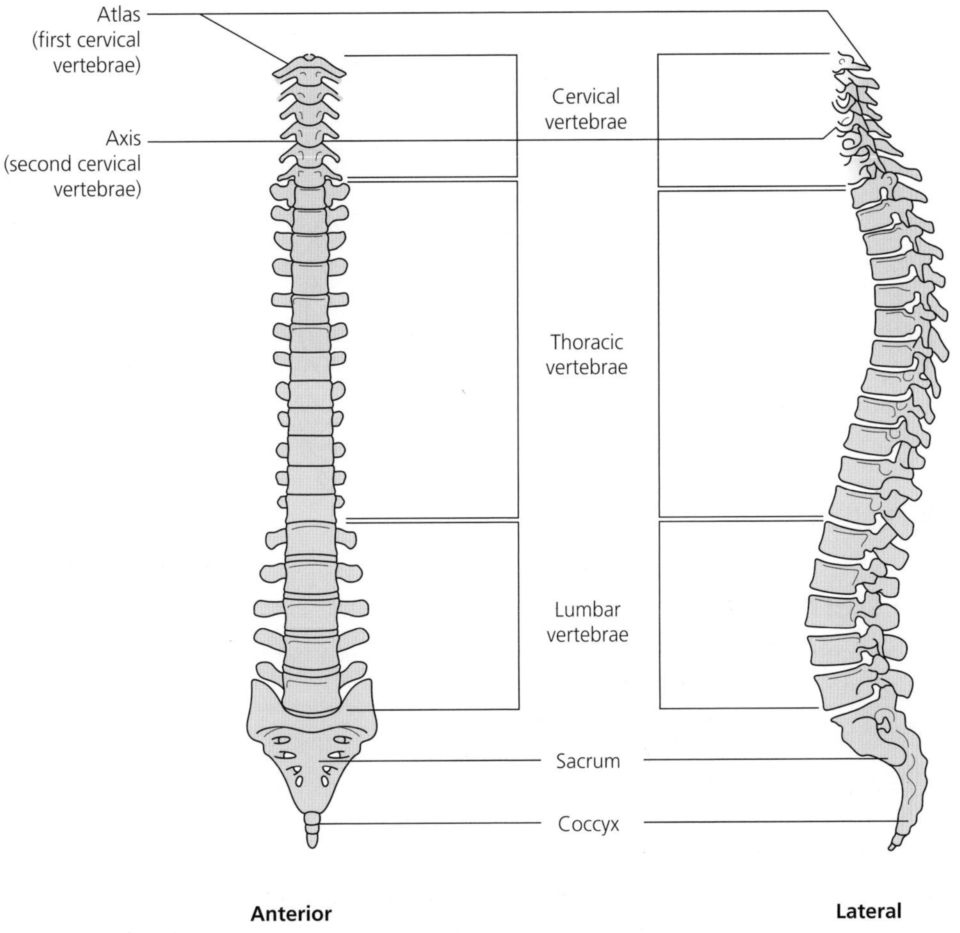

▲ Figure 2.25 Vertebrae of the spine

Vertebrae of the lower back

There are five vertebrae that lie in the lower back; they are much larger than the vertebrae above them as they are designed to support body weight.

Sacrum

The sacrum is made up of five fused vertebrae that form a flat, triangular-shaped bone lying between the pelvic bones.

Coccyx

The coccyx is made of four coccygeal vertebrae fused together.

The thoracic cavity

This is the area of the body enclosed by the ribs, providing protection for the heart and lungs.

Essential bones found in the thoracic cavity include:

- the sternum
- the ribs
- 12 thoracic vertebrae.

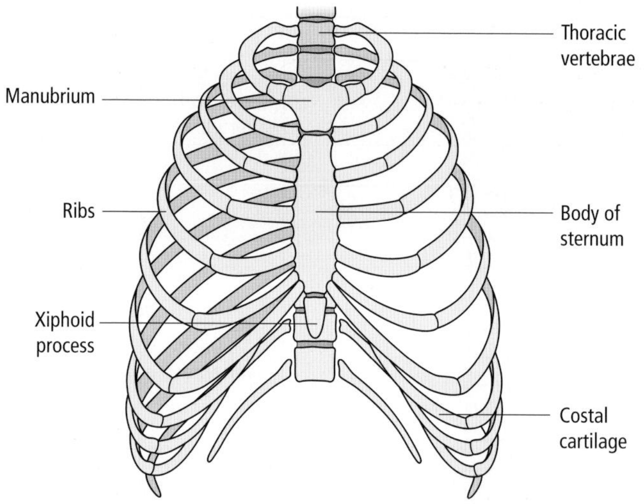

▲ Figure 2.26 The thoracic cavity

The sternum

This is commonly referred to as the breastbone and is a flat bone lying just beneath the skin in the centre of the chest.

The sternum is divided into three parts:

- the manubrium, the top section
- the main body, the middle section
- the xiphoid process, the bottom section.

The top section of the sternum articulates with the clavicle and the first rib. The middle section articulates with the costal cartilages that link the ribs to the sternum. The bottom section provides a point of attachment for the muscles of the diaphragm and the abdominal wall.

The ribs

There are 12 pairs of ribs. They articulate with the thoracic vertebrae posteriorly. Anteriorly, the first ten pairs attach to the sternum via the costal cartilages, the first seven directly (known as the true ribs), and the remaining three indirectly (known as the false ribs). The last two ribs have no anterior attachment and are called the floating ribs.

Bones of the shoulders

The shoulder girdle connects the upper limbs with the thorax and consists of four bones:

- two clavicles
- two scapulae.

The **clavicle** forms the anterior part of the shoulder girdle. It is a long, slender bone with a double curve, which is located at the base of the neck and runs horizontally between the sternum and the shoulders. It articulates with the sternum at its medial end and with the scapula at its lateral end. The clavicle acts as a brace for the scapula, helping to hold the shoulders in place.

The **scapulae** form the posterior part of the shoulder girdle and are located on either side of the upper back. The scapula is a large, flat bone, triangular in outline, which articulates with the clavicle and the humerus. The scapula has several prominent processes that serve as attachments for muscles and ligaments. The combined action of scapula, clavicle, humerus and associated muscles allows for a considerable amount of movement of the shoulder and upper limbs.

To access a drag and drop labelling exercise on bones of the neck, chest and shoulder girdle visit www.hodderplus.co.uk/indianhead/chapter-2.

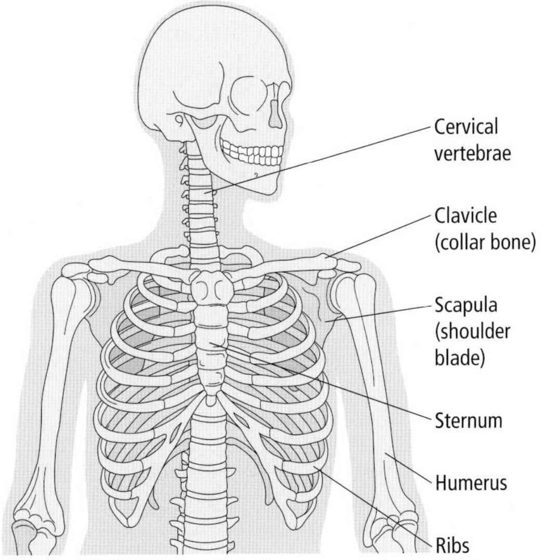

▲ Figure 2.27 Bones of the neck, chest and shoulder girdle

Bones of the upper limb

The upper limb consists of the following bones:

- humerus
- radius
- ulna

- carpals
- metacarpals
- phalanges.

Humerus

The humerus is the long bone of the upper arm. The head of the humerus articulates with the scapula, forming the shoulder joint. The distal end of the bone articulates with the radius and ulna to form the elbow joint.

The radius and ulna

The ulna and radius are the long bones of the forearm. The two bones are bound together by a fibrous ring, which allows a rotating movement in which the bones pass over each other. The ulna is the bone of the little finger side and is the longer of the two forearm bones. The radius is situated on the thumb side of the forearm. The joint between the ulna and the radius permits a movement called pronation. This is when the radius moves obliquely across the ulna so that the thumb side of the hand is closest to the body. The movement called supination takes the thumb side of the hand to the lateral side. The radius and the ulna articulate with the humerus at the elbow and the carpal bones at the wrist.

The wrist and hand

Carpals

The wrist consists of eight small bones of irregular size that are collectively called carpals. They fit closely together and are held in place by ligaments. The carpals are arranged in two groups of four; those of the upper row articulate with the ulna and the radius, and those of the lower row articulate with the metacarpals. The upper row nearest the forearm consists of the scaphoid, lunate, triquetral and pisiform; the lower row consists of the trapezium, trapezoid, capitate and hamate.

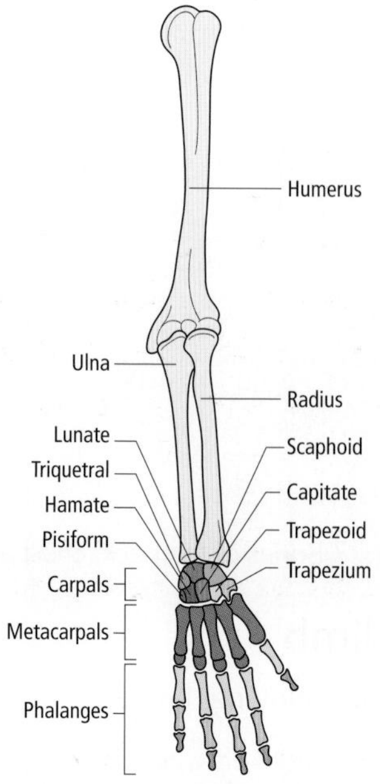

▲ Figure 2.28 Bones of the upper limb

Metacarpals

There are five long metacarpal bones in the palm of the hand; their proximal ends articulate with the wrist bones and the distal ends articulate with the finger bones.

Phalanges

There are 14 phalanges, which are the finger bones, two of which are in the thumb or pollex, and three in each of the other digits.

Bones of the skull

The skull rests on the upper end of the vertebral column and weighs around 11 pounds! It consists of 22 bones: 8 bones that make up the cranium and 14 forming the facial skeleton. The cranium encloses and protects the brain and provides a surface attachment for various muscles of the skull.

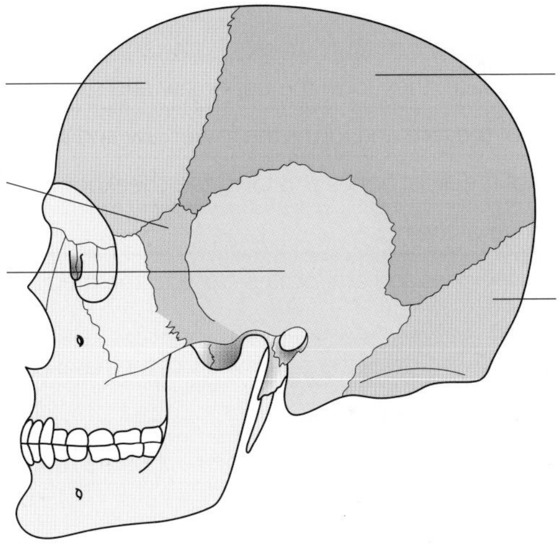

▲ Figure 2.29 Bones of the skull

Name of bone/s	Position
Frontal × I	Forms the anterior part of the roof of the skull, the forehead and the upper part of the orbits or eye sockets
Parietal ×2	Form the upper sides of the skull and the back of the roof of the skull
Temporal ×2	Form the sides of the skull below the parietal bones and above and around the ears
Sphenoid × I	Located in front of the temporal bone and serves as a bridge between the cranium and the facial bones
Ethmoid × I	Forms part of the wall of the orbit, the roof of the nasal cavity and part of the nasal septum
Occipital × I	Forms the back of the skull

▲ Table 2.11 The eight bones of the cranium

Note: The hyoid bone (1) is a U-shaped bone located in the neck. It anchors the tongue and is associated with swallowing.

To access a drag and drop labelling exercise on bones of the skull visit www.hodderplus.co.uk/indianhead/chapter-2.

Bones of the face

There are 14 facial bones in total. These are mainly in pairs, one on either side of the face.

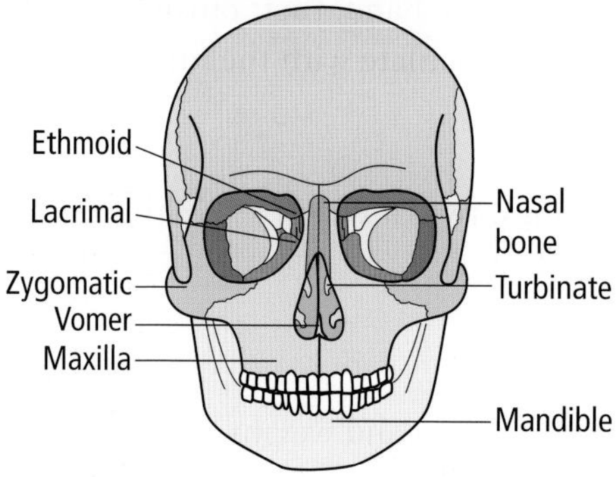

▲ Figure 2.30 Bones of the face

Name of bone/s	Position
Maxilla × 2	These are the largest bones of the face; they form the upper jaw and support the upper teeth.
Mandible × 1	This is the only moveable bone of the face and forms the lower jaw and supports the lower teeth.
Zygomatic × 2	These are the most prominent of the facial bones and form the cheekbones.
Nasal × 2	These small bones form the bridge of the nose.
Lacrimal × 2	These are the smallest of the facial bones and are located close to the medial part of the orbital cavity.
Turbinate × 2	These are layers of bone located either side of the outer walls of the nasal cavities.
Vomer × 1	This is a single bone at the back of the nasal septum.
Palatine × 2	These are L-shaped bones that form the anterior part of the roof of the mouth.

▲ Table 2.12 Bones of the face

Key fact

There are many openings present in the bones of the skull that act as passages for blood vessels and nerves entering and leaving the cranial cavity. For instance, there is a large opening at the base of the skull called the foramen magnum, through which the spinal cord and blood vessels pass to and from the brain.

The sinuses

There are four pairs of air-containing spaces in the skull and face called the sinuses. The function of the sinuses is to lighten the head, provide mucus and act as a resonance chamber for sound. The pairs of sinuses are named according to the facial bones by which they are located. They are the frontal sinuses, the sphenoidal sinuses, the ethmoidal sinuses, and the maxillary sinuses (which are the largest).

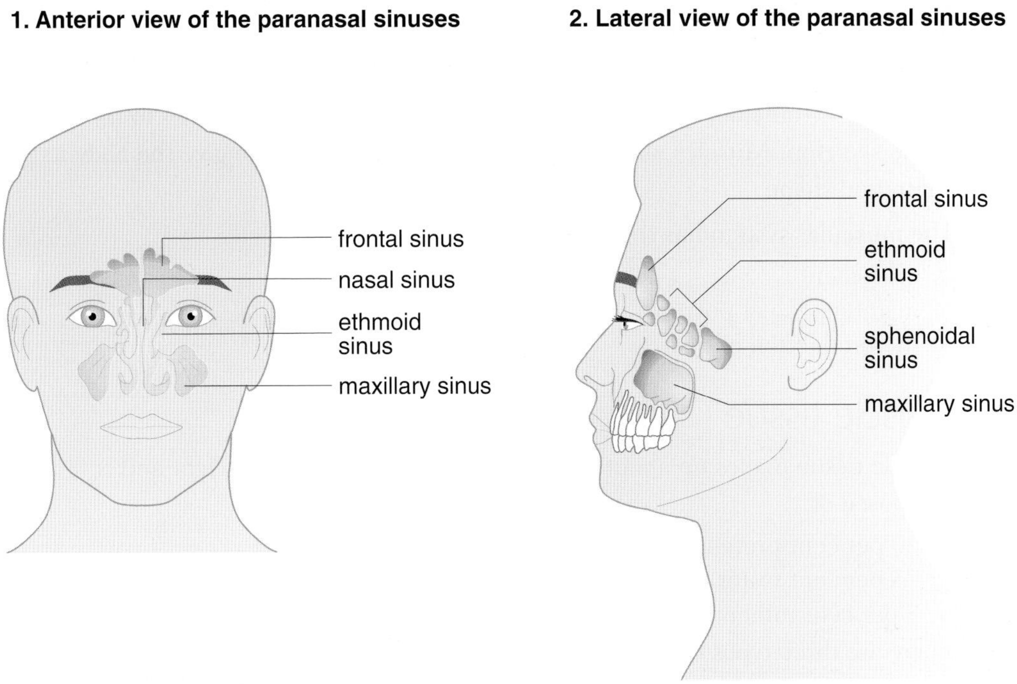

▲ Figure 2.31 The sinuses

Key fact

Indian head massage can help to make parts of the skeletal system, such as the shoulders and neck, more mobile by reducing restrictions in the joints, muscles and their fascia.

Knowledge check 5

1. List the eight bones of the skull.
2. Name the facial bone that forms the lower jaw.
3. Which facial bones form the cheekbones?
4. Which facial bones form the upper jaw and support the upper teeth?
5. List the bones of the shoulder girdle.

To see the answers to this knowledge check, scan the QR code below or visit www.hodderplus.co.uk/indianhead/chapter-2.

To access interactive exercises for bones and the skeletal system visit www.hodderplus.co.uk/indianhead.

The muscular system

There are over 600 skeletal or voluntary muscles in the body that collectively help to create body movement, stabilise joints and maintain body posture. Some skeletal muscles lie superficially, while those layered beneath them are known as deep muscles.

The functions of the muscular system

The muscular system consists largely of skeletal muscle tissue, which covers the bones on the outside, and connective tissue, which attaches muscles to the bones of the skeleton. Muscles, along with connective tissue, help to give the body its contoured shape.

The muscular system has three main functions:

- movement
- maintenance of posture
- the production of heat.

Muscle tissue

Muscle tissue makes up about 50 per cent of your total body weight and is composed of:

- 20 per cent protein
- 75 per cent water
- 5 per cent mineral salts, glycogen and fat.

There are three types of muscle tissue in the body:

1. **skeletal** or **voluntary** muscle tissue, which is primarily attached to bone
2. **cardiac** muscle tissue, which is found in the walls of the heart
3. **smooth** or **involuntary** muscle tissue, which is found inside the digestive and urinary tracts, as well as in the walls of blood vessels.

All three types of muscle tissue differ in their structure and functions and the degree of control the nervous system has on them.

Type of muscle tissue	Description	Location	Function
Voluntary/skeletal	Striped appearance Has many nuclei Held together by connective tissue	Attached to bones, skin or other muscles	Facilitates movement of bones Moves blood and lymph Heat production Maintenance of posture
Cardiac	Striped appearance Branched structure Has a single nucleus Has intercalated discs between each cardiac muscle cell	Heart	Provides a consistent flow of blood throughout the body
Smooth/involuntary	Non-striated Shaped like spindles Has a single nucleus	In walls of stomach, intestines, bladder, uterus and in blood vessels	Move substances through the various tracts (digestive, genito-urinary)

▲ Table 2.13 Types of muscle tissue

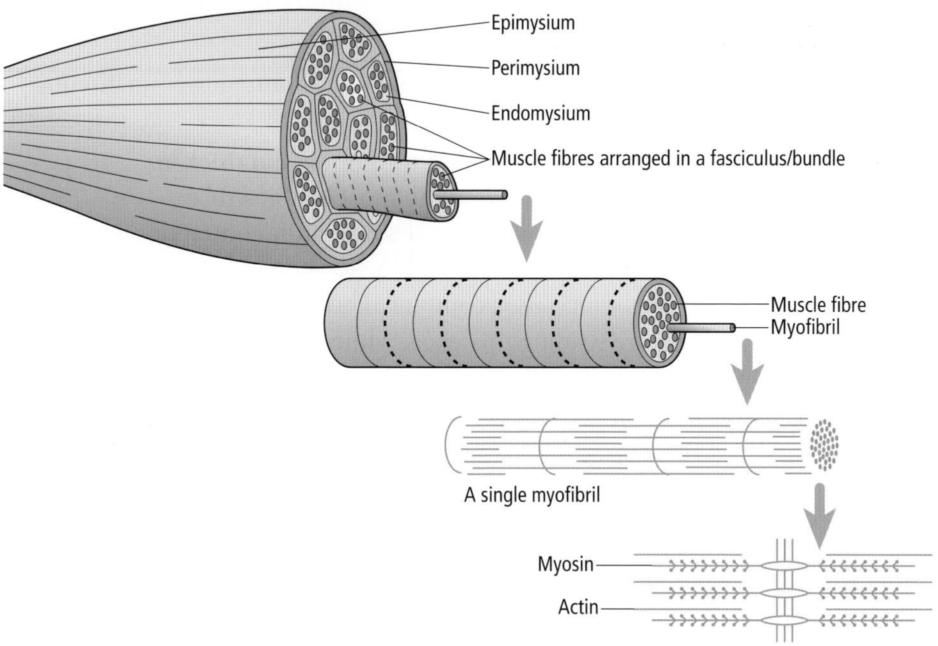

▲ Figure 2.32 The structure of voluntary muscle tissue

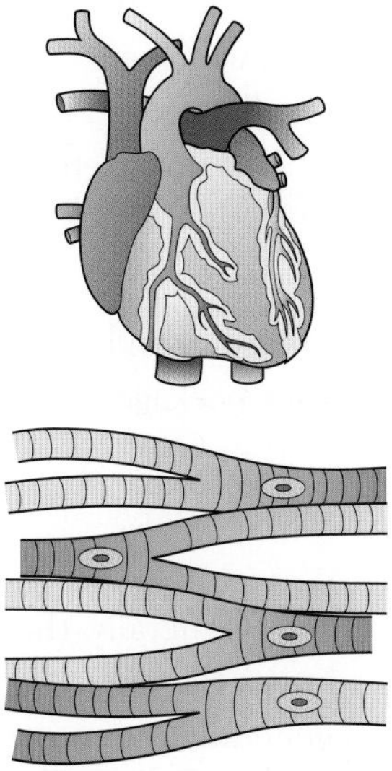

▲ Figure 2.33 Cardiac muscle tissue

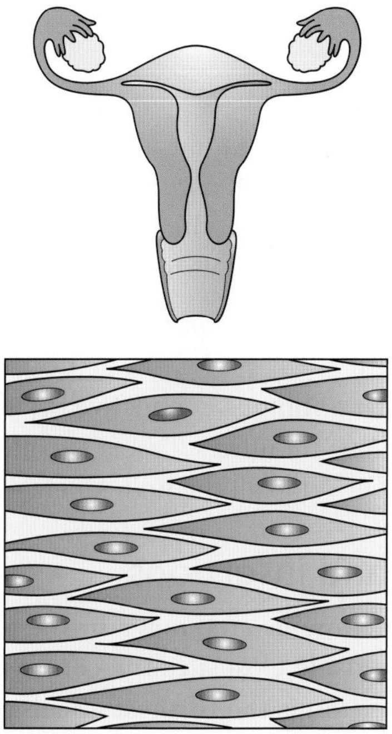

▲ Figure 2.34 Smooth/involuntary muscle tissue

Muscle contraction

Muscle tissue has several characteristics that help contribute to the functioning of a muscle:

- contractibility – the capacity of the muscle to shorten and thicken
- extensibility – the ability to stretch when the muscle fibres relax
- elasticity – the ability to return to its original shape after contraction
- irritability – the response to stimuli provided by nerve impulses.

Muscles vary in the speed at which they contract. The muscle in your eyes will be moving very fast as you are reading this page, while the muscles in your limbs assisting you in turning the pages will be contracting at a moderate speed. The speed of a muscle contraction is therefore modified to meet the demands of the action concerned and the degree of nervous stimulus it has received.

Muscle attachments

In order to understand how skeletal muscles produce movement, it is helpful first to understand how muscles are attached to the rest of the body.

Tendons

Tendons are tightly woven, white, glistening, tough, fibrous bands or cords that link muscle to bone. They do not stretch or contract the way muscles do, so they are not at all elastic.

Ligaments

Ligaments are strong, fibrous, elastic tissues that are usually cord-like in nature. They are placed parallel with or closely interlaced with one another, which creates a white, shining, silvery effect. A ligament is pliant and flexible, to allow good freedom of movement, but is also strong, tough and inextensible (does not stretch).

Fascia

Fascia consist of fibrous connective tissue that envelops certain muscles and then forms partitions for others. Fascia are all-encompassing in that they package, support and envelop all the body's muscles and organs.

Origins and insertions

Muscle attachments are known by the terms origin and insertion. Generally, the end of the muscle closest to the centre of the body is referred to as the origin, and the insertion is the furthest attachment. The insertion is generally the most moveable point and is therefore the point at which the muscle work is done.

Muscle movement

In the coordination of movement, muscles work in pairs or groups. Muscles are classified by functions as:

- agonists (prime movers)
- antagonists

- synergists
- fixators (stabilisers).

Although muscles are usually described as performing a particular action, they do not act alone. Any movement is the result of cooperation between a large number of muscles, and is coordinated in the brain for smooth, efficient actions.

Antagonists

This is when two muscles or sets of muscles pull in opposite directions. They do not actually work against each other, but work in a reciprocal, complementary way, with one relaxing to allow the other to contract.

Agonists/prime movers

This is known as the main activating muscle. An example is the action of the biceps and triceps of the upper arm. The biceps is the agonist in flexion of the elbow joint, and the triceps is the antagonist. In relation to extending or straightening the elbow the roles are reversed.

Synergysts

This term refers to muscles on the same side of a joint that work together to perform the same movement. An example of this is flexing the elbow. The biceps actually works synergistically with the brachialis muscle that lies underneath.

Fixators

These are muscles that stabilise a bone to give a steady base from which the agonist works. For the biceps and triceps to flex and extend the elbow joint, muscles around the shoulder and upper back control the position of the arm.

Muscle contraction

Biomechanically, muscles do one of two things – stretch or contract. Muscular contractions can be isometric or isotonic. Isotonic contractions may be further classified as either concentric or eccentric. The opposite of contracting is stretching, which extends the muscles.

Isometric contraction

This is when the muscle works without actual movements (*iso* means same and *metric* means length). Postural muscles work by isometric contraction.

Isotonic contraction

This is when the muscle's force is considered to be constant (tonic meaning the same tone or tension), but the muscle length changes. There are two types of isotonic contraction:

- concentric contractions (towards the centre) occur when the muscle shortens to move the attachments closer, such as when the biceps bends up the forearm
- eccentric contractions (away from the centre) occur when a muscle is stretched as it tries to resist a force pulling the bones of attachment away from one another, such as when someone pulls your forearm straight while you are tensing the biceps.

Anatomical term	Description	Illustration
Flexion	Bending of a body part at a joint, so that the angle between the bones is decreased	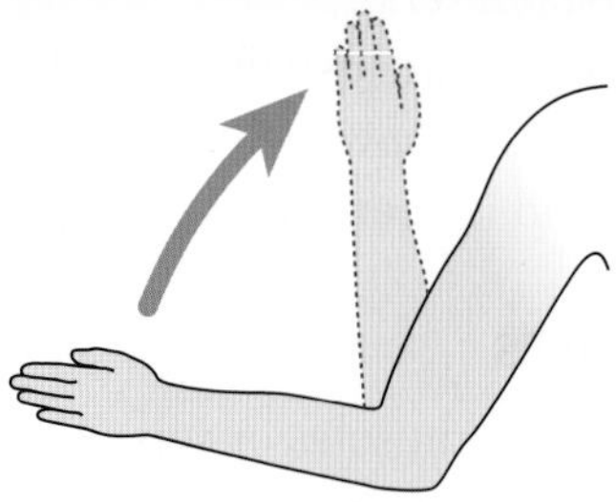
Extension	straightening of a body part at a joint so that the angle between the bones is increased	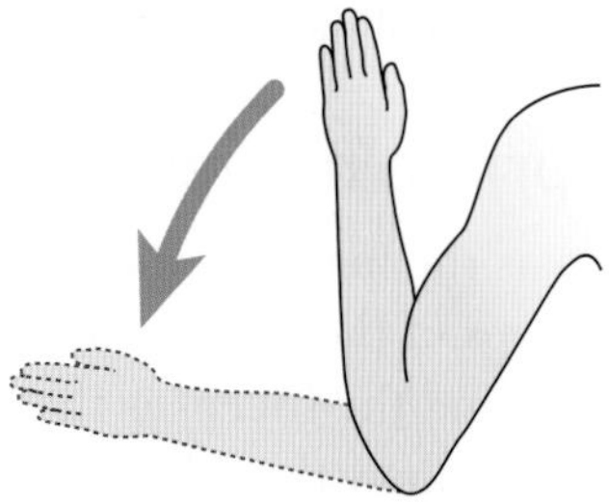
Plantar flexion	Downward movement of the foot so that feet face downwards towards the ground	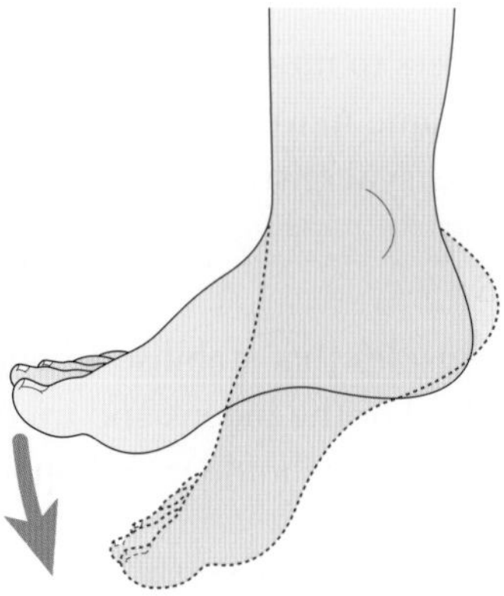
Adduction	movement of a limb towards the midline	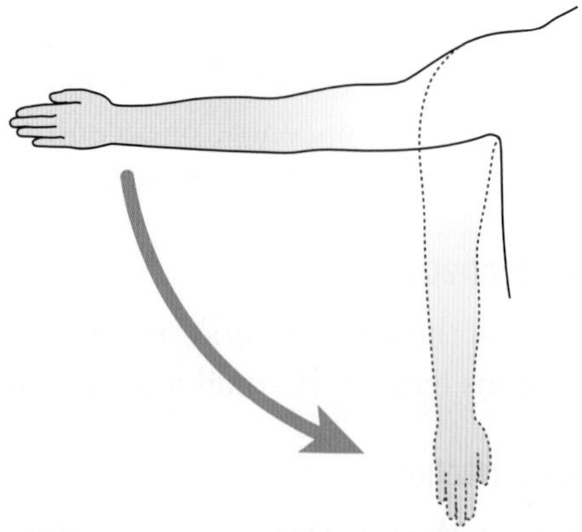

▲ Table 2.14 Muscle/joint movements

Anatomical term	Description	Illustration
Abduction	movement of a limb away from the midline	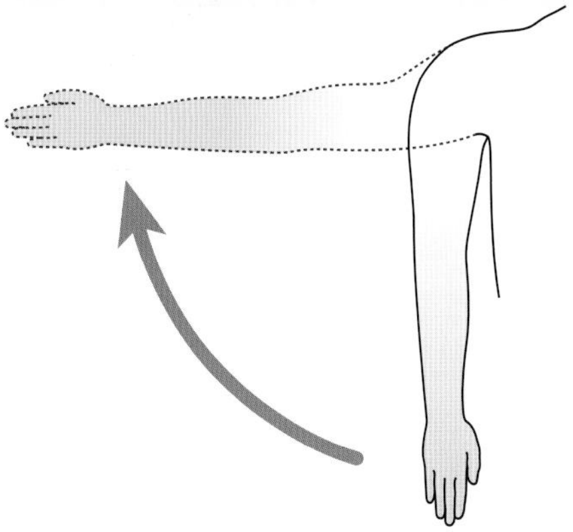
Rotation	movement of a bone around an axis (180 degrees)	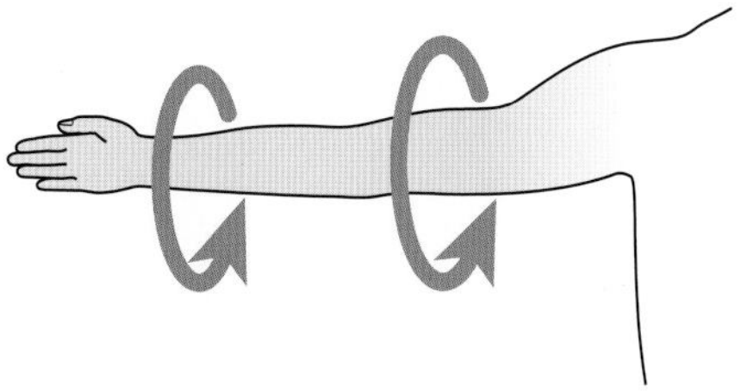
Circumduction	a circular movement of a joint (360 degrees)	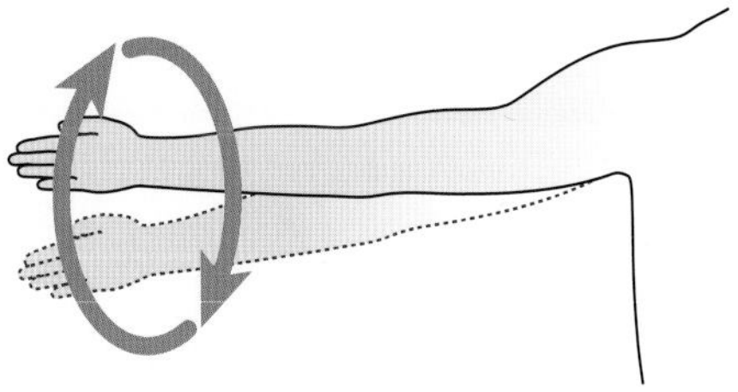
Supination	turning the hand so that the palm is facing upwards	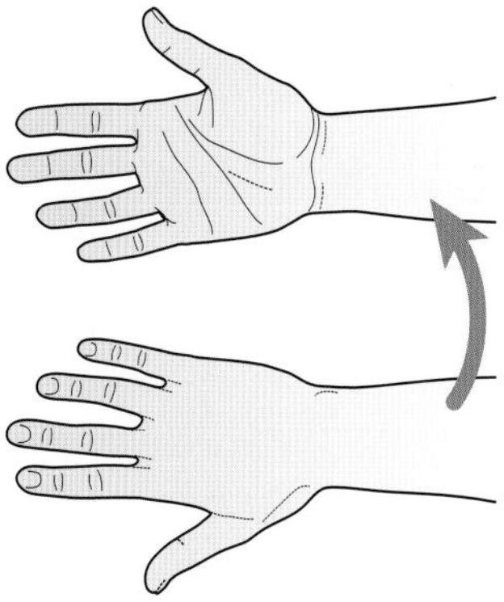

▲ Table 2.14 *Continued*

Anatomical term	Description	Illustration
Pronation	turning the hand so that the palm is facing downwards	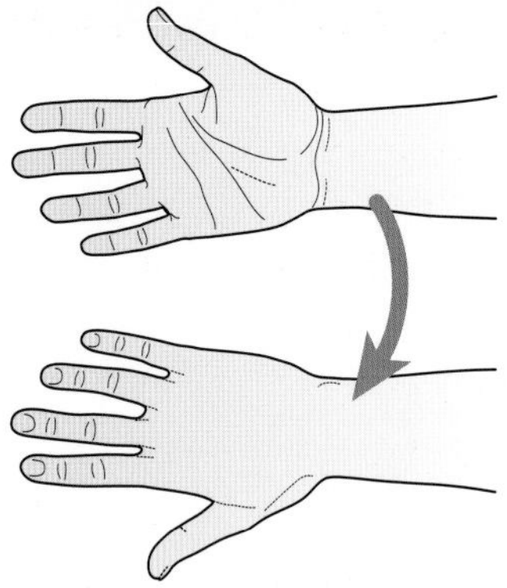
Eversion	soles of the feet face outwards	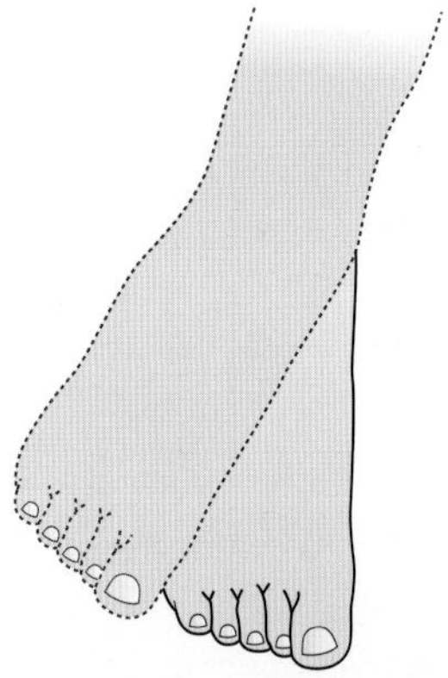
Inversion	soles of the feet face inwards	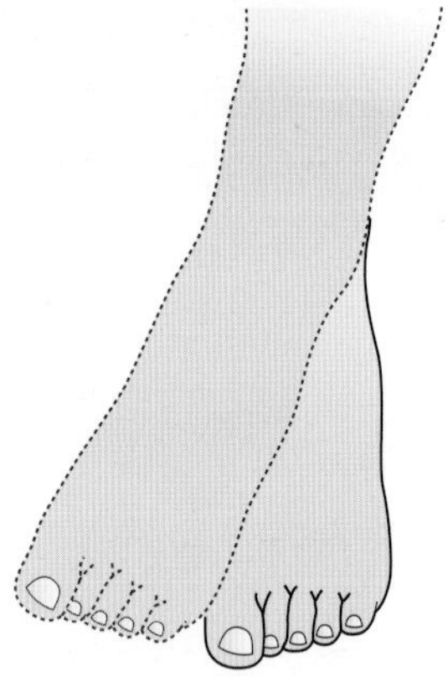

▲ Table 2.14 *Continued*

Muscle fatigue

Muscles require fuel or energy in the form of carbohydrates (glucose), and oxygen is needed to help burn the glucose to release the energy.

After vigorous exercise or activities, the oxygen and energy supply becomes depleted.

This results in a waste product called lactic acid being released into the bloodstream, which causes the muscle to ache.

This is known as muscle fatigue and is defined as the loss of the ability of a muscle to contract efficiently due to insufficient oxygen, exhaustion of the energy supply and the accumulation of lactic acid.

Muscle tone

Even in a relaxed muscle, a few muscle fibres remain contracted to give the muscle a certain degree of firmness. At any given time, a small number of motor units in a muscle are stimulated to contract and cause tension in the muscle, rather than full contraction and movement, while the others remain relaxed. This state of partial contraction of a muscle is known as muscle tone and is important for maintaining body posture. The group of motor units functioning in this way change periodically, so that muscle tone is maintained without fatigue.

Good muscle tone may be recognised by the muscles appearing firm and rounded. Poor muscle tone may be recognised by the muscles appearing loose and flattened.

Muscles with less than the normal degree of tone are said to be flaccid, and when the muscle tone is greater than normal the muscles become spastic and rigid.

Key fact

Muscle tone will vary from person to person and will largely depend on the amount of exercise undertaken. Muscles with good tone have a better blood supply as their blood vessels will not be inhibited by fat.

Knowledge check 6

1. What are the three main functions of the muscular system?
2. List the three types of muscle tissue in the body and where they may be found.
3. Out of the following attachments, which is the most moveable part of a muscle: the origin or the insertion?
4. What is meant by the following terms in relation to joint/muscle movements?
   i. flexion
   ii. extension
   iii. adduction
   iv. rotation.
5. What is the waste product that is released into the bloodstream causing the muscle to ache?
6. How would you recognise muscles with good tone?

To see the answers to this knowledge check, scan the QR code below or visit www.hodderplus.co.uk/indianhead/chapter-2.

Study tip

Learning muscles can be daunting. It is helpful to break the information down into manageable chunks and learn a few muscles at a time.

The following may help you when studying muscles:

1. Is there are clue in the name of the muscle as to where it is located in the body – for example, the frontalis muscle is located across the frontal bone of the forehead?
2. Try to visualise where the muscle is on your body or on a client's body.
3. Look for information that will help you remember the muscle's action (see the Key facts column in Tables 2.15–2.18).

If you know where the muscle is located and attached, you can work out its action by moving that body part and feeling the muscle contracting!

Name of muscle	Position	Origin	Insertion	Action/s	Key facts
Frontalis (front-ta-lis)	Extends over the forehead	Galea aponeurosis (tendon between frontalis and occipitalis)	Fascia and skin above the nose and eyes	Wrinkles the forehead and raises the eyebrows	Used when expressing surprise
Occipitalis (ok-sip-it-ta-lis)	Base/back of skull	Occipital bone and mastoid process	Galea aponeurosis (tendon between frontalis and occipitalis)	Moves the scalp backwards	Is united to the frontalis muscle by a broad tendon called the epicranial aponeurosis, which covers the skull like a cap
Temporalis (tem-po-ra-lis)	Fan-shaped muscle situated on the side of the skull, above and in front of the ear	Temporal and frontal bones	Mandible	Raises the lower jaw when chewing	Muscle becomes tightened with a tension headache
Orbicularis oculi (or-bik-you-la-ris ock-you-ly)	Circular muscle surrounding the eye	Medial wall or orbit of eye	Circular path around the orbit of eye	Closes the eye	Used when blinking or winking Also compresses the lacrimal gland, aiding the flow of tears
Orbicularis oris (or-bik-you-la-ris or-ris)	Circular muscle that surrounds the mouth	Maxilla and mandible bones, muscle fibres surrounding the mouth	Corner of mouth	Closes the mouth	Used when shaping the lips for speech and when kissing Also contracts the lips when tense
Corrugator (kor-u-gay-tor)	Located in between the eyebrows	Frontal bone	Inner edge of eyebrow	Brings the eyebrows together	Used when frowning
Procerus (pro-ser-rus)	Located in between the eyebrows	Nasal bones and cartilage	Skin between eyebrows	Draws the eyebrows inwards	Creates a puzzled expression
Nasalis (nay-sa-lis)	Located at sides of the nose	Maxillae bones and the nostrils	Bridge and tip of nose	Dilates and compresses the nostrils	Used when blowing the nose
Zygomatic major and minor/ zygomaticus (zi-go-mat-ik-us)	Lies in the cheek	Zygomatic bone	Corner of the mouth	Draws the angle of the mouth upwards and laterally	Used when laughing or smiling
Levator labii superioris (le-vay-tor lay-be-eye soo-pee-ri-o-ris)	Above the lip, located towards the inner cheek beside the nose	Maxilla and zygomatic bones	Upper lip and corner of mouth	Raises the upper lip and the corner of mouth	Used to create a snarling expression

▲ Table 2.15 Muscles of the head and neck

Name of muscle	Position	Origin	Insertion	Action/s	Key facts
Levator anguli oris (le-vay-tor ang-you-lie o-ris)	Above the lip, located at a angle above the side of the mouth	Maxilla	Corner of mouth	Raises the corner of mouth	Used when smiling Also known as the caninus (kay-ni-nus), as its contraction can result in the teeth, especially the canine tooth, becoming visible
Depressor anguli oris (dee-pres-or ang-you-lie o-ris)	Side of chin extending down at an angle from the side of mouth	Mandible	Corner of mouth	Draws the corners of the mouth downwards	Used when expressing sadness or uncertainty
Depressor labii inferioris (dee-pres-or lay-be-eye in-fee-ri-o-ris)	Side of chin, extending down from lower lip	Mandible	Lower lip	Pulls the lower lip downwards	Used when expressing sorrow, doubt or irony
Risorius (ri-sor-ri-us)	Triangular-shaped muscle extending diagonally from the corners of the mouth (lies above the buccinator)	Fascia of parotid (salivary) gland	Corner of mouth	Pulls the corner of the mouth sideways and outwards	Used when grinning
Buccinator (buk-sin-a-tor)	Main muscle of the cheek	Maxilla and mandible	Muscles of lips	Compresses the cheeks when sucking or blowing	Used when blowing up a balloon or blowing a trumpet Helps hold food in contact with the teeth when chewing
Mentalis (men-ta-lis)	Radiates from the lower lip over the centre of the chin	Mandible	Chin	Elevates the lower lip and wrinkles the skin of the chin	When expressing displeasure and when pouting
Masseter (ma-sa-ter)	Thick, flattened muscle at sides of cheek/jaw	Maxilla and zygomatic	Mandible	Raises the jaw and exerts pressure on the teeth when chewing	Main muscle of mastication Can be felt just in front of the ear when the teeth are clenched
Lateral pterygoids (lat-er-al ter-i-goyds)	Outer part of cheeks	Sphenoid bone	Mandible and temporomandibular joint	Opens the jaw and moves mandible when chewing	Tension in these muscles may be associated with dysfunction of the temporomandibular joint (TMJ syndrome)

▲ Table 2.15 *Continued*

Name of muscle	Position	Origin	Insertion	Action/s	Key facts
Medial pterygoids (mee-dee-al ter-i-goyds)	Outer part of cheeks	Sphenoid and maxilla	Mandible	Closes the jaw and moves mandible when chewing	Tension in these muscles may be associated with dysfunction of the temporomandibular joint (TMJ syndrome)
Levator palpebrae (le-vay-tor pal-pray)	Across the eyelids	Roof or orbit of eye	Skin of upper eyelid	Opening the eyes	Assists the orbicularis oculi in moving the eyelids and protecting the eye
Sternocleido-mastoid (ster-no-kli-do-mas-toyd)	Long muscle that lies obliquely across each side of the neck	Sternum and clavicle mastoid process (back of the ear)	Mastoid process (back of the ear)	When working together, they flex the neck (pull the chin down towards the chest), and when working individually, they rotate the head to the opposite side	Spasm of the sternocleidomastoid muscle results in a condition known as torticollis or wryneck. Sternocleidomastoid is the only muscle that moves the head but is not attached to any vertebrae
Platysma (pla-tiz-ma)	Superficial muscle that covers the front of the neck	Fascia covering the upper part of pectoralis major and deltoid	Mandible, facial and muscles of chin and jaw	Depresses the lower jaw and lower lip	Used in yawning and when creating a pouting expression

▲ Table 2.15 *Continued*

To access a drag and drop labelling exercise on muscles of the head and neck visit www.hodderplus.co.uk/indianhead/chapter-2.

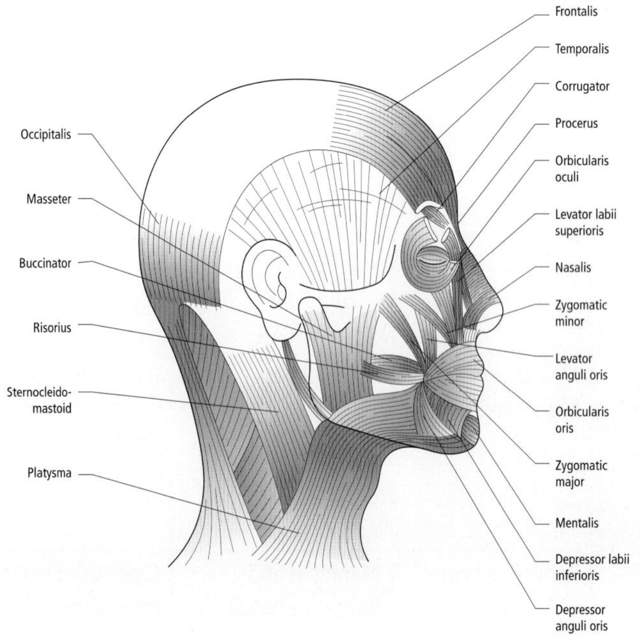

▲ Figure 2.35 Muscles of the head and neck

Name of muscle	Position	Origin	Insertion	Action/s	Key facts
Trapezius (tra-pee-zee-us)	Large, triangular-shaped muscle in upper back Its fibres are arranged in three groups – upper, middle and lower	Occipital bone, 7th cervical vertebrae and 12th thoracic vertebrae	Clavicle and scapula	The upper fibres raise the shoulder girdle; the middle fibres pull the scapula towards the vertebral column; the lower fibres draw the scapula and shoulder downwards	One of the most commonly found muscles to hold upper body tension, causing discomfort and restrictions in the neck and shoulders
Levator scapula (le-vay-tor skap-you-la)	Strap-like muscle that runs almost vertically through the neck	Cervical vertebrae	Scapula	Elevates and adducts the scapula	Due to its attachments, tension in the levator scapula can affect mobility of both the neck and the shoulders
Deltoid (del-toid)	Thick, triangular muscle that caps the top of the humerus and shoulder	Clavicle and the spine of the scapula	Humerus	Abducts arm, draws the arm backwards and forwards	The deltoid has anterior, lateral and posterior fibres, and these give the shoulder its characteristic shape

▲ Table 2.16 Muscles of the upper back and shoulders

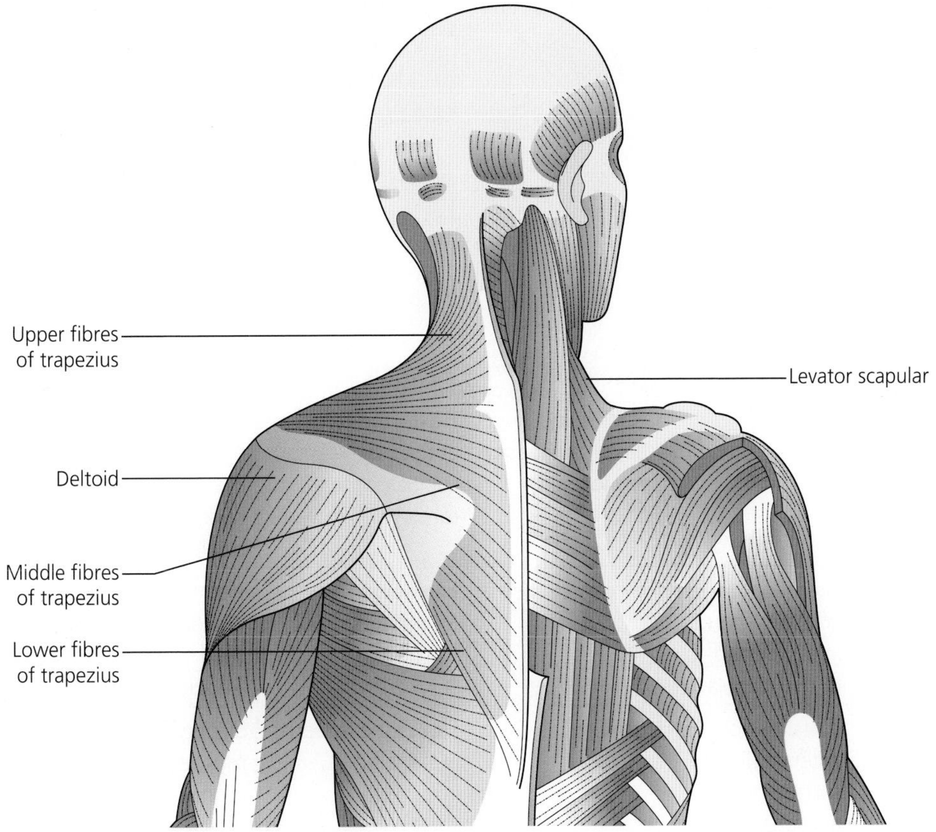

▲ Figure 2.36 Muscles of the upper back/shoulders

Name of muscle	Position	Origin	Insertion	Action/s	Key facts
Pectoralis major (pek-to-ra-lis may-jor)	Thick, fan-shaped muscle covering the anterior surface of the upper chest	Clavicle, sternum and ribs (2nd–6th)	Humerus	Adducts arm, medially (inwardly) rotates arm	Tightness in this muscle can cause restrictions of the chest and postural distortions (rounded shoulders)
Pectoralis minor (pek-to-ra-lis my-nor)	Thin muscle that lies beneath the pectoralis major	Ribs (3rd–5th)	Scapula	Draws the shoulder downwards and forwards	Involved in forced expiration; an accessory respiratory muscle

▲ Table 2.17 Muscles of the chest

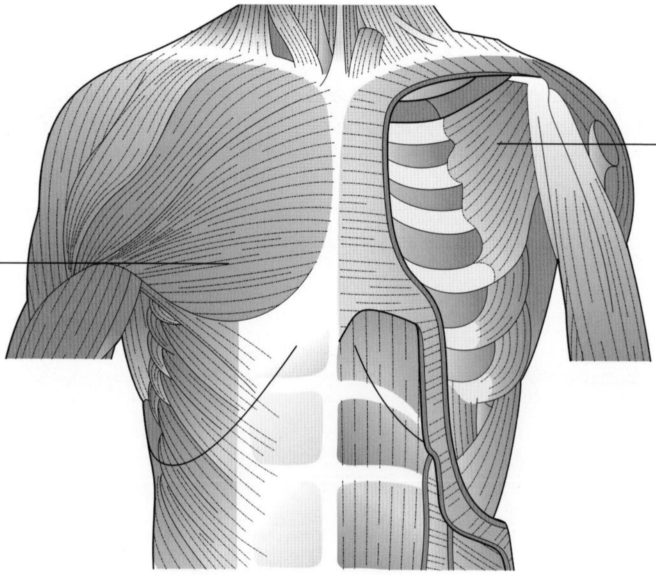

▲ Figure 2.37 Muscles of the chest

Name of muscle	Position	Origin	Insertion	Action/s	Key facts
Biceps (by-seps)	Anterior surface of upper arm (humerus)	Scapula	Radius and flexor muscles of the forearm	Flexes the forearm at the elbow and supinates the forearm	The actions of the biceps muscle are likened to the action of removing a corkscrew from a wine bottle
Triceps (try-seps)	Posterior surface of the upper arm	Posterior (back) of the humerus and outer edge of the scapula	Ulna	Extension (straightening) of the forearm	Also referred to as the 'boxer's muscle', as it is used when delivering a 'knock-out' punch
Brachialis (bray-key-al-is)	Lies beneath the biceps	Distal half of the anterior (front) surface of the humerus	Ulna	Flexes the forearm at the elbow	Strong and fairly large muscle, which accounts for much of the contour of the biceps muscle

▲ Table 2.18 Muscles of the upper limbs

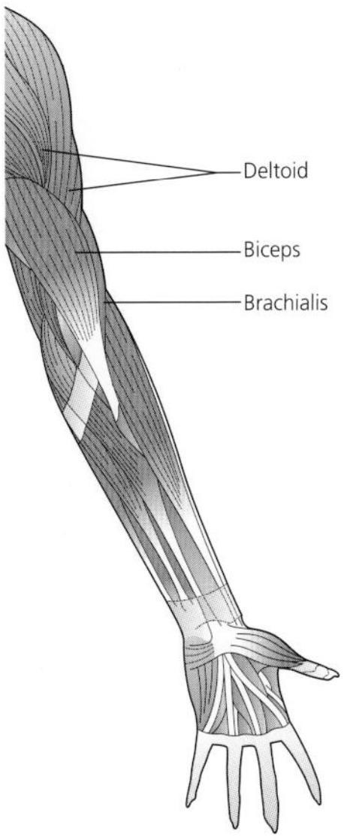

▲ Figure 2.38 Muscles of the upper limbs (anterior)

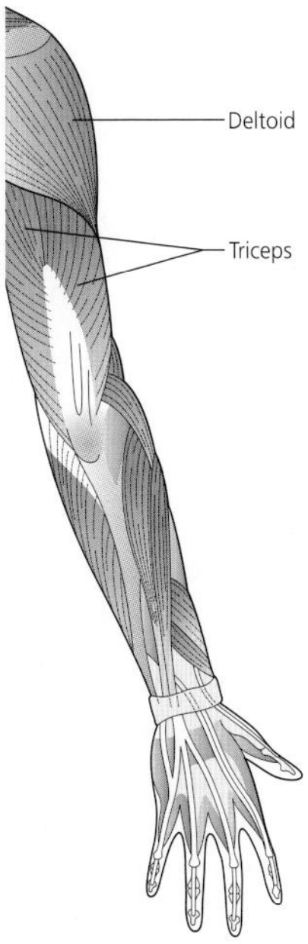

▲ Figure 2.39 Muscles of the upper limbs (posterior)

Knowledge check 7

1. Name the muscle that extends over the forehead.
2. Name the muscle that raises the lower jaw when chewing.
3. Which muscle closes the mouth?
4. Which muscle is used when laughing?
5. Which muscle depresses the lower jaw and lip?

To see the answers to this knowledge check, scan the QR code opposite or visit www.hodderplus.co.uk/indianhead/chapter-2.

To access interactive exercises for the muscles visit www.hodderplus.co.uk/indianhead/chapter-2.

Key fact

Muscular tension is often a sign of emotional as well as physical stress. Indian head massage can help to relieve pain from tight, sore muscles, as well as relieve muscular fatigue, by increasing blood flow, which increases the amount of oxygen and nutrition into the muscles and encourages elimination of waste, absorbing the products of fatigue.

Posture

Posture is a measure of balance and body alignment, and is the maintenance of strength and tone of the body's muscles against gravity. Good posture is said to be when the maximum efficiency of the body is maintained with the minimum effort. When evaluating posture, an imaginary line is drawn vertically through the body and called the centre of gravity line. From the front or back, this line should divide the body into two symmetrical halves:

- with feet together, the ankles and knees should touch
- the hips should be the same height
- the shoulders should be level
- the sternum and vertebral column should run down the centre of the body, in line with the centre of gravity line
- the head should be erect and not tilted to one side.

Posture varies considerably in individuals and is influenced by factors such as body frame size, heredity, occupation, habits and personality. Additional factors that may also affect posture include clothing, shoes and furniture.

Good posture is important as it:

- allows a full range of movement
- improves physical appearance
- keeps muscle action to a minimum, thereby conserving energy and reducing fatigue
- reduces the susceptibility of injuries
- aids the body's systems to function efficiently.

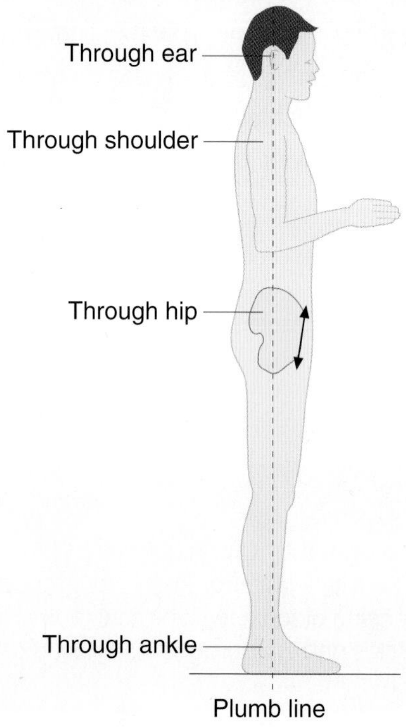

▲ Figure 2.40 Postural alignment

Postural defects

Lordosis

This is an abnormally increased inward curvature of the lumbar spine. In this condition, the pelvis tilts forwards, and as the back is hollow the abdomen and buttocks protrude, and the knees may be hyperextended. Typical problems associated with this condition are tightening of the back muscles followed by a weakening of the abdominal muscles. Because of the anterior tilt of the pelvis, hamstring problems are common. An increase in weight or pregnancy may cause or exacerbate this condition.

Kyphosis

This is an abnormally increased outward curvature of the thoracic spine. In this condition, the back appears round, as the shoulders point forwards and the head moves forwards. A tightening of the pectoral muscles is common in this condition.

Scoliosis

This is a lateral curvature of the vertebral column, which may be to the left or right side.

Evidence of this condition include unequal leg length, distortion of the ribcage, unequal position of the hips or shoulders and curvature of the spine (usually in the thoracic region).

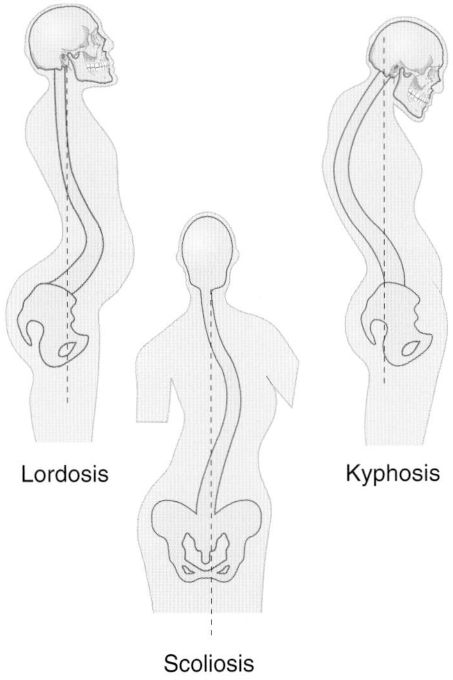

▲ Figure 2.41 Postural defects

Poor posture may have the following effects on the body:

- produce alterations in body function and movement
- waste energy
- increase fatigue
- increase the risk of backache and headaches
- impair breathing
- increase the risk of muscular, ligament or joint injury
- affect circulation
- affect digestion
- give a poor physical appearance.

Blood

Blood is the fluid tissue or medium in which all materials are transported to and from individual cells in the body. Blood is therefore the chief transport system of the body.

The percentage composition of blood

Fifty-five per cent of blood is fluid or plasma, which is a clear, pale yellow, slightly alkaline fluid:

- 91 per cent of plasma is water
- 9 per cent consists of dissolved blood proteins, waste, digested food materials, mineral salts and hormones.

Forty-five per cent of blood is made up of the blood cells: erythrocytes, leucocytes and thrombocytes.

Type of blood cell	**Description**	**Function**
Erythrocyte	Disc-shaped structures Non-nucleated Red in colour due to protein haemoglobin	Transport the gases of respiration
Leucocytes	Largest of all the blood cells White due to lack of haemoglobin	Protect the body against infection and disease
Thrombocytes/ platelets	Granular, disc-shaped, small fragments of cells	Blood clotting

▲ Table 2.19 Summary of the three types of blood cells

Functions of blood

There are four main functions of blood:

- transport
- defence
- regulation
- clotting.

Transport

Blood is the primary transport medium for a variety of substances that travel throughout the body.

- Oxygen is carried from the lungs to the cells of the body in red blood cells.
- Carbon dioxide is carried from the body's cells to the lungs.
- Nutrients, such as glucose, amino acids, vitamins and minerals, are carried from the small intestine to the cells of the body.
- Cellular wastes, such as water, carbon dioxide, lactic acid and urea, are carried in the blood to be excreted.
- Hormones, which are internal secretions that help to control important body processes, are transported by the blood to target organs.

Defence

White blood cells are collectively called leucocytes and they play a major role in combating disease and fighting infection.

Regulation

Blood helps to regulate the body's temperature by absorbing large quantities of heat produced by the liver and the muscles; this is then transported around the body to help maintain a constant internal temperature. Blood also helps to regulate the body's pH balance.

Clotting

If the skin becomes damaged, specialised blood cells called thrombocytes clot to prevent the body from losing too much blood and to prevent the entry of bacteria.

Blood vessels

Blood flows round the body due to the pumping action of the heart and is carried in vessels known as arteries, veins and capillaries.

Arteries	Carry blood away from heart
Veins	Carry blood towards the heart
Capillaries	Unite arterioles and venules, forming a network in the tissues

▲ Table 2.20 Overview of arteries, veins and capillaries

Key facts about blood vessels

Arteries

- Arteries carry blood away from the heart.
- Blood is carried under high pressure.
- Arteries have thick, muscular and elastic walls to withstand pressure.
- Arteries have no valves, except at the base of the pulmonary artery, where they leave the heart.
- Arteries carry oxygenated blood (except the pulmonary artery to the lungs).

- Arteries are generally deep-seated, except where they cross over a pulse spot.
- Arteries give rise to small blood vessels called arterioles, which deliver blood to the capillaries.

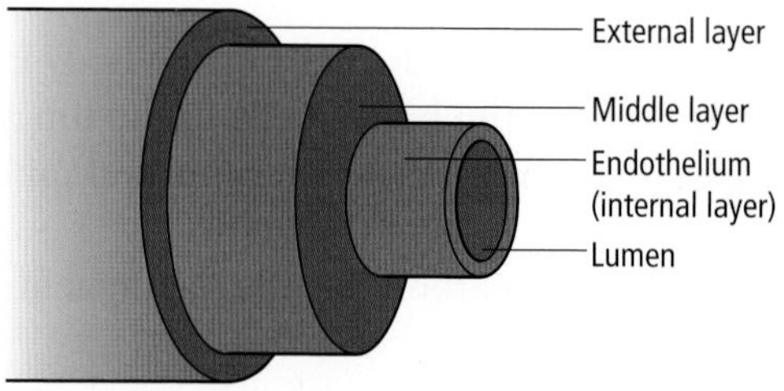

▲ Figure 2.42 Structure of an artery

Veins

- Veins carry blood towards the heart.
- Blood is carried under low pressure.
- Vein walls are thinner and less muscular.
- Veins have valves at intervals to prevent the backflow of blood.
- Veins carry deoxygenated blood (except the pulmonary veins from the lungs).
- Veins are generally superficial, not deep-seated.
- Veins form finer blood vessels called venules, which continue from capillaries.

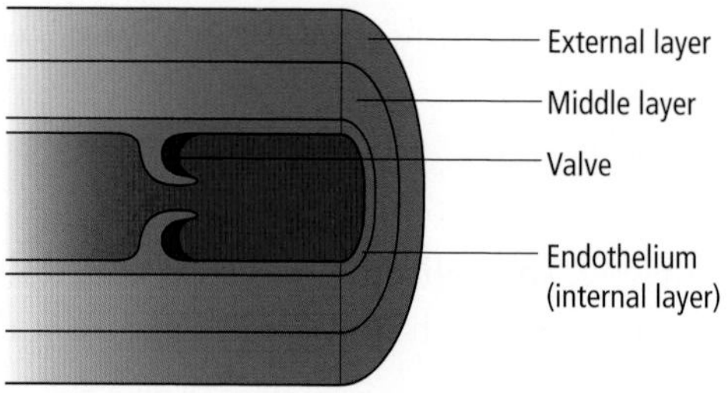

▲ Figure 2.43 Structure of a vein

Key fact

Both arteries and veins have three layers (external, middle and internal layers), but because an artery must contain the pressure of blood pumped from the heart, its walls are thicker and more elastic.

Capillaries

- Capillaries are the smallest vessels.
- Capillaries unite arterioles and venules, forming a network in the tissues.
- The wall of a capillary vessel is only a single layer of cells thick. It is therefore sufficiently thin to allow the process of diffusion of dissolved substances to and from the tissues to occur.
- Capillaries have no valves.
- Blood is carried under low pressure, but higher than in veins.
- Capillaries are responsible for supplying the cells and tissues with nutrients.

Key fact

The key function of a capillary is to permit the exchange of nutrients and waste between the blood and tissue cells. Substances such as oxygen, vitamins, minerals and amino acids pass through to the tissue fluid to nourish the nearby cells, and substances such as carbon dioxide and waste are passed out of the cells. This exchange of nutrients can only occur through the semipermeable membrane of a capillary, as the walls of arteries and veins are too thick.

Oxygenated blood flowing through the arteries appears bright red in colour due to the oxygen pigment haemoglobin; as it moves through capillaries it offloads some of its oxygen and picks up carbon dioxide. This explains why the blood in veins appears darker.

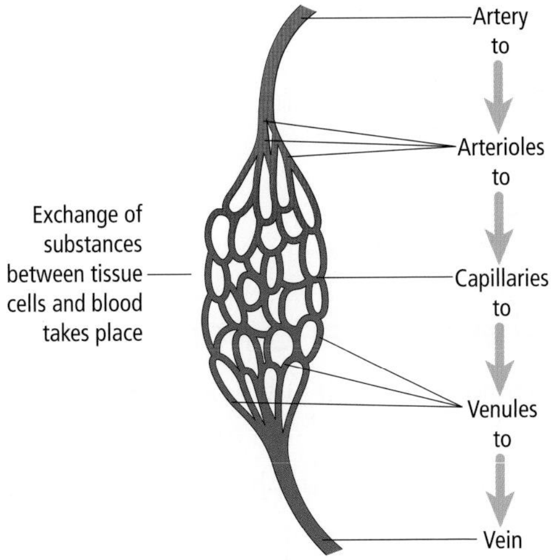

▲ Figure 2.44 Blood flow from an artery to a vein

The circulatory system

The circulatory system comprises blood, the heart and the vast network of circulatory vessels known as arteries, veins and capillaries. The primary function of the circulatory system is transportation. Within the cardiovascular system there are two circuits: the pulmonary circulation and the systemic circulation.

The pulmonary circulation brings deoxygenated blood from the right ventricle of the heart to the alveoli of the lungs, to release carbon dioxide and to regain oxygen. Oxygenated blood returns to the left atrium of the heart and moves into the systemic circuit with the contraction of the left ventricle.

The systemic circuit carries oxygenated blood around the body via the body's main artery: the aorta. On leaving the left ventricle, the aorta emerges from the top of the heart. It passes superiorly for a short distance as the ascending aorta, and curves to form the arch of the aorta before it passes inferiorly as the descending aorta.

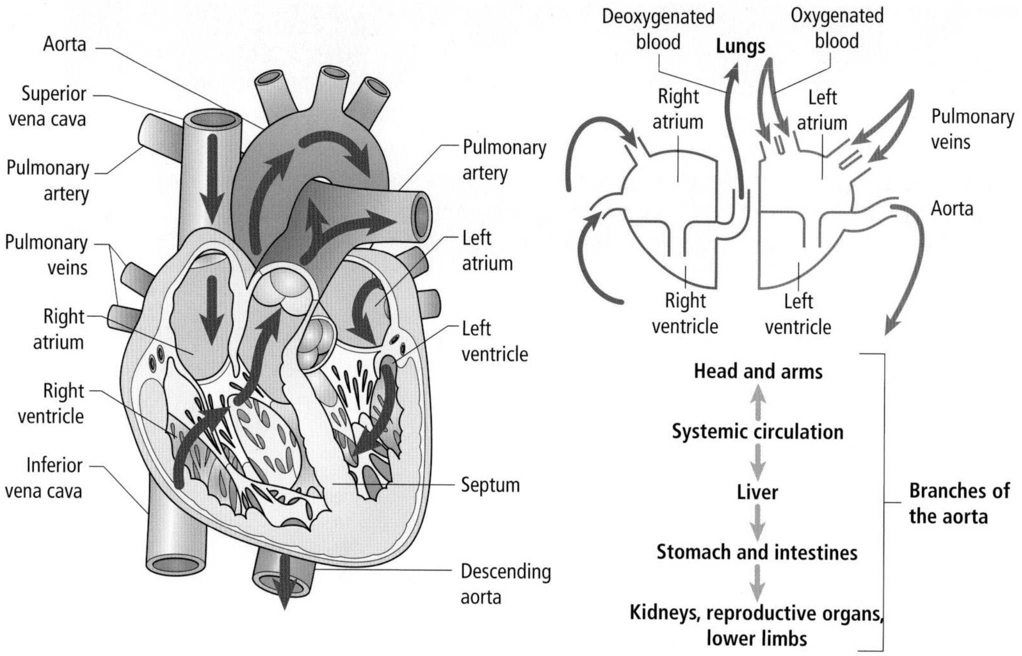

▲ Figure 2.45 Blood circulation and the heart

Blood flow to the head and neck

As the aorta emerges from the heart, it subdivides to form the main trunk called the brachiocephalic trunk, which splits and forms:

- the common carotid artery, which supplies oxygenated blood to the head, face and neck
- the subclavian artery, which supplies blood to the shoulders, chest wall, arms, back and central nervous system.

Arterial blood supply to the head and neck

Blood is supplied to parts within the neck, head and brain through branches of the subclavian and common carotid arteries.

The common carotid artery extends from the brachiocephalic trunk, extends on each side of the neck and divides at the level of the larynx into two branches:

- the internal carotid artery
- the external carotid artery.

The internal carotid artery passes through the temporal bone of the skull to supply oxygenated blood to the brain, eyes, forehead and part of the nose.

The external carotid artery is divided into branches (facial, temporal and occipital), which supply the skin and muscles of the face, sides and back of the head respectively. This vessel also supplies more superficial structures of the head and neck; these include the salivary glands, scalp, teeth, nose, throat, tongue and thyroid gland.

The vertebral arteries are a main division of the subclavian artery. They arise from the subclavian arteries in the base of the neck, near the tip of the lungs. They pass upwards through the openings (foramina) of transverse processes of the cervical vertebrae and unite to form a single basilar artery. The basilar artery then terminates by dividing into two posterior cerebral arteries that supply the occipital and temporal lobes of the cerebrum.

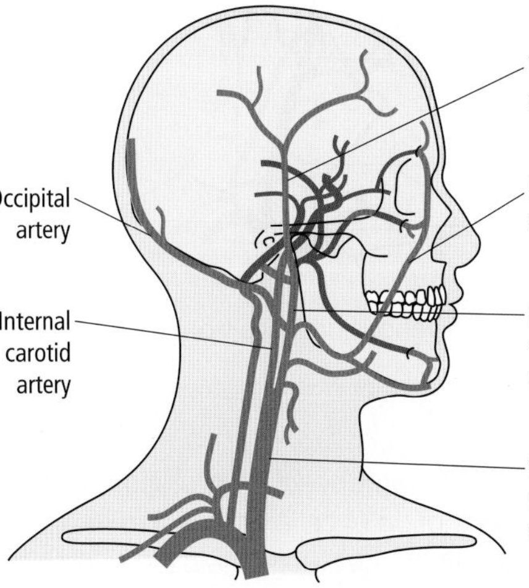

▲ Figure 2.46 Arterial blood supply to the head and neck

To access a drag and drop labelling exercise on arterial blood vessels to the head and neck visit www.hodderplus.co.uk/indianhead.

Venous drainage from the head and neck

The majority of blood draining from the head is passed into three pairs of veins: the external jugular veins, the internal jugular veins and the vertebral veins. Within the brain, all veins lead to the internal jugular veins.

The external jugular vein is smaller than the internal jugular and lies superficial to it. It receives blood from superficial regions of the face, scalp and neck. The external jugular veins descend on either side of the neck, passing over the sternocleidomastoid muscles and beneath the platysma. They empty into the right and left subclavian veins in the base of the neck.

The internal jugular veins form the major venous drainage of the head and neck and are deep veins that parallel the common carotid artery. They collect deoxygenated blood from the brain, passing downwards through the neck beside the common carotid arteries and joining the subclavian veins.

The vertebral veins descend from the transverse openings (or foramina) of the cervical vertebrae and enter the subclavian veins. The vertebral veins drain deep structures of the neck, such as the vertebrae and muscles.

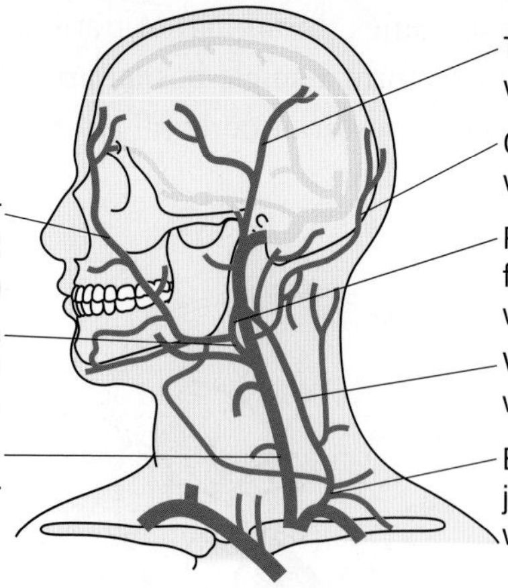

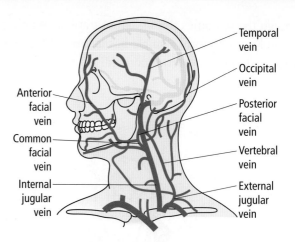

▲ Figure 2.47 Venous drainage from the head and neck

To access a drag and drop labelling exercise for venous drainage from the head and neck visit www.hodderplus.co.uk/indianhead/chapter-2.

Key fact

Indian head massage can help to enhance the circulation of blood, and hence increase cell nutrition and elimination of cellular waste to and from the head and neck. The improved circulation to the head also helps to refresh the brain, helping to relieve stress, tension and fatigue.

To access interactive exercises for the blood circulatory system visit www.hodderplus.co.uk/indianhead.

Blood pressure

Blood pressure is the amount of pressure exerted by blood on an arterial wall due to the contraction of the left ventricle. The pressure in the arteries varies during each heartbeat.

The maximum pressure of the heartbeat is known as the systolic pressure and represents the pressure exerted on the arterial wall during active ventricular contraction. Systolic pressure can therefore be measured when the heart muscle contracts and pushes blood out into the body through the arteries.

The minimum pressure, or diastolic pressure, represents the static pressure against the arterial wall during rest or pause between contractions. Therefore, the minimum pressure is when the heart muscle relaxes and blood flows into the heart from the veins. Blood pressure may be measured with the use of a sphygmomanometer.

Factors affecting blood pressure

As blood pressure is the result of the pumping of the heart in the arteries, anything that makes the heart beat faster will raise the blood pressure. Factors affecting blood pressure include:

- excitement
- anger
- stress
- fright
- pain
- exercise
- smoking and drugs.

A normal blood pressure reading is between 100 and 140 mmHg systolic and between 60 and 90 mmHg diastolic. Blood pressure is measured in millimetres of mercury and is expressed as 120/80 mmHg.

Pulse

The pulse is a pressure wave that can be felt in the arteries which corresponds to the beating of the heart. The pumping action of the left ventricle of the heart is so strong that it can be felt as a pulse in arteries a considerable distance from the heart. The pulse can be felt at any point where an artery lies near the surface. The radial pulse can be found by placing two or three fingers over the radial artery below the thumb. Other sites where the pulse may be felt include the carotid artery at the side of the neck and over the brachial artery at the elbow.

The average pulse in an adult is between 60 and 80 beats per minute. Factors affecting the pulse rate include:

- exercise
- heat
- strong emotions, such as grief, fear, anger or excitement.

? Knowledge check 8

1. List the four main functions of blood.
2. What is the function of the following in circulation?
   - i. artery
   - ii. vein
   - iii. capillary
3. List the two main circulatory pathways that carry blood around the body.
4. Which blood vessels supply oxygenated blood to the head, face and neck?
5. Which veins form the major venous drainage of the head and neck?
6. What is meant by the term blood pressure?
7. List four factors affecting blood pressure.
8. What is the average pulse rate in an adult?

To see the answers to this knowledge check, scan the QR code below or visit www.hodderplus.co.uk/indianhead/chapter-2.

The lymphatic system

The lymphatic system is a one-way drainage system in that it removes excess fluid from the body's tissues and returns it to the circulatory system. It is also important in helping the body to fight infection.

Lymphatic vessels form a network of tubes that extend all over the body. The smallest of the vessels, lymphatic capillaries, end blindly in the body's tissues. Here they collect a liquid called lymph, which leaks out of the body capillaries and accumulates in the tissues. Once collected, lymph flows in one direction along progressively larger lymphatic vessels. Along the network of lymphatic vessels are lymphatic nodes, which filter bacteria and micro-organisms from the lymph as it passes through them. The cleansed lymph is then collected by two main lymphatic ducts (the thoracic and the right lymphatic ducts), which empty the lymph into the bloodstream.

The lymphatic system therefore returns the excess fluid that accumulates in the body's tissues into the bloodstream, while at the same time filtering micro-organisms and releasing antibodies to help the body to fight infection.

Functions of the lymphatic system

Drainage of excess fluid from the tissues

The lymphatic system is important for the distribution of fluid and nutrients in the body because it drains excess fluid from the tissues and returns to the blood protein molecules that are unable to pass back through the blood capillary walls because of their size.

Fighting infection

The lymphatic nodes help to fight infection by filtering lymph and destroying invading micro-organisms. Lymphocytes are reproduced in the lymph node and, following infection, they generate antibodies to protect the body against subsequent infection. Therefore, the lymphatic system plays an important part in the body's immune system.

Absorption of products of fat digestion

The lymphatic system also plays an important part in absorbing the products of fat digestion from the villi of the small intestine. While the products of carbohydrate and protein digestion pass directly into the bloodstream, fats pass directly into the intestinal lymphatic vessels, known as lacteals.

What is lymph?

Lymph is a transparent, colourless, watery liquid that is derived from tissue fluid and is contained within lymphatic vessels. It resembles blood plasma in composition, except that it has a lower concentration of plasma proteins. This is because some large protein molecules are unable to filter through the cells forming the capillary walls, so they remain in blood plasma. Lymph contains only one type of cell: these are called lymphocytes.

How is lymph formed?

As blood is distributed to the tissues, some of the plasma escapes from the capillaries and flows around the tissue cells, delivering nutrients such as oxygen and water to the cells, and picking up cellular waste such as urea and carbon dioxide. Once the plasma is outside the capillary and is bathing the tissue cells, it becomes tissue fluid.

Some of the tissue fluid passes back into the capillary walls to return to the bloodstream via the veins, and some is collected by lymphatic vessels, where it becomes lymph.

The connection between blood and lymph

The lymphatic system is often referred to as a secondary circulatory system, as it consists of a network of vessels that assist the blood in returning fluid from the tissues back to the heart. In this way, the lymphatic system is a complementary system for the circulatory system. After draining the tissues of excess fluid, the lymphatic system returns this fluid to the cardiovascular system. This helps to maintain blood volume and blood pressure and prevent oedema.

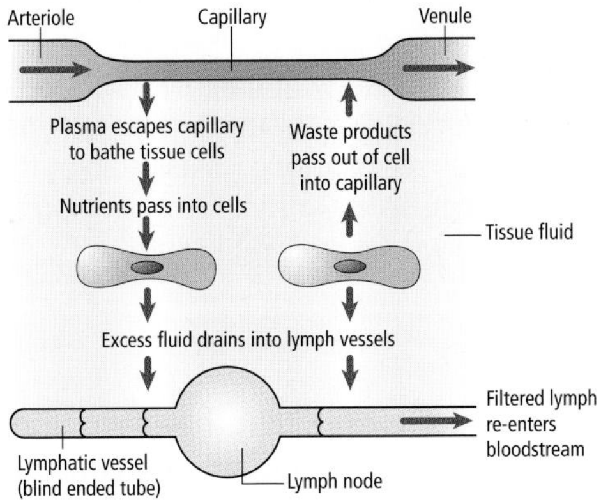

▲ Figure 2.48 The connection between blood and lymph

Structures of the lymphatic system

The lymphatic system contains the following structures:

- lymphatic capillaries
- lymphatic vessels
- lymphatic nodes
- lymphatic collecting ducts.

Structure	Description	Function
Lymphatic capillaries	Minute blind-end tubes, similar in structure to blood capillaries	Drain away excess fluid and waste products from the tissue spaces of the body
Lymphatic vessels	Similar in structure to veins; have one-way valves and thin, collapsible walls	Carry the lymph towards the heart
Lymphatic nodes	Oval or bean-shaped structures, covered by a capsule of connective tissue; they are made up of lymphatic tissue	Filter lymph of micro-organisms, cell debris or harmful substances
Lymphatic ducts (thoracic and right lymphatic)	The thoracic duct is the largest lymphatic vessel in the body and extends from second lumbar vertebra up through the thorax to the root of the neck. The right lymphatic duct is very short in length. It lies in the root of the neck.	Collect lymph from the whole body and return it to the blood via the subclavian veins

▲ Table 2.21 Overview of the structures of the lymphatic system

Lymphatic capillaries

Lymphatic vessels commence as lymphatic capillaries in the tissue spaces of the body as minute, blind-end tubes, as the lymphatic system is a one-way circulatory pathway. The walls of the lymphatic capillaries are like those of the blood capillaries in that they are a single-cell thick, to make it possible for tissue fluid to enter them. However, they are permeable to substances of larger molecular size than those of the blood capillaries.

The lymphatic capillaries mirror the blood capillaries and form a network in the tissues, draining away excess fluid and waste products from the tissue spaces of the body. Once the tissue fluid enters a lymphatic capillary it becomes lymph and is gathered up into larger lymphatic vessels.

Key fact

The movement of lymph throughout the lymphatic system is known as lymphatic drainage and it begins in the lymphatic capillaries. The movement of lymph out of the tissue spaces and into the lymphatic capillaries is assisted by the pressure exerted by the compression of skeletal muscles. This explains why techniques such as Indian head massage are an effective way of draining lymph.

Lymphatic vessels

Lymphatic vessels are similar to veins in that they have thin, collapsible walls and their role is to transport fluid (lymph) along its circulatory pathway. They have a considerable number of valves, which help to keep the lymph flowing in the right direction and prevent backflow. Superficial lymphatic vessels tend to follow the course of veins by draining the skin, whereas the deeper lymphatic vessels tend to follow the course of arteries and drain the internal structures of the body.

The lymphatic vessels carry the lymph towards the heart under steady pressure; about two to four litres of lymph pass into the venous system every day. Once lymph has passed through the lymph vessels, it drains into at least one lymphatic node before returning to the blood circulatory system.

Key fact

As the lymphatic system lacks a pump, lymphatic vessels have to make use of contracting muscles to assist the movement of lymph. Therefore, lymphatic flow is at its greatest during exercise, due to the increased contraction of muscle.

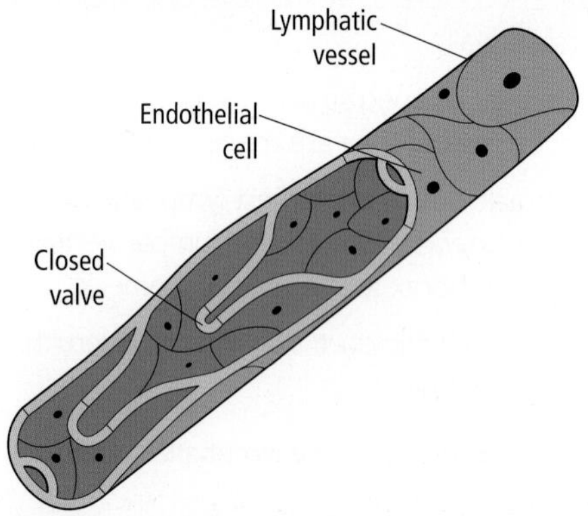

▲ Figure 2.49 A lymphatic vessel

Lymphatic nodes

At intervals along the lymphatic vessels, lymphatic nodes occur. A lymphatic node is an oval- or bean-shaped structure, covered by a capsule of connective tissue. It is made up of lymphatic tissue and is divided into two regions: an outer cortex and an inner medulla.

There are more than a hundred lymphatic nodes, placed strategically along the course of lymphatic vessels. They vary in length between 1 and 25 mm and are massed in groups; some are superficial and lie just under the skin, while others are deeply seated and are found near arteries and veins.

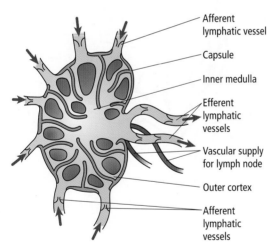

Each lymphatic node receives lymph from several afferent lymphatic vessels, and blood from small arterioles and capillaries. Valves of the afferent lymphatic vessels open towards the node; therefore, lymph in these vessels can only move towards the node. Lymph flows slowly through the node, moving from the cortex to the medulla, and leaves through an efferent vessel that opens away from the node.

- The afferent vessels enter a lymphatic node.
- The efferent vessels drain lymph from a node.

The function of a lymphatic node is to act as a filter, to remove or trap any micro-organisms, cell debris or harmful substances that may cause infection, so that when lymph enters the blood, it has been cleared of any foreign matter. When lymph enters a node, it comes into contact with two specialised types of leucocytes:

- macrophages – these are phagocytic in action. They engulf and destroy dead cells, bacteria and foreign material in the lymph.
- Lymphocytes – these are reproduced within the lymphatic nodes and can neutralise invading bacteria, and produce chemicals and antibodies to help fight disease.

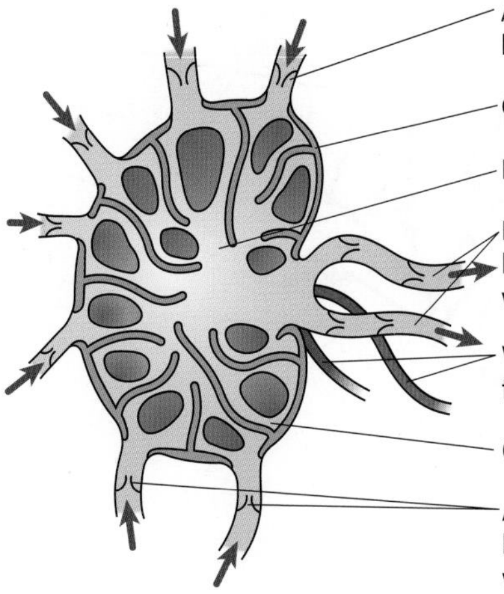

▲ Figure 2.50 A lymphatic node

Once filtered, the lymph leaves the node by one or two efferent vessels, which open away from the node. Lymphatic nodes occur in chains, so that the efferent vessel of one node becomes the afferent vessel of the next node in the pathway of lymph flow. Lymph drains through at least one lymphatic node, then passes into two main collecting ducts before it is returned to the blood.

Key fact

If an area of the body becomes inflamed or otherwise diseased, the nearby lymph nodes will swell up and become tender, indicating that they are actively fighting the infection.

Lymphatic ducts

From each chain of lymphatic nodes, the efferent lymph vessels combine to form lymphatic trunks, which empty into two main ducts: the thoracic and the right lymphatic ducts. These ducts collect lymph from the whole body and return it to the blood via the subclavian veins.

The thoracic duct

This is the main collecting duct of the lymphatic system. It is the largest lymphatic vessel in the body and extends from the second lumbar vertebra, up through the thorax to the root of the neck. The thoracic duct collects lymph from the left side of the head and neck, the left arm, the lower limbs and abdomen, and drains into the left subclavian vein to return the fluid to the bloodstream.

The right lymphatic duct

This duct is very short in length. It lies in the root of the neck and collects lymph from the right side of the head and neck and the right arm, and drains into the right subclavian vein, to return the fluid to the bloodstream.

Lymphatic drainage of the head and neck

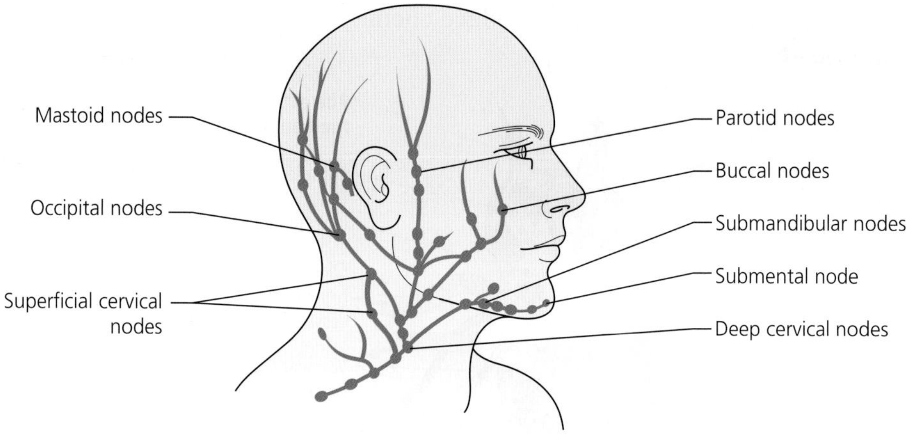

▲ Figure 2.51 Lymphatic nodes of the head and neck

To access a drag and drop labelling exercise on lymph nodes of the head and neck visit www.hodderplus.co.uk/indianhead/chapter-2.

Lymphatic node	Position	Areas from which lymph is drained
Cervical nodes (deep)	Deep within the neck, located along the path of the larger blood vessels (carotid artery and internal jugular vein)	Drain lymph from the larynx, oesophagus, posterior of the scalp and neck, superficial part of chest and arm
Cervical nodes (superficial)	Located at the side of the neck, over the sternocleidomastoid muscle	Drain lymph from the lower part of the ear and the cheek region
Submandibular nodes	Beneath the mandible	Drain chin, lips, nose, cheeks and tongue

▲ Table 2.22 Lymphatic nodes of the head and neck

Lymphatic node	Position	Areas from which lymph is drained
Occipital nodes	At the base of the skull	Drain back of scalp and the upper part of the neck
Mastoid nodes (post-auricular)	Behind the ear in the region of the mastoid process	Drain the skin of the ear and the temporal region of the scalp
Parotid nodes	At the angle of the jaw, below the parotid gland	Drain nose, eyelids and ear
Buccal nodes	In the cheeks above the buccinator muscle	Drain lymph on its journey to the submandibular nodes
Submental nodes	Below the chin	Drain the teeth, tip of the tongue, centre of the lower lip and chin

▲ Table 2.22 *Continued*

To see the answers to this knowledge check, scan the QR code below or visit www.hodderplus.co.uk/indianhead/chapter-2.

Knowledge check 9

1. List three functions of the lymphatic system.
2. What is the function of each of the following?
   i. lymphatic capillaries
   ii. lymphatic vessels
   iii. lymphatic nodes
   iv. lymphatic ducts.
3. State the name of the lymphatic nodes situated below the chin.
4. State the name of the lymphatic nodes that drain lymph on its journey to the submandibular nodes.
5. Which lymphatic nodes are located at the base of the skull?
6. State the area/s the submandibular nodes drain lymph from.

To access interactive exercises for the lymphatic system visit www.hodderplus.co.uk/indianhead/chapter-2.

The nervous system

The nervous system comprises the brain, spinal cord and nerves (neurones), which together form a communication network to coordinate the various actions of the body.

The nervous system works on the same principle as a computer, in that it receives information, processes the information and produces an output. The information received reaches the brain from the sensory organs and internal organs; the information is then processed within the brain. The output is through the action of organs, muscles or glands.

The nervous system contains billions of interconnecting neurones, which are designed to transmit nerve impulses. There are three types of neurones:

- **Sensory neurones** receive stimuli from sensory organs and receptors, and transmit the impulse to the spinal cord and brain. Sensations transmitted by sensory neurones include heat, cold, pain, taste, smell, sight and hearing.
- **Motor neurones** conduct impulses away from the brain and the spinal cord to muscles and glands, to stimulate them into carrying out their activities.

- **Association (mixed) neurones** link sensory and motor neurones, helping to form the complex pathways that enable the brain to interpret incoming sensory messages, decide what should be done and send out instructions in response, in order to keep the body functioning properly.

Organisation of the nervous system

The nervous system has two main parts:

- the **central nervous system** (the main control system), consisting of the brain and the spinal cord
- the **peripheral nervous system**, consisting of 31 pairs of spinal nerves, 12 pairs of cranial nerves and the autonomic nervous system.

Key fact

It is important for therapists to have a basic knowledge of the nervous system to understand its effects, in relation to Indian head massage, of inducing relaxation and minimising pain.

Clients will experience the effects of massage on their muscle tension via the sensory nerves in their muscles. Techniques used in Indian head massage help clients to become aware of specific areas of tension and can thereby initiate relaxation and reduce the unconscious motor message (of tension) to the muscles.

The central nervous system

The brain

The brain is an extremely complex mass of nervous tissue lying within the skull. It is the main communication centre of the nervous system and its function is to coordinate the nerve stimuli received and effect the correct responses.

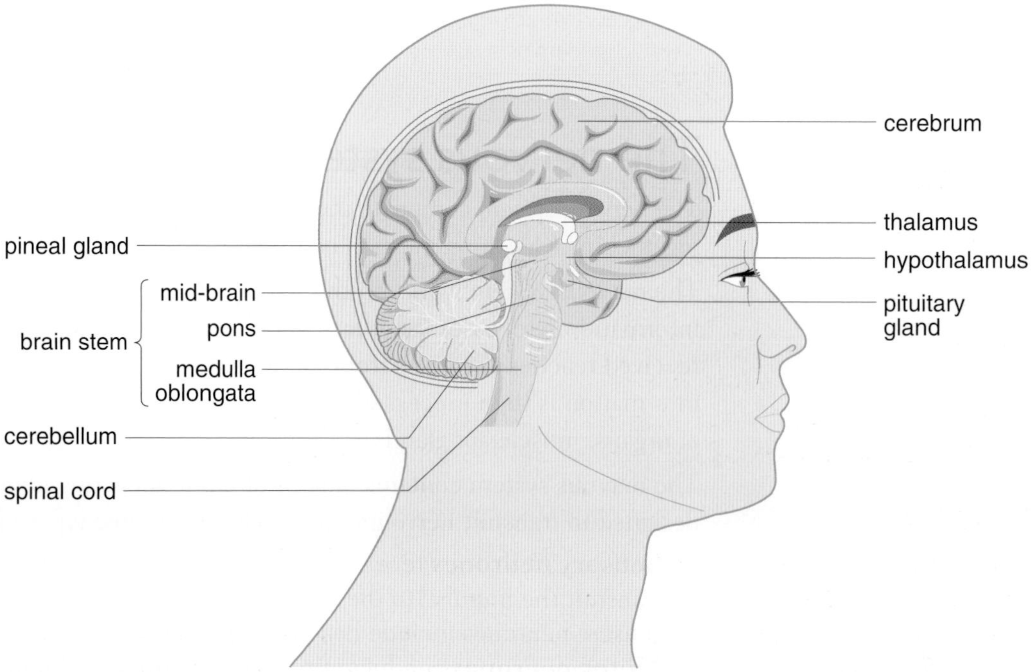

▲ Figure 2.52 Principal parts of the brain

Part of brain	Location	Function
Cerebrum	Largest part of brain Makes up front and top part of brain	Intelligence, emotions
Thalamus	Lies either side of forebrain	Relays sensory impulses to the cerebral cortex
Hypothalamus	Small structure lies beneath the thalamus	Governs many important homeostatic functions (hunger, thirst, temperature regulation, anger, aggression, hormones, sexual behaviour, sleep patterns and consciousness)
Pineal gland	Pea-sized mass of nervous tissue attached by a stalk in the central part of the brain; attached to the upper portion of the thalamus	Secretes melatonin and regulates circadian rhythms
Cerebellum	Cauliflower-shaped structure located at the posterior of the cranium, below the cerebrum	Coordination of skeletal muscles, posture and balance
Brain stem	Enlarged continuation of the spinal cord	Connects the brain with the spinal cord; contains control centres for heart, lungs and intestines

▲ Table 2.23 The main parts of the brain

The spinal cord

The spinal cord is an extension of the brain stem, extending from an opening at the base of the skull down to the second lumbar vertebra. Its function is to relay impulses to and from the brain. Sensory tracts conduct impulses to the brain and motor tracts conduct impulses from the brain.

Within the spinal cord there are two pathways for sensory information to reach the brain.

- The fast pathway transmits impulses rapidly and relates to receptors sensitive to light pressure, vibration and touch.
- The slow pathway transmits information about pain, temperature and pressure.

When the fast pathway is activated – that is, through massage to the skin – the pain pathway is inhibited, as pleasant sensations from the massage arrive at the brain before the pain sensation, thereby helping to displace the awareness of pain.

The peripheral nervous system

The peripheral nervous system contains all the nerves outside of the central nervous system. It consists of cable-like nerves that link the central nervous system to the rest of the body. The peripheral nervous system can be subdivided into the somatic nervous system and the autonomic nervous system.

The somatic nervous system contains:

- **31 pairs of spinal nerves** (nerves originating from the spinal cord)
- **12 pairs of cranial nerves** (nerves originating from the brain).

Spinal nerves

The 31 pairs of spinal nerves pass out of the spinal cord; each has two thin branches, which link it with the autonomic nervous system. Spinal nerves receive sensory impulses from the body and transmit motor signals to specific regions of the body, thereby providing two-way communication between the central nervous system and the body.

Each spinal nerve is numbered and named according to the level of the spinal column from which it emerges. There are:

- 8 cervical nerves
- 12 thoracic nerves
- 5 lumbar nerves
- 5 sacral nerves
- 1 coccygeal spinal nerve.

Each spinal nerve is divided into several branches, forming a network of nerves or plexuses that supply different parts of the body.

Nerve plexus	Location	Area/s of the body it supplies
Cervical	Neck	Skin and muscles of the head, neck and upper region of the shoulders
Brachial	Top of shoulder	Skin and muscles of the arm, shoulder and upper chest
Lumbar	Between waist and hip	Front and sides of the abdominal wall and part of the thigh
Sacral	Base of the abdomen	Skin and muscles and organs of the pelvis
Coccygeal	Base of spine	Skin in the area of the coccyx and the muscles of the pelvic floor

▲ Table 2.24 Nerve plexuses

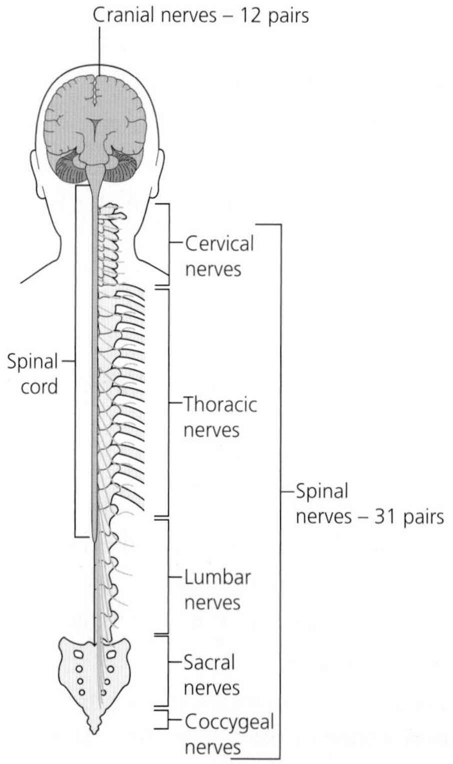

▲ Figure 2.53 Nerves of the body

Cranial nerves

The 12 pairs of cranial nerves connect directly to the brain. Between them they provide a nerve supply to sensory organs, muscles and skin of the head and neck. Some of the nerves are mixed, containing both motor and sensory nerves, while others are either sensory or motor.

Cranial nerve	Type of nerve	Description
Olfactory	Sensory	Nerve of olfaction
Optic	Sensory	Nerve of vision
Oculomotor	Mixed	Innervates both internal and external muscles of the eye and a muscle of the upper eyelid
Trochlear	Motor	Smallest of the cranial nerves Innervates the superior oblique muscle of the eyeball, which helps you look upwards
Abducens	Mixed	Innervates only the lateral rectus muscle of the eye, which helps you look to the side
Facial	Mixed	Conducts impulses to and from several areas in the face and neck. The sensory branches are associated with the taste receptors on the tongue, and the motor fibres transmit impulses to the muscles of facial expression
Vestibulocochlear	Sensory	Transmits impulses generated by auditory stimuli and stimuli related to equilibrium, balance and movement
Glossopharyngeal	Mixed	Supplies motor fibres to part of the pharynx and to the parotid salivary glands, and sensory fibres to the posterior third of the tongue and the soft palate
Vagus	Mixed	Has branches to numerous organs in the thorax and abdomen, as well as the neck Supplies motor nerve fibres to the muscles of swallowing and to the heart and organs of the chest cavity Sensory fibres carry impulses from the organs of the abdominal cavity and the sensation of taste from the mouth
Accessory	Motor	Innervating muscles in the neck and upper back, such as the trapezius and the sternocleidomastoid, as well as muscles of the palate, pharynx and larynx
Hypoglossal	Motor	Innervates the muscles of the tongue
Trigemenal (has three main branches: ophthalmic; maxillary; mandibular)	Mixed	Contains motor and sensory nerves that conduct impulses to and from several areas in the face and neck Also controls the muscles of mastication (the masseter, temporalis and pterygoids)

▲ Table 2.25 Cranial nerves

Autonomic nervous system

This is the part of the nervous system that controls the automatic body activities of smooth and cardiac muscle, and the activities of glands. It is divided into the sympathetic and parasympathetic divisions, which possess complementary responses.

Effects of the sympathetic and parasympathetic nervous systems

The activity of the sympathetic system is to prepare the body for expending energy and dealing with emergency situations.

The parasympathetic nervous system balances the action of the sympathetic division by working to conserve energy and create the conditions needed for rest and sleep. It slows down the body processes, except digestion and the functions of the genito-urinary system.

In general, the actions of the parasympathetic system oppose those of the sympathetic system and the two systems work together to regulate the internal workings of the body.

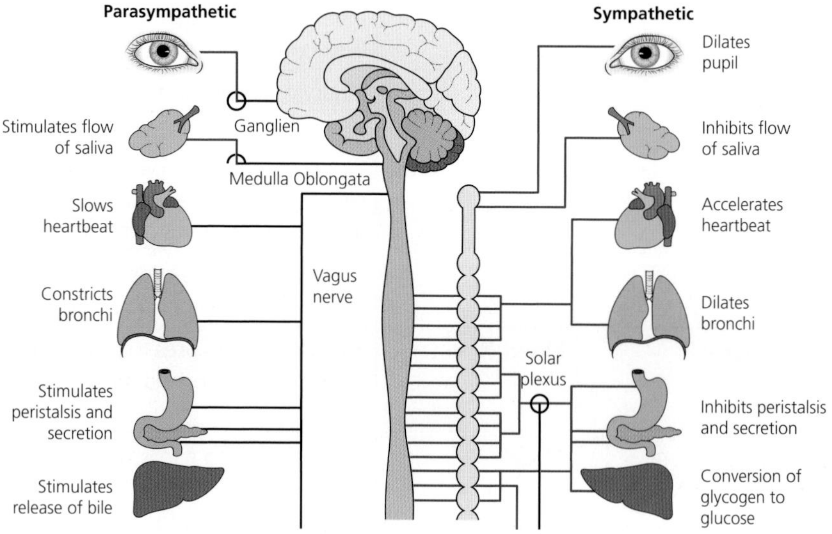

▲ Figure 2.54 The autonomic nervous system

Part of body	Effects of sympathetic stimulation	Effects of parasympathetic stimulation
Heart	Increases heart rate	Slows down heart rate
Lungs	Dilates bronchi to increase respiration	Slows down breathing rate
Blood vessels	Dilates blood vessels	Constricts blood vessels
Adrenal glands	Stimulates release of adrenalin	
Sweat glands	Stimulates/increases secretion of sweat	
Digestive	Reduces peristalsis	Increases peristalsis
Liver	Increases conversion of glycogen to glucose	Increases conversion of glucose to glycogen
Bladder	Relaxes bladder	Contracts bladder
Skin	Constricts arterioles so less blood flows near skin surface (skin looks pale)	
Eyes	Dilates pupils	Constricts pupils

▲ Table 2.26 Effects of sympathetic and parasympathetic stimulation

Study tip

The effects of the sympathetic nervous system increase most body activity (except digestion), while the parasympathetic nervous system slows everything down (apart from digestion).

Key fact

The sympathetic nervous system is activated at times of anger, fright, anxiety or any type of emotional upset, whether real or imagined. The relaxing effects of an Indian head massage can help to *decrease* the effects of the sympathetic nervous system, while *stimulating* parasympathetic activity to promote relaxation and reduce stress levels. It can also help to reduce stress hormones such as cortisol, by activating the relaxation process.

Indian head massage is also thought to increase serotonin levels, which can help to decrease stress levels and depression.

Knowledge check 10

1. What are the two main parts in the organisation of the nervous system?
2. What is the autonomic nervous system and what does it control?
3. State four effects of the sympathetic and parasympathetic nervous systems on the body.

To see the answers to this knowledge check, scan the QR code below or visit www.hodderplus.co.uk/indianhead/chapter-2.

Respiration

Oxygen is needed by every cell of the body for survival and delivery. Respiration is the process by which the living cells of the body receive a constant supply of oxygen and remove carbon dioxide and other gases. The respiratory system consists of the nose, pharynx, larynx, trachea, bronchi and lungs, which provide the passageway for air in and out of the body.

During inhalation, air is drawn in through the nose, pharynx, trachea and bronchi, into the lungs. Inside the lungs, each bronchus divides to form a tree of tubes called bronchioles, which progressively decrease in diameter and end in microscopic air sacs called alveoli. Oxygen from the inhaled air that reaches the alveoli diffuses through the alveolar walls and into the surrounding blood capillaries. This oxygen-rich blood is carried first to the heart and is then pumped to cells throughout the body. Carbon dioxide diffuses out of the blood, into the alveoli, and is removed from the body during exhalation.

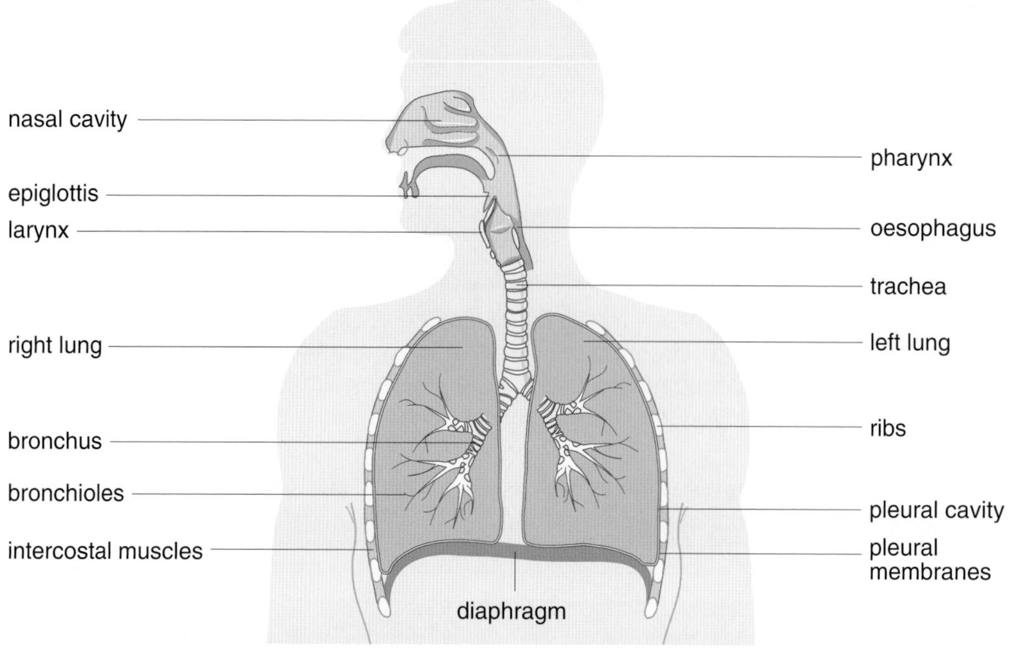

▲ Figure 2.55 The respiratory tract

> **Key fact**
>
> Breathing affects both our physiological and psychological states. By freeing tight respiratory muscles, Indian head massage can help to increase the vital capacity and function of the lungs.

The mechanism of respiration

The mechanism of respiration is the means by which air is drawn in and out of the lungs. It is an active process where the muscles of respiration contract to increase the volume of the thoracic cavity.

The major muscle of respiration is the diaphragm. During inspiration, the diaphragm contracts and flattens, increasing the volume of the thoracic cavity, and is responsible for 75 per cent of air movement into the lungs. The external intercostals are also involved in respiration, and on contraction they increase the depth of the thoracic cavity by pulling the ribs upwards and outwards. The external intercostal muscles are responsible for bringing approximately 25 percent of the volume of air into the lungs.

The combined contraction of the diaphragm and the external intercostals increases the thoracic cavity, which decreases the pressure inside the thorax, so that air from outside the body is pulled into the lungs.

Other accessory muscles that assist in inspiration include the sternocleidomastoid, serratus anterior, pectoralis minor, pectoralis major and the scalene muscles in the neck.

During normal respiration, the process of expiration is passive and is brought about by the relaxation of the diaphragm and the external intercostal muscles.

This increases the internal pressure inside the thorax, so that air is pushed out of the lungs. In forced expiration, the process of expiration becomes active and is assisted by muscles such as the internal intercostals, which help to depress the ribs. Abdominal muscles, such as the external and internal obliques, rectus abdominus and the transversus abdominus, help to compress the abdomen and force the diaphragm upwards, thus assisting expiration.

Rib movements in breathing

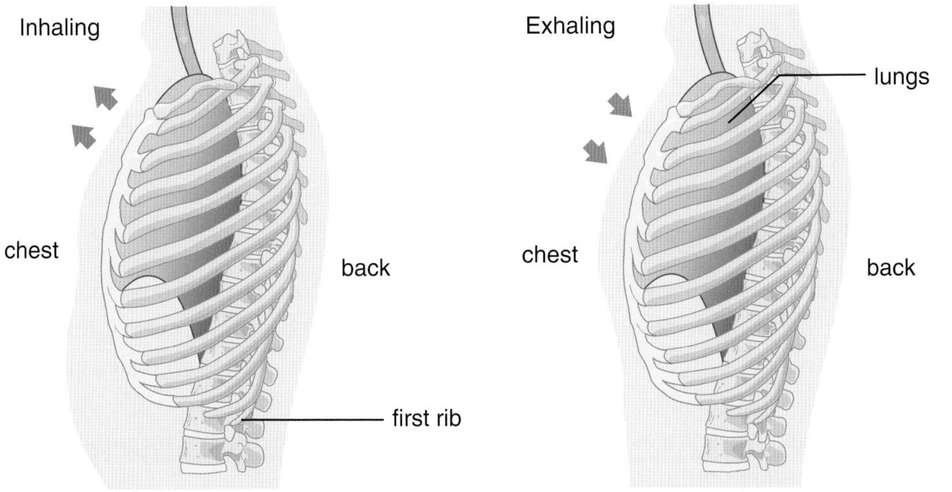

Inhaling. The diaphragm and intercostal muscles contract, pulling the ribs upward. This increases the volume of the chest cavity, drawing air into the lungs.

Exhaling. The contracted muscles relax, the ribs fall slightly and decrease the volume of the chest. Air is forced out of the lungs.

How the diaphragm works

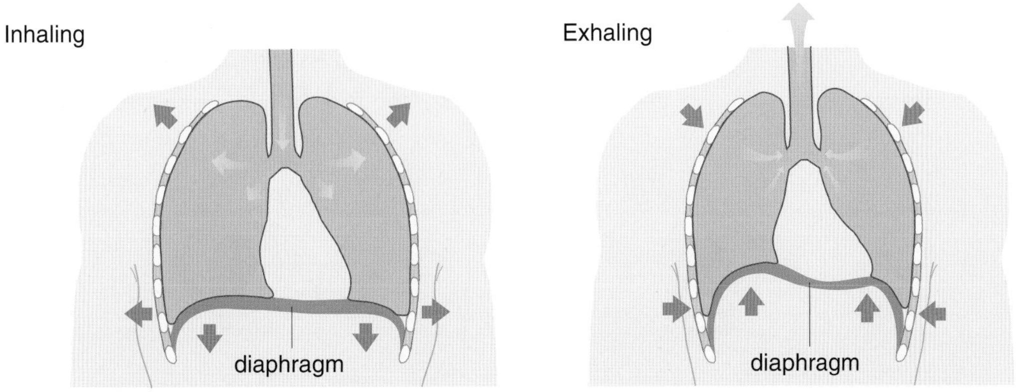

Inhaling. As the rib cage expands *(arrows, above)*, the diaphragm contracts and flattens downwards, enlarging the chest cavity.

Exhaling. The diaphragm relaxes and is pressed up by the abdominal organs, returning to its dome shape. The chest narrows, driving air out of the lungs.

▲ Figure 2.56 The mechanism of respiration

To see the answers to this knowledge check, scan the QR code below or visit www.hodderplus.co.uk/indianhead/chapter-2.

Knowledge check 11

1. List the parts of the respiratory tract.
2. What are the main muscles involved in the mechanism of respiration?

The endocrine system

The endocrine system comprises a series of internal secretions called hormones, which help to regulate body processes by providing a constant internal environment.

Hormones are chemical messengers and act as catalysts in that they affect the physiological activities of other cells in the body.

The endocrine system works closely with the nervous system. Nerves enable the body to respond rapidly to stimuli, whereas the endocrine system causes slower and longer-lasting effects.

What is a hormone?

A hormone is a chemical messenger or regulator, secreted by an endocrine gland that reaches its destination by the bloodstream and has the power of influencing the activity of other organs. Some hormones have a slow action over a period of years, such as the growth hormone from the anterior pituitary, while others have a quick action, such as adrenaline from the adrenal medulla. Hormones therefore regulate and coordinate various functions in the body.

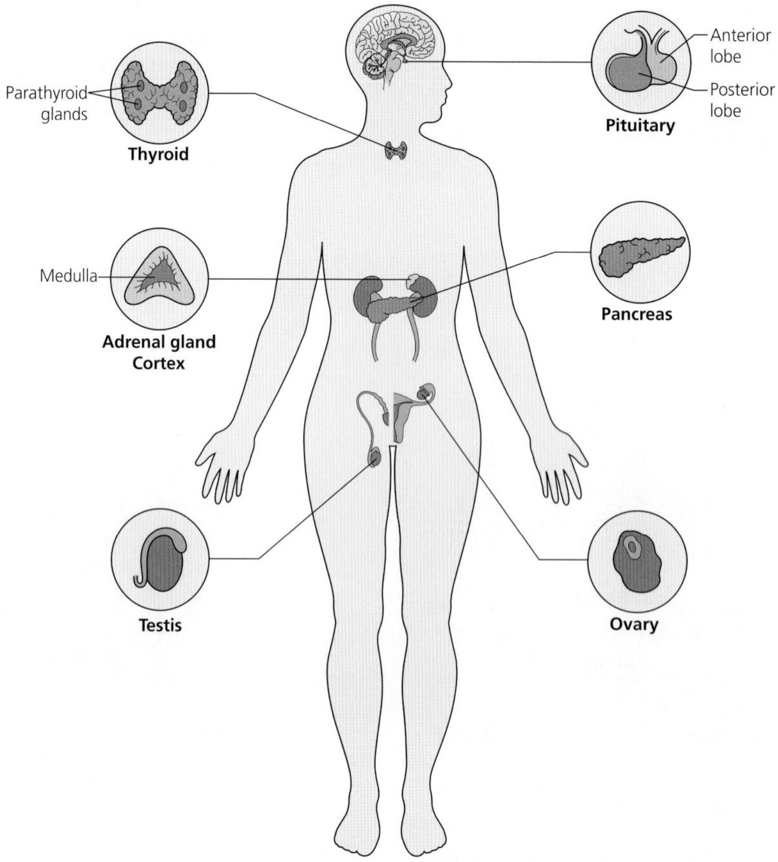

▲ Figure 2.57 The endocrine glands

The endocrine glands

The endocrine glands are ductless glands, as the hormones they secrete pass directly into the bloodstream to influence the activity of another organ or gland.

Endocrine gland	Location
Pituitary gland	Attached by a stalk to the hypothalamus of the brain
Thyroid gland	In the neck on either side of the trachea
Parathyroid glands	Four small glands situated on the posterior of the thyroid gland
Adrenal glands	Two triangular-shaped glands that lie on top of each kidney
Pancreas	Situated behind the stomach, between the duodenum and the spleen
Ovaries	Situated in the lower abdomen below the kidneys
Testes	Situated in the groin in a sac called the scrotum

▲ Table 2.27 Overview of the endocrine glands

Knowledge check 12

1. What is a hormone?
2. What is the main function of the endocrine system?
3. List the seven main endocrine glands in the body.

To see the answers to this knowledge check, scan the QR code below or visit www.hodderplus.co.uk/indianhead/chapter-2.

Multiple-choice self-assessment questions

1. In which of the following layers are epidermal cells constantly being reproduced?
   a Horny layer
   b Granular layer
   c Clear layer
   d Basal cell layer
2. How many layers make up the epidermis?
   a 4
   b 5
   c 3
   d 6
3. Which is the thinnest layer of the skin?
   a Dermis
   b Epidermis
   c Subcutaneous layer
   d Subdermal layer
4. How many layers does the dermis have?
   a 3
   b 1
   c 2
   d 5
5. Three functions of the skin include
   a protection, movement and sensitivity
   b sensitivity, protection and temperature regulation
   c attachment, movement and protection
   d protection, fights infection and temperature regulation.
6. Key indicators of dehydration in the skin are
   a flakiness, visible fine lines and a feeling of tightness
   b open pores
   c blocked pores
   d dilated capillaries.
7. The functions of hair are
   a contraction and protection
   b insulation and protection
   c storage and protection
   d vasodilation and vasoconstriction.
8. Hair growth occurs from the
   a cuticle
   b cortex
   c medulla
   d matrix.
9. Hair grows from a sac-like depression called the
   a hair shaft
   b hair root
   c hair follicle
   d hair bulb.
10. Hair colour is due to the presence of melanin in which parts of the hair shaft?
    a Cortex and medulla
    b Cuticle and cortex
    c Cuticle and medulla
    d Medulla only
11. The correct order of the hair growth cycle from growing to resting is
    a anagen, telogen, catagen
    b catagen, anagen, telogen
    c telogen, anagen, catagen
    d anagen, catagen, telogen.
12. The sebaceous glands produce an oily substance called
    a sweat
    b lactic acid
    c sebum
    d keratin.
13. Which lies beneath the subcutaneous layer of the skin?
    a Papillary layer
    b Reticular layer
    c Clear layer
    d Subdermal muscle layer
14. The bacterial infection that appears as a pustule at the base of a hair follicle is known as
    a impetigo
    b boil
    c sebaceous cyst
    d folliculitis.
15. Which of the following is a fungal infection of the skin?
    a Impetigo
    b Herpes simplex
    c Ringworm
    d Scabies
16. Which of the following skin disorders are caused by a parasitic infection?
    a Tinea capitis, tinea corporis
    b Herpes simplex, herpes zoster
    c Scabies and pediculosis
    d Acne vulgaris, acne rosacea

17. A condition where there is an inherited absence of pigmentation in the skin, hair and eyes is
- a chloasma
- b albinism
- c lentigo
- d vitiligo.

18. A papule is
- a a small, raised elevation on the skin
- b a lump under the skin containing pus
- c a small growth of fibrous tissue
- d a mark left on the skin after the skin has healed.

19. How many bones are located in the neck?
- a 8
- b 10
- c 12
- d 7

20. The bone forming the posterior (back) part of the shoulder girdle is the
- a clavicle
- b scapula
- c sternum
- d manubrium.

21. The long bone of the upper arm is the
- a radius
- b ulna
- c humerus
- d scaphoid.

22. The bone forming the back of the skull is the
- a parietal
- b temporal
- c occipital
- d vomer.

23. A bone of the skull that forms the sides of the skull above and around the ears is called the
- a frontal
- b temporal
- c occipital
- d ethmoid.

24. The bone of the face that forms the lower jaw is called the
- a maxilla
- b zygomatic
- c mandible
- d lacrimal.

25. The facial sinuses are designed to
- a lighten the head, provide mucus and act as a resonance chamber for sound
- b lighten air quality and reduce the volume of mucus
- c reduce sound and the volume of mucus excreted
- d lighten the head and assist with air inhalation and exhalation.

26. Which of the following is the only type of muscle under voluntary control?
- a Skeletal
- b Smooth
- c Cardiac
- d Anaerobic

27. What is the muscle that causes movement referred to as?
- a Synergist
- b Agonist
- c Antagonist
- d Fixator

28. The state of partial contraction of a muscle is known as
- a hypertrophy
- b muscle spasm
- c muscle tone
- d muscular atrophy.

29. The condition muscle fatigue is caused by
- a insufficient oxygen, exhaustion of energy and accumulation of lactic acid
- b excessive oxygen, exhaustion of energy and accumulation of lactic acid
- c insufficient carbon dioxide, exhaustion of energy and accumulation of lactic acid
- d excessive oxygen and carbon dioxide, exhaustion of energy and accumulation of lactic acid.

30. The muscle that extends from the chest, up the sides of the neck to the chin is called the
- a pectoralis major
- b occipitalis
- c temporalis
- d platysma.

31. The position of the corrugator muscle is
- a between the eyebrows
- b around the eyes
- c sides of nose
- d in the cheek.

32. The fan-shaped muscle on the side of the skull, above and in front of the ear, is called the
- a occipitalis
- b buccinator
- c mentalis
- d temporalis.

33. The muscle that surrounds the eye is called the
- a orbicularis oris
- b risorius
- c masseter
- d orbicularis oculi.

34. The action of the risorius muscle is to
- a raise the corner of the mouth
- b close the mouth
- c draw the end corners of the mouth laterally
- d elevate the lower lip.

35. The facial expression associated with the mentalis muscle is
- a pouting
- b smiling
- c laughing
- d grinning.

36. The action of the sternocleidomastoid muscles is to
- a depress the mandible
- b extend the head
- c elevate and retract the lower jaw
- d flex the neck and turn the head to one side.

37. The action of the triceps muscle is
- a flexion of the forearm
- b extension of the forearm
- c flexion of the wrist
- d extension of the wrist.

38. The action of the buccinator muscle is to
- a raise the lower jaw
- b compress the cheek
- c elevate and retract the lower jaw
- d elevate the lower lip.

39. The muscle responsible for the action abduction of the arm is
- a deltoid
- b biceps
- c brachialis
- d triceps.

40. The blood cells responsible for fighting infection in the body are
- a erythrocytes
- b thrombocytes
- c leucocytes
- d platelets.

41. The function of an artery is to
- a carry oxygenated blood
- b carry deoxygenated blood
- c prevent backflow of blood
- d carry blood under low pressure.

42. What in a vein's structure prevents backflow of blood?
- a Thick, elastic walls
- b Valves
- c Thick, muscular walls
- d Capillaries

43. The average pulse in an adult is between
- a 50 and 70 beats per minute
- b 60 and 80 beats per minute
- c 90 and 120 beats per minute
- d 40 and 50 beats per minute.

44. Blood pressure is the amount of pressure exerted by blood on an arterial wall due to the contraction of the
- a left atrium
- b right ventricle
- c left ventricle
- d right atrium.

45. Upon injury, blood prevents the severe loss of blood by
- a clotting and forming a network of platelets
- b forming a network of white blood cells
- c forming a network of red blood cells
- d vasodilation of blood capillaries.

46. Blood follows two circulatory pathways around the body, known as
- a arterial and venous
- b pulmonary and portal
- c pulmonary and systemic
- d systemic and general.

47. The name of the blood vessels that are responsible for supplying oxygenated blood to the head and neck is the
- a brachiocephalic arteries
- b subclavian arteries
- c jugular veins
- d carotid arteries.

48. The name of the blood vessels responsible for draining deoxygenated blood from the head and neck is the
- a jugular veins
- b superior vena cava
- c brachiocephalic veins
- d vertebral veins.

49. The lymphatic system has the following functions
- a fights infection, drains excess fluid, absorbs products of fat digestion
- b produces fat, fights infection and drains blood
- c fights infection, reduces fat digestion and increases fluid retention
- d produces fat, produces blood cells and reduces fluid retention.

50. Lymph is formed when plasma escapes from the blood capillaries and becomes
- a cellular waste
- b tissue fluid
- c carbon dioxide
- d oxygen.

51. The name of the structure that carries lymph towards the heart under steady pressure is a
- a lymphatic capillary
- b lymphatic node
- c lymphatic vessel
- d lymphatic duct.

52. The lymph nodes that drain lymph from the back of the scalp and the upper part of the neck are called
- a submandibular nodes
- b deep cervical nodes
- c occipital nodes
- d parotid nodes.

53. The lymph nodes that drain lymph from the larynx, oesophagus, posterior of the scalp and neck, and superficial part of the chest and arm are called
- a superficial cervical nodes
- b mastoid nodes
- c deep cervical nodes
- d occipital nodes.

54. Which of the following nodes drains lymph on its journey to the submandibular nodes?
- a Parotid
- b Submental
- c Buccal
- d Post-auricular

55. The central nervous system consists of the
- a sympathetic and parasympathetic nervous systems
- b facial and spinal nerves
- c brain and spinal cord
- d autonomic nervous system.

56. The autonomic nervous system controls
- a smooth and cardiac muscle
- b voluntary muscle
- c blood and lymphatic flow
- d reflex actions from the brain.

57. Which of the following is an effect of the sympathetic nervous system?
- a Pupil constriction
- b Increased gastrointestinal activity
- c Constriction of skeletal blood vessels
- d Increased heartbeat

58. The correct order of respiratory organs is

a nose, pharynx, larynx, trachea, bronchi and lungs
b nose, larynx, pharynx, trachea, bronchi and lungs
c nose, trachea, pharynx, larynx, bronchi and lungs
d nose, pharynx, trachea, larynx, bronchi and lungs.

59. The process of inspiration is brought about by the

a combined relaxation of the diaphragm and the internal intercostal muscles
b combined contraction of the diaphragm and the external intercostal muscles
c combined relaxation of the diaphragm and the external intercostal muscles
d combined contraction of the diaphragm and the internal intercostal muscles.

60. The endocrine system is concerned with

a regulation of blood
b producing hormones
c respiration
d sensory function.

To see the answers, scan the QR code opposite or visit www.hodderplus.co.uk/indianhead/chapter-2. To access an interactive version of these multiple-choice self-assessment questions visit www.hodderplus.co.uk/indianhead/chapter-2.

To access an interactive crossword for this chapter visit www.hodderplus.co.uk/indianhead/chapter-2.

3 Conditions affecting the head, neck and shoulders

Introduction

A considerable increase in stress levels in sophisticated present-day life has led to a great deal of interest in holistic therapies such as Indian head massage, which continues to grow in popularity. More and more people are seeking the benefits of an Indian head massage treatment to help improve their emotional and physical well-being.

Therapists practising Indian head massage need to be knowledgeable within the sphere of their chosen therapy, but also be sufficiently familiar with conditions affecting the head, neck and shoulders in order to design a safe and effective treatment plan that is adapted to the client's needs.

Learning objectives

By the end of this chapter, you will be able to relate the following to your practical work:

- knowledge of common conditions of the head, neck and shoulders
- the cautions, recommendations and restrictions involved in treatment applications.

This knowledge will help to empower therapists to make an informed decision as to a suitable treatment plan that is within safe and ethical medical guidelines. It is very important that a therapist never diagnoses a client's medical condition, and refers the client to their GP before any form of treatment is commenced.

Study tip

It should be noted that while the information given reflects an accurate representation of the condition in generic terms, all clients will vary in the severity of their condition. Each client should be assessed individually as to their condition at the time of the proposed treatment and reassessed on subsequent treatments. The guidelines given are meant as a general guide and thus therapists are encouraged to seek further clarification of a client's medical condition from the GP and from the client themselves.

Alopecia

A term used to describe temporary baldness or severe hair loss, which may follow illness, shock, a period of extreme stress, or may be the side effect of drug therapy – for example, chemotherapy. It is important to distinguish temporary baldness from male pattern baldness, which is progressive and permanent and is unlikely to be helped by therapies such as Indian head massage.

Patchy hair loss, or alopecia areata, is a relatively common disorder. The onset is fairly sudden and presents with a round or oval bald area; the loss of hair may be complete, or so-called 'exclamation mark hairs' may be seen in the bald patches or at the edges. Occasionally the scalp is erythematous (red) in the part affected. The skin itself is not scaly, unlike the bald areas seen in fungal infection of the scalp. In alopecia areata there may be one or several bald patches. The most frequent course for alopecia areata to take is for the hair to regrow after a period of time (frequently two to three months). When regrowth occurs, the hair is often white, but usually repigments in time.

Cautions, restrictions and recommendations

- Concentrate on massaging the scalp to increase the local circulation, using almond or coconut oil.
- Wrap a warm towel round the head after the treatment to help aid the absorption.
- Encourage the client to use the oils and massage the scalp at home twice a week, leaving the oils to absorb for about two hours before shampooing.
- Advise the client of the importance of dietary requirements for healthy hair (adequate protein and essential fatty acids to promote healthy growth, and vitamin B complex and vitamin C to provide nourishment for the hair follicles; vitamin B5 helps to relieve stress).

Angina

This is pain in the left side of the chest and usually radiating to the left arm. It is caused by insufficient blood to the heart muscle, usually on exertion or excitement. The pain is often described as constricting or suffocating, and can last for a few seconds or minutes. The patient may become pale and sweaty. This condition indicates ischaemic heart disease.

Health and safety note

As sudden exposure to extreme heat or cold can bring on an attack, keep the client warm and avoid extreme fluctuations in temperature.

It is important that clients have their necessary medications with them when they attend for treatment, in the event of an emergency.

Cautions, restrictions and recommendations

- Stress predisposes an angina attack. Indian head massage can help to reduce stress levels by reducing the activity of the sympathetic nervous system.

Ankylosing spondylitis

This systemic joint disease is characterised by inflammation of the intervertebral disc spaces, costovertebral and sacroiliac joints. Fibrosis, calcification, ossification and stiffening of joints are common and the spine becomes rigid. Typically, a client will complain of persistent or intermittent lower back pain. Kyphosis is present when the thoracic or cervical regions of the spine are affected and the weight of the head compresses the vertebrae and bends the spine forwards. This condition can cause muscular atrophy, loss of balance and falls. Typically, ankylosing spondylitis affects young male adults.

Health and safety note

Avoid forcibly mobilising ankylosed joints; and in the case of cervical spondylitis, avoid hyperextending the neck.

Cautions, restrictions and recommendations

- Position the client according to individual comfort – extra cushioning and support may be required.

- Gentle massage may be very beneficial and the heat generated may help to ease the pain.
- Advise the client to do breathing exercises regularly in order to help mobilise the thorax.

Anxiety

This can be defined as fear of the unknown, but as an illness it can vary from a mild form to panic attacks and severe phobias that can be disabling socially, psychologically and, at times, physically. It presents with a feeling of dread that something serious is likely to happen, and is associated with palpitations, rapid breathing, sweaty hands, tremor (shakiness), dry mouth and general pains in the muscles. It can present with similar features of mild to moderate depression of the agitated type. The causes of anxiety can be related to personality, with some genetic and behavioural predisposition, or a traumatic experience or physical illness – for example, hyperthyroidism.

Cautions, restrictions and recommendations

- Clients are likely to present with various symptoms; therefore a thorough assessment is required.
- Indian head massage and relaxation exercises are likely to be a valuable source of help and support.
- Clients with anxiety are more likely to become emotionally dependent on their therapist and may need to be referred to another professional for help.

Arthritis: osteoarthritis

This is a joint disease characterised by the breakdown of articular cartilage, growth of bony spikes, swelling of the surrounding synovial membrane and stiffness and tenderness of the joint. It is also known as degenerative arthritis. It is common in the elderly and takes a progressive course. This condition involves varying degrees of joint pain, stiffness, limitation of movement, joint instability and deformity. It commonly affects the weight-bearing joints: the hips, knees, lumbar and cervical vertebrae.

Cautions, restrictions and recommendations

- Passive and gentle friction movements around the joint may be beneficial where there is minimal pain, but excessive movement may cause joint pain and damage.
- Gentle massage may help with muscle spasms, joint stiffness and muscle atrophy.

Health and safety note

Always ask the client to demonstrate the range of movement possible in their shoulder and neck; this will guide you as to the limitations of treatment possible.

Arthritis: rheumatoid

Chronic inflammation of peripheral joints results in pain, stiffness and potential damage to joints. It can cause severe disability. Joint swellings and rheumatoid nodules are tender.

> **Health and safety note**
>
> In the acute stage, avoid massaging, but encourage passive movement of the affected joints. In the chronic stage, massage movements can help to reduce the thickening that occurs in and around the articular cartilage.
>
> Always ensure there is no pain and that care is taken when gently mobilising a joint.

Cautions, restrictions and recommendations

- Although Indian head massage cannot cure arthritis, it can help to prevent its progress through relaxation and reduction of discomfort.
- In the early stages of diagnosis, clients should be encouraged to have treatment in order to maintain the range of joint movements and help prevent contractures.

Asthma

This condition involves attacks of shortness of breath and difficulty in breathing caused by spasm or swelling of the bronchial tubes, in turn caused by hypersensitivity to allergens, such as the pollens of various plants, grass, flowers, pet hair, dust mites and various proteins in foodstuffs, such as shellfish, eggs and milk. Asthma may be exacerbated by exercise, anxiety, stress or smoking. It runs in families and can be associated with hay fever and eczema.

Cautions, restrictions and recommendations

- Indian head massage is ideally suited as a treatment for asthma sufferers as clients are seated in an upright position.
- Relaxation provided by the treatment, in conjunction with deep breathing exercises, can help to reduce bronchiospasm and should be encouraged.

> **Health and safety note**
>
> Always obtain a detailed history during the consultation stage, specifically the triggers that bring on an asthma attack. If the client has a history of allergies, then ensure that the client is not allergic to any preparations or substances you may be proposing to use.
>
> It is advisable for the client to have their required medications handy, in the event of an attack.

Bell's palsy

This is a disorder of the seventh cranial nerve (facial nerve) that results in paralysis on one side of the face. The disorder usually comes on suddenly and is commonly caused by inflammation around the facial nerve as it travels from the brain to the exterior. It may be caused by pressure on the nerve caused by tumours, injury to the nerve, infection of the meninges or inner ear, or dental surgery. Diabetes, pregnancy and hypertension are other causes.

The condition may present with a drooping of the mouth on the affected side, caused by flaccid paralysis of the facial muscles, and there may be difficulty in puckering the lips because of paralysis of the orbicularis oris muscle. Taste may be diminished or lost if the nerve proximal to the branch that carries taste sensations has been affected. The condition also presents with the individual having difficulty in closing the eye tightly and creasing the forehead. The buccinator muscle is also affected, which prevents the client from puffing the cheeks and is the cause of food getting caught between the teeth and cheeks. There is also excessive tearing from the affected eye. Pain may be present near the angle of the jaw and behind the ear. Eighty to 90 per cent of individuals recover spontaneously and completely in around one to eight weeks. Corticosteroids may be used to reduce the inflammation of the nerve.

Cautions, restrictions and recommendations

- Use light strokes, in an upward direction, from the middle of the face to the sides (towards the ears).

- To help increase tone on the affected side of the face, use kneading movements with the fingertips.
- Light tapotement (tapping) and vibration movements may be used to help stimulate paralysed muscles.
- To help maintain tone, the face massage can be performed two to three times a day.
- The client may also be shown suitable facial exercises to help reduce the atrophy of the affected muscles.

Health and safety note

Be aware that cold and chills are known to trigger Bell's palsy.

Bronchitis

A chronic or acute inflammation of the bronchial tubes. Chronic bronchitis is common in smokers and may lead to emphysema, which is caused by damage to lung structure. Acute bronchitis can result from a recent cold or flu.

Cautions, restrictions and recommendations

- Clients with bronchitis may find Indian head massage more comfortable because of the fact that they are seated.
- Encourage the client to breathe slowly and deeply throughout the treatment.

Health and safety note

As sufferers of chronic bronchitis are prone to respiratory infection, therapists should avoid treating such clients if they have even the mildest form of acute chest infection.

Cerebral palsy

This condition is caused by damage to the central nervous system of the baby during pregnancy, delivery or soon after birth. The damage could be caused by bleeding, lack of oxygen or other injuries to the brain.

The signs and symptoms of this condition depend on the area of the brain affected. Speech is impaired in most individuals and there may be difficulty in swallowing. There may or may not be mental retardation. Muscles may increase in tone to become spastic, making coordinated movements difficult. The muscles are hyperexcitable, and even small movements, touch, stretch of muscle or emotional stress can increase the spasticity.

The posture is abnormal because of muscle spasticity, and the gait is also affected. Some individuals may have abnormal involuntary movements of the limbs that may be exaggerated on voluntarily performing a task. Weakness of muscles may also be associated with the condition, along with seizures. There may also be problems with hearing and vision.

Cautions, restrictions and recommendations

- Seek the support of the client's doctors, nurses, physiotherapist and family before proceeding.
- Indian head massage can help to reduce stress, prevent contractures, improve the circulation to the skin and muscles that are unused and provide tremendous emotional support.
- Since any form of stress increases the symptoms, concentrate on relaxation, as this will help to reduce muscular spasms and involuntary movements.
- Also be aware that the spasticity in an individual may change from day to day, with changes in posture, and is related to emotional stress.

Health and safety note

If treatment is suitable, perform a shorter treatment (15 to 20 minutes), using mild to moderate pressure.

Be aware that some clients may have reduced sensations and may be unable to give adequate feedback regarding pressure and pain.

> **Health and safety note**
> Place a clean towel over the client's shoulders when proceeding to the scalp massage to prevent dead skin cells from the scalp falling on to their clothing.

Dandruff (pityriasis capitis)

This extremely common condition presents with visible scaling from the surface of the scalp and is associated with the presence of the yeast pityrosporum ovale. It is the precursor of seborrhoeic eczema of the scalp, in which there is a degree of inflammation in addition to the greasy scaling.

Cautions, restrictions and recommendations

- Regular scalp massage and use of oils helps to remove dead skin cells and increase the circulation.
- Vitamin A is useful to improve a dry, scaly scalp.

Depression

This combines symptoms of lowered mood, loss of appetite, poor sleep, lack of concentration and interest, lack of a sense of enjoyment, occasional constipation and loss of libido. On occasions there can be suicidal thinking, death wish or active suicide attempts.

Depression can be the result of chemical imbalance, usually related to serotonin and noradrenaline. There might be no medical cause for the depression; instead it might be linked to genetic predisposition, the result of physical illness, actual loss of a close relative, object or limb, or loss of a relationship. A depressed person looks miserable, hunchbacked and downcast, and will usually avoid eye contact. The severity, as suggested above, can be variable, but may become severe enough to become psychotic, manifested by hallucinations, delusions, paranoia or thought disorders.

Cautions, restrictions and recommendations

> **Health and safety note**
> If there is any indication of suicidal thinking at any time, the client should be referred to their GP.

- A depressed client can present with physical ailments including backache, gastrointestinal symptoms (usually constipation) and headaches.
- Physical illness can present with depression and can include, for example, long-term illness, terminal illness, Parkinson's disease and arthritis.
- Therapists need to ensure that clients do not become emotionally dependent on them; they may need to be referred to another professional.
- Indian head massage is thought to help increase levels of serotonin from the brain and may be effective in helping to lift depression.

Epilepsy

This is a neurological disorder that makes the individual susceptible to recurrent and temporary seizures. Epilepsy is a complex condition, and classifications of types of epilepsy are not definitive.

Generalised

This may take the form of major or tonic-clonic seizures (formerly known as grand mal), in which at the onset the patient falls to the ground, unconscious, with their muscles in a state of spasm (tonic phase). This is then replaced by convulsive movements (the clonic phase), when the tongue may be bitten and urinary incontinence may occur. Movements gradually cease and the patient may rouse in a state of confusion, complaining of a headache, or may fall asleep.

Partial

This may be idiopathic or a symptom of structural damage to the brain. In one type of partial idiopathic epilepsy, often affecting children, seizures may take the form of absences (formerly known as petit mal), in which there are brief spells of unconsciousness lasting for a few seconds. The eyes stare blankly and there may be fluttering movements of the lids and momentary twitching of the fingers and mouth. This form of epilepsy seldom appears before the age of three or after adolescence. It often subsides spontaneously in adult life, but may be followed by the onset of generalised or partial epilepsy.

Focal

This is partial epilepsy caused by brain damage (either local or caused by a stroke). The nature of the seizure depends on the location of the damage in the brain. In a Jacksonian motor seizure, the convulsive movements may spread from the thumb to the hand, arm and face.

Psychomotor

This type of epilepsy is caused by dysfunction of the cortex of the temporal lobe of the brain. Symptoms may include hallucinations of smell, taste, sight and hearing. Throughout an attack, the patient is in a state of clouded awareness and afterwards may have no recollection of the event.

Cautions, restrictions and recommendations

- As epilepsy is a complex condition and Indian head massage involves stimulation of the brain, caution is advised.
- If the client is on controlled medication, the chances of a seizure are minimal; however, caution is advised because of the complexity of this condition.
- It has never been reported that holistic therapies have ever provoked the onset of epilepsy, although there is a theoretical risk to be considered in that deep relaxation or overstimulation could provoke an attack (although this has never been proven in practice).

Health and safety note

Always refer to the client's GP regarding the type and nature of epilepsy.

Fibromyalgia

This chronic condition produces musculoskeletal pain. Predominant symptoms include widespread musculoskeletal pain, lethargy and fatigue. Other characteristic features include a non-refreshing sleep pattern, in which the patient wakes feeling exhausted and more tired than later in the day, and interrupted

> **Health and safety note**
> Avoid deep massage on localised tender areas, which include base of skull, cervical vertebrae C5–C7, midpoint of the upper border of the trapezius and above the spine of the scapula.

sleep. Other recognised symptoms include early morning stiffness, pins and needles sensation, unexplained headaches, poor concentration, memory loss, low mood, urinary frequency, abdominal pain and irritable bowel syndrome. Anxiety and depression are also common.

Cautions, restrictions and recommendations

- Caution is advised regarding stiffness.
- Relaxation is integral to reduce muscle spasm and feeling of stress.

Frozen shoulder (adhesive capsulitis)

In this chronic condition there is pain, stiffness and reduced mobility, or locking, of the shoulder joint. This may follow an injury, a stroke or myocardial infarction, or may develop because of incorrect lifting or a sudden movement.

> **Health and safety note**
> If the condition is severe, refer the client to a physiotherapist.
>
> Avoid massaging the affected areas while there is acute inflammation.

Cautions, restrictions and recommendations

- This condition can cause neck pain and pain at the base of the skull, which result in a headache.
- Be aware that the synovial capsule of the shoulder joint will be tender, and surrounding muscles and tendons will also be affected.
- The client will benefit from gentle stretching exercises to help mobilise the shoulder joint.

Headache (tension)

This is the most common type of headache. It involves contraction and spasm of the neck and scalp muscles. The pain is produced by the pressure of the contracted muscle on the nerves and blood vessels in the area. The resultant blood flow increases the accumulation of waste products (such as lactic acid) in the area, which perpetuate the pain. The sufferer will usually complain of a dull, persistent ache and a feeling of tightness around the head, temple, forehead and occiput. Factors that may precipitate an attack include mental strain, noise, bright lights, alcohol consumption, menstruation and fatigue.

> **Health and safety note**
> It is important to try to identify the precipitating cause of the headache.
>
> Remember that clients may be taking painkillers and therefore may give inadequate feedback.

Cautions, restrictions and recommendations

- Indian head massage is usually very successful in helping to relieve this type of headache, particularly if it is stress-induced.
- Encourage the client to relax the shoulder and neck muscles with relaxation exercises before commencing the massage.
- Concentrate on relaxing areas that are less tense with effleurage (smoothing/stroking) and gentle kneading, and then move on to muscles that are in spasm with frictions (it is likely that these will be the neck muscles, trapezius, levator scapula and rhomboids).
- Massage of the scalp and face can be helpful (concentrating on the temporalis muscle, the masseters and the frontalis).

Kyphosis

This is a deformity of the spine that produces a rounded back. The condition presents with a rounded back and a flattened chest. There may be difficulty in breathing because of shortening of the pectoral muscles, and the back muscles become weakened. In this condition the scapula tends to be pulled forwards and the head is pushed forwards.

Cautions, restrictions and recommendations

- A postural assessment is required in order to identify range of motion.
- Concentrate on relaxing the muscles of the shoulders and neck.
- Gentle stretching exercises for the back and neck may help to improve posture.
- The aim of the treatment will be to relax and reduce pain in tense muscles.
- Deep, diaphragmatic breathing should be encouraged to help mobilise the thorax.

Health and safety note

Take care with the positioning of the client and, if necessary, offer supporting cushions/pillows.

Avoid joint mobilisation if the condition is caused by changes in bone or connective tissue.

Migraine

This is a specific form of headache, usually unilateral (one side of the head), associated with nausea or vomiting and visual disturbances (usually scintillating light waves or zigzag patterns). Clients may experience a visual aura before an attack actually happens. This is usually called a classical migraine. On occasions they cause painful, red and watery eyes, classified as ophthalmoplegic migraine.

Another form of migraine can cause one-sided paralysis and weakness of the face and body; this is called neuropathic migraine. Abdominal migraine can affect children, who present with recurring attacks of abdominal pain, with or without nausea/vomiting. Migraine can be treated with simple analgesics or more specialised medication.

Cautions, restrictions and recommendations

- Indian head massage is well known in helping migraine sufferers, as the relaxation and relief from stress and tension can help to reduce the frequency of attacks.
- Remember that women are likely to have more attacks during premenstrual periods, when they are taking the contraceptive pill, during the menopause or when starting HRT.
- Tension headaches can be a variant of migraine. Indian head massage is an ideal therapy in this event.

Health and safety note

Avoid treatment during acute attacks, especially if the condition has not yet been diagnosed.

Myalgic encephalomyelitis (chronic fatigue syndrome)

This condition is characterised by extreme disabling fatigue that has lasted for at least six months and is made worse by physical or mental exertion and is not resolved by bed rest. The symptom of fatigue is often accompanied by some of the following: muscle pain or weakness, poor coordination, joint pain, slight fever, sore throat, painful lymph nodes in the neck and armpits, depression, inability to concentrate and general malaise. It can happen in any age group, but recently a higher incidence has been noticed in children and adolescents.

Health and safety note

Be aware of tenderness in the muscles and joints.

Cautions, restrictions and recommendations

- This is a condition that can benefit from Indian head massage, but avoid any claim that could be misinterpreted as curative.
- Relaxation can help the client to cope.
- Clients may require a lot of support and understanding.

Multiple sclerosis

This is a disease of the central nervous system in which the myelin (fatty) sheath covering the nerve fibres is destroyed and various functions become impaired, including movement and sensations. Multiple sclerosis is characterised by relapses and remissions. It can present with blindness or reduced vision and can lead to severe disability within a short period. It can also cause incontinence, loss of balance, tremor and speech problems. Depression and mania can occur.

Health and safety note

Temperature extremes may make the symptoms worse.

Be aware of loss of sensation.

Be aware that massage and joint movement may trigger muscle spasm.

Cautions, restrictions and recommendations

- Relaxation therapies and exercises may be helpful in decreasing tone in rigid muscles and preventing stiffness and contractures.
- Treatments should be slow and gentle and of short duration, as clients may tire easily.

Psoriasis (of the scalp)

This chronic skin disease presents as erythematous (red) scaly lesions on the scalp (other common areas affected include the knees, elbows, hands, nails and sacral area). The client with psoriasis of the scalp may complain of a severe case of dandruff. However, unlike dandruff, scalp psoriasis can easily be felt as thick plaques occurring in patches. It may cause some hair thinning, which tends to recover with successful treatment of the psoriasis.

Health and safety note

Caution is advised regarding the application of oils – avoid oils that are too hot or too stimulating to the scalp (almond and coconut are good choices).

Cautions, restrictions and recommendations

- See dandruff (pityriasis capitis) on page 112.
- Acute flare-up of psoriasis can cause painful and tender lesions of the skin, and care is needed during massage.
- As psychological stress is a considerable cause of the exacerbation of psoriasis, Indian head massage can help clients to cope with their condition.

Seborrhoeic eczema (or dermatitis)

This condition presents with redness and diffuse scaling of the scalp (see dandruff on page 112), which may be mild or severe. Red scaly areas may also occur on the face, especially in the eyebrows and the nasolabial folds. A similar rash may occur behind the ears.

Cautions, restrictions and recommendations

See dandruff (page 112) and psoriasis (page 116).

Sinusitis

This is a condition involving inflammation of the paranasal sinuses. It is usually caused by a viral or bacterial infection, or may be associated with a common cold or allergy. The congestion of the nose results in a blockage in the opening of the sinus into the nasal cavity and a build-up of pressure in the sinus.

The condition presents with nasal congestion, followed by a mucous discharge from the nose. The pain is located in specific areas, depending on the sinuses affected. If the frontal sinuses are affected, a major symptom is a headache over one or both eyes. If the maxillary sinuses are affected, one or both cheeks will hurt and it may feel as if there is toothache in the upper jaw.

Cautions, restrictions and recommendations

- Pressures around the eyes and around the zygomatic bones can help to drain the sinuses and relieve pain.
- Encourage the client to drink plenty of water after the treatment to increase elimination; encourage them to consider a cleansing diet.

Health and safety note

Be aware of the site of inflammation, where there will be pain and swelling.

Stroke

This is a blocking of blood flow to the brain by an embolus in a cerebral blood vessel. A stroke can result in a sudden attack of weakness affecting one side of the body, caused by the interruption of the flow of blood to the brain. A stroke can vary in severity, from a passing weakness or tingling in a limb to a profound paralysis and a coma if severe. Sometimes the term is used to describe cerebral haemorrhage when an artery or congenital cyst of blood vessels in the brain bursts, resulting in damage to the brain and causing similar signs to thrombus of cerebral vessels. Haemorrhage is usually associated with severe headaches and can cause neck stiffness.

Cautions, restrictions and recommendations

- Therapists will normally deal with clients who have recovered or are recovering from a stroke. Indian head massage can aid recovery.

Health and safety note

Be aware of muscle spasm and jerking movements in a paralysed limb.

Neck massage is best avoided.

Temporomandibular joint tension

Also known as TMJ syndrome, this collection of symptoms and signs is produced by disorders of the temporomandibular joint. It is characterised by bilateral or unilateral muscle tenderness and reduced motion. It presents with a dull, aching pain around the joint, often radiating to the ear, face, neck or shoulder. The condition may start off as clicking sounds in the joint. There may be protrusion of the jaw or hypermobility and pain on opening the jaw. It slowly progresses to decreased mobility of the jaw, and locking of the jaw may occur.

Causes include chewing gum, biting nails, biting off large chunks of food, habitual protrusion of the jaw, tension in the muscles of the neck and back and clenching of the jaw. It may also be caused by injury and trauma to the joint or by a whiplash injury.

Cautions, restrictions and recommendations

- The muscles of the neck, base of skull and shoulders should be massaged thoroughly to help reduce tension and spasms.
- The client needs to be educated on relaxing the muscles of the jaw. Ask the client to clench the jaw firmly and concentrate on the feeling of tightness in the jaw, then relax and let the jaw fall open.
- Clients may benefit from a posture assessment and breathing exercises.
- Clients should be encouraged to consult their dentist and a physiotherapist for specific treatment techniques.

Health and safety note

Be aware that the masseter, temporalis and pterygoid muscles may be in spasm and will be tender.

Tinnitis

This condition involves the sensation of sounds in the ears or head in the absence of an external sound source. The most common cause is ordinary age-related hair cell loss in the cochlear. Other causes include wax blocking the ear canal, damage to the eardrum, diseases of the inner ear such as Ménière's disease, and abnormalities of the auditory nerve.

Cautions, restrictions and recommendations

- Indian head massage has been known to be effective in clearing congestion in the head and may help to relieve the symptoms.
- Concentrate on relaxing the neck muscle and work thoroughly above, in front of and behind the ears, to increase lymph drainage.

Health and safety note

Be aware that some clients may experience dizziness and loss of balance when getting up.

Trigeminal neuralgia

This painful condition is caused by irritation of the fifth cranial nerve (the trigeminal nerve). The condition is characterised by excruciating intermittent pain, confined to one or both sides of the face, along the distribution of the trigeminal nerve. The pain may be triggered by any touch or movement, such as eating, chewing or swallowing. Exposure to hot or cold may also trigger an attack. Some cases of facial neuralgia are caused by a previous attack of shingles that has left a predisposition to lifelong pain.

Cautions, restrictions and recommendations

- Obtain a detailed history of the signs and symptoms and refer the client to their GP before proceeding.
- The client may not allow you to touch the affected side of the face.
- If the client finds massage beneficial, use smoothing movements and light frictions over the skull. Then stroke gently from the middle of the face towards the temples, starting in the least sensitive area and moving gradually towards the more sensitive areas.
- Treatment may be scheduled every other day initially.

Health and safety note

Avoid overworking the area, as it may irritate the nerve and induce pain and discomfort.

Whiplash

This condition is produced by damage to the muscles, ligaments, intervertebral discs or nerve tissues of the cervical region by sudden hyperextension and/or flexion of the neck. The most common cause is a road traffic accident, when acceleration/deceleration causes a sudden stretch of the tissue around the cervical spine. It may also occur as a result of hard-impact sports. It can present with pain and limitation of neck movements and muscle tenderness, which can start hours to days after the accident and may take months to subside. The condition is usually affected by complicated physical, psychological and legal issues.

Cautions, restrictions and recommendations

- The condition may last for a few months or many years.
- Consider compensation as a reason for delayed healing, and therefore avoid making any comments about reasons, prognosis or suitability of the therapy.
- Ascertain that the client is not seeking a cure; neither should the client receive any promise to be cured.
- Relaxation exercises can help.
- Holistic therapies such as Indian head massage may help clients to cope with the condition.
- Remember that clients with this condition would have seen many professionals and there may be legal issues you may want to avoid becoming involved with.

Health and safety note

Take care when massaging the neck and avoid manipulation or moving vigorously.

Knowledge check

State what precautions and adaptations may be necessary in the treatment of a client with

1. alopecia
2. dandruff (pityriasis capitis)
3. migraine
4. kyphosis
5. sinusitis
6. psoriasis of the scalp.

To see the answers to this knowledge check, scan the QR code opposite or visit www.hodderplus.co.uk/indianhead/chapter-3.

Multiple-choice self-assessment questions

1. **Which of the following statements is correct?**
   - a Alopecia is a term used to describe temporary baldness with scaly patches.
   - b Alopecia is a term used to describe permanent baldness with scaly patches.
   - c Alopecia is a term used to describe temporary baldness without scaly patches.
   - d Alopecia is a term used to describe permanent baldness without scaly patches.
2. **Rheumatoid arthritis is**
   - a a progressive disease affecting the rhomboids
   - b a chronic inflammation of peripheral joints
   - c a condition present only in elderly clients
   - d a condition also known as degenerative arthritis.
3. **Which of the following conditions involves a sensation of sounds in the ears?**
   - a Earache
   - b Bell's palsy
   - c Rhinitis
   - d Tinnitus
4. **Which of the following statements is correct?**
   - a Psychomotor epilepsy seizure depends on the location of the damage in the brain.
   - b Psychomotor epilepsy was formerly known as grand mal seizure.
   - c Psychomotor epilepsy is caused by dysfunction of the cortex of the temporal lobe of the brain.
   - d Psychomotor epilepsy was formerly known as petit mal seizure.
5. **For a client with multiple sclerosis**
   - a treatments should be quick and firm and of short duration, as clients may tire easily
   - b treatments should be slow and gentle and of short duration, as clients may tire easily
   - c treatments should be quick and firm and of longer duration, to increase clients' stamina
   - d treatments should be slow and gentle and of longer duration, to increase clients' stamina.
6. **If a client is suffering with sinusitis**
   - a avoid pressure around the eyes
   - b it may feel as if there is a toothache if the frontal sinuses are affected
   - c one or both cheeks will hurt if the maxillary sinuses are affected
   - d the congestion of the nose results in a blockage in the pharynx.
7. **A deformity of the spine that produces a rounded back is known as**
   - a lordosis
   - b fibromyalgia
   - c osteoarthritis
   - d kyphosis.
8. **The condition pityriasis capitis is otherwise known as**
   - a seborrhoeic dermatitis
   - b seborrhoeic eczema
   - c dandruff
   - d psoriasis.
9. **Which of the following is NOT a symptom of psoriasis of the scalp?**
   - a Hair thinning
   - b Red scaly lesions
   - c Loss of sensation
   - d Thick plaques in patches
10. **In the case of treatment for a client with migraine**
    - a avoid treatment during acute attacks
    - b only avoid treatment if the client feels nauseous
    - c only avoid treatment if the client has visual disturbances
    - d avoid treatment altogether.

To see the answers, scan the QR code opposite or visit www.hodderplus.co.uk/indianhead/chapter-3. To access an interactive version of these multiple-choice self-assessment questions visit www.hodderplus.co.uk/indianhead/chapter-3.

To access an interactive crossword for this chapter visit www.hodderplus.co.uk/indianhead/chapter-3.

4 Consultation for Indian head massage

Introduction

A client consultation involves professional communication between a client and a therapist; it is a critical skill that helps to establish a positive and trusting therapeutic relationship between both parties.

The time spent in establishing a professional relationship with the client will often result in client satisfaction and their continued patronage. Therapists therefore need to have effective communication skills, which involve both talking and listening to clients in order to be able record and respond positively to the information elicited.

Learning objectives

By end of this chapter you will be able to:

- carry out a consultation for Indian head massage
- understand how contraindications and precautions may affect the proposed treatment
- formulate a treatment plan for Indian head massage
- liaise with other health care professionals.

Client consultation skills

As with all holistic therapy treatments, a consultation for Indian head massage involves one-to-one communication. During a consultation, a therapist's contact with the client involves talking, listening and non-verbal communication, as well as the recording of written information.

When carrying out a consultation, therapists need to adopt a warm, calm, open and understanding attitude towards the client, in order to facilitate a channel of positive communication. Clients presenting for treatment may be nervous or apprehensive about the treatment, so it is important for a therapist to adopt a sensitive, respectful and friendly attitude to the client at all times.

Although talking is an important part of a consultation, one of the most important skills a therapist can develop is to listen. Through effective listening, a therapist can customise the treatment, with the aim of meeting the client's needs and expectations. It is important for therapists to realise that clients often communicate without the spoken word, and non-verbal messages may be projected without the client's awareness. Therapists therefore need to be aware of what a client may be communicating in the tone of their words, gestures they may make, the posture they may present or their facial expressions. With this in mind, therapists may realise that there might be a difference between what a client is expressing in words and what their body language may indicate.

It is also important to be aware of how to adjust communication skills to suit clients from different walks of life. Clients may have different cultural and religious backgrounds, based on their upbringing, and their individual beliefs will need to be considered respectfully in the consultation. For instance, a client may have specific religious beliefs that prevent the use of certain products (massage oils containing essential oils), or their religion may restrict them being massaged by a member of the opposite sex.

Study tip

It is essential when carrying out a consultation that all clients are treated equally, regardless of any differences in their culture, background or religion, and that you avoid discrimination of any sort. As well as being a legal requirement to ensure compliance with antidiscrimination legislation, it is a moral requirement to respect a client's individuality and differences.

Consultation environment

In order to facilitate a positive approach to a consultation, it is important to be aware of the environment in which it is undertaken. The environment for a consultation should ideally be private, in order to respect the client's privacy and dignity in disclosing personal information.

Attention to aspects such as lighting, smell, temperature and comfort of a consultation area can all help to aid client relaxation and decrease apprehension.

Client education

Consultations provide an ideal opportunity for therapists to educate clients on what Indian head massage involves, its potential benefits and the costs and time involved. Clients do not usually want to become passive recipients of the treatment, and if they are to invest time and money in a therapy they need to be educated so that they become partners in their healing process.

Consultations also provide the client with the opportunity to ask questions about the treatment, for reassurance and clarification. Based on the information and the education provided about the service, the client is then responsible for making a decision about the treatment objectives. It is the therapist's responsibility to provide a treatment to suit the client's needs, but to accurately inform them if their objectives and expectations are unrealistic. It is essential for therapists to stress to clients the importance of regular treatments to maintain long-term benefits.

Clients may also be empowered to take charge of their own healing, through client education of adjustments to lifestyle, posture and the correct use of ergonomics (the positioning of furniture at work).

Client confidentiality

Client confidentiality is an important factor in a therapeutic relationship between a client and a therapist. Clients should be reassured that all information recorded will remain confidential and is stored securely, and that no information will be disclosed to a third party without the client's written consent. Maintaining client confidentiality will also help to establish a trusting professional relationship between a client and a therapist.

Key fact

Client information recorded on a consultation form should always be stored in a secure area following treatment, in accordance with the Data Protection Act (1998), which is the legislation designed to protect the client's confidentiality.

Written documentation

Written documentation is essential in a consultation, as it provides a systematic and continued record of the client's progress. Consultation documents should always be used as a guide to facilitate communication, and questions may need to be phrased in a certain way to maximise communication and receive qualitative information. For instance, when asked about their stress levels, a client may merely reply 'high'. In order to gain more information, a therapist may pose the question, 'In which part of the body do you feel stress most often?' or 'What factors are involved in your stress levels being high at the moment?'

Study tip

Always remember to use open-ended questions in a consultation (using words such as 'how', 'what', 'when' and 'where'), as these will enable you to gain more information from the client in order to be able to help them in the most effective way.

It is important for therapists to realise that information received from the client is largely subjective in that it is from their viewpoint, and this information may differ from the evaluation of the therapist. Important information to be discussed during the consultation includes any factors that may affect the client's physical and emotional health, such as medical history, diet, lifestyle, occupation, sleep patterns, exercise and relaxation, which may all contribute to an overall picture of the client from a holistic point of view.

Besides talking, listening and recording information on a client's records, client consultation involves other assessment skills, such as:

- visual assessment – this commences from the first point of contact with the client. Observations as to the client's mood, rate and depth of breathing, posture and gait may all help to contribute to the state of the client's physical and emotional health.
- manual assessment of the tissues – the most effective form of communication a therapist can facilitate is in touch, and throughout the Indian head massage treatment the therapist can assess the tissues for tension, restrictions, temperature changes, and so on.

Assessing posture

Posture may be assessed by observing your client from all aspects (front, back and sides). It is also helpful to observe the client's sitting, standing and walking stance. Be aware of any exaggerated curves in the spine or alignment imbalances (see page 76 on good posture).

Remember that areas exhibiting postural imbalance may result in client discomfort, muscle fatigue, muscle strain and muscular tension.

Therefore, some form of postural education may be needed – that is, the client may need to be aware of the problem area and how to correct it – and you may need to adapt the treatment in some way due to the client's physical condition (it may mean a change of position or extra cushioning in order to facilitate client comfort).

In the case of poor posture that has developed as a result of the client's occupation, the condition may be improved through a combination of strengthening and stretching exercises and avoiding factors that increase it – for example, sitting hunched over a desk for long periods without a break. In some cases, the postural condition may be genetic and may be associated with a spinal disorder, which will also need medical help.

To see the answers to this knowledge check, scan the QR code below or visit www.hodderplus.co.uk/indianhead/chapter-4.

Study tip

Remember that a client's posture may be influenced by their occupation, physical health, stress levels and their psychological state.

Knowledge check 1

1. What is one of the most important skills to have when carrying out a client consultation?
2. What steps need to be taken in a consultation to protect a client's confidentiality?
3. State three factors to be taken into consideration in a consultation environment.
4. State three ways in which clients may be assessed for treatment.

Related medical history/general health	Enables you to establish the client's suitability for Indian head massage, and whether medical advice is necessary before treatment commences
Medication	The effects of some medication may affect the client adversely, either during or after the treatment
Date of birth	Indicates client's age group, and may be relevant in terms of the stage in their life hormonally, or medically
Occupation	May be a relevant factor in contributing to stress levels and an increase in muscle tension/poor posture
Hobbies and interests	May be a relevant factor in assessing how and when (how often) a client relaxes
Exercise undertaken	The nature and regularity of exercise will give you an indication of the client's overall health and energy levels, and their ability to cope with stress
Dietary and fluid intake	An indication of how healthy/balanced a diet the client has will be indicative as to their general health and energy levels
Alcohol consumption	Excessive alcohol consumption can have a dehydrating effect on the body, as well as depriving the body of vital nutrients
Smoking habits	Being a toxic substance, nicotine can affect cell renewal, circulation, cause serious health-related problems and contribute to premature ageing of the skin
Sleep patterns	Poor sleep patterns are usually indicative of increased stress levels
Skin and hair condition	The condition of the client's skin and hair will often reflect their general health, and may be associated with a disorder
Postural condition	Areas of postural imbalance may be causing the client discomfort, muscle fatigue, muscle strain and muscular tension
Muscle tone	Whether the muscle tone is good or poor may be indicative of the client's lifestyle and exercise patterns, and will be a factor to consider when adapting/modifying the techniques used in treatment

▲ Table 4.1 Relevant factors to be considered in a consultation

Contraindications for Indian head massage

Despite Indian head massage being an extremely safe and effective treatment, it is important for therapists to be aware of:

- conditions that are totally contraindicated and for which treatment cannot be provided
- conditions that require referral to the client's GP or another professional before treatment may be given
- conditions that present as localised contraindications; therefore treatment should be avoided in the affected area
- additional cautions that may affect the proposed treatment plan.

Conditions that are totally contraindicated

These include:

- fever/high temperature – this is a contraindication due to the risk of spreading infection as a result of the increased circulation. During fever, the body temperature rises as a result of infection.
- acute infectious diseases (for example, colds, flu, measles, mumps, tuberculosis, chicken pox) – acute infectious diseases are contraindicated due to the fact that they are highly contagious
- skin or scalp infections – these should be avoided due to the risk of cross-infection; some of the most common skin diseases that may be encountered on the head and neck include herpes simplex (cold sores), herpes zoster (shingles), impetigo, ringworm, scabies, conjunctivitis, folliculitis, pediculosis capitis (head lice) and tinea capitis (ringworm of the scalp) – see pages 36–52 for more detail on these and other skin and scalp disorders

Study tip

In order to assess signs of skin and scalp infections, it may be helpful to use a magnifying lamp.

- recent haemorrhage – haemorrhaging is excessive bleeding which may be either internal or external

Health and safety note

In the case of a recent haemorrhage, Indian head massage should be avoided due to increasing the risk of blood spillage from blood vessels.

- intoxication with alcohol or drugs

Health and safety note

It is inadvisable to carry out treatment if a client is under the influence of alcohol, as the increase of blood flow to the head could make them feel dizzy and nauseous.

Health and safety note

Male clients should be advised to avoid consuming in excess of four units of alcohol a day; for women it is just three units a day. A unit is equivalent to one small glass of wine, half a pint of lager or beer, or a single measure of a spirit.

Health and safety note

Correct knowledge of contraindications and precautions enables a therapist to work safely and effectively, thereby avoiding risks to either client or therapist.

Health and safety note

It is essential to assess the skin, hair and scalp for any diseases and disorders prior to treatment, in order to avoid cross-infection. Skin, hair and scalp conditions will usually present with visible recognition signs, such as the skin appearing inflamed or infected (there may be pus present), or there may be signs of hair breakage or loss of hair.

- acute migraine attack

Health and safety note

It is inadvisable to carry out treatment if a client indicates the onset of an attack of migraine, due to the fact they may become nauseous, dizzy, experience visual disturbances, with severe headache and possible vomiting. In reality, clients experiencing an acute attack of migraine will usually be incapacitated from its effects and would be unable to receive treatment, let alone desire a treatment, at the time of the attack. *However, Indian head massage may help as a preventative treatment, particularly if the migraine is stress-induced.*

- recent head or neck injury

Health and safety note

In the case of a recent blow to the head with concussion, or an acute neck injury due to a recent accident, such as whiplash, it would be inadvisable to treat due to the risk of exacerbating the condition and increasing the inflammation and pain. However, if there is an old injury, massage may help to reduce scar tissue, decrease pain and increase mobility. Always obtain medical advice to ensure the client's condition is suitable for treatment.

Conditions that require medical advice

Conditions that may be contraindicated to Indian head massage, but require medical advice before deciding whether treatment is advisable include:

- severe circulatory disorders/heart conditions

Health and safety note

Medical advice should always be sought before massaging a client with a severe heart condition or circulatory problem, as the increased circulation from the massage may overburden the heart and can increase the risk of a thrombus or embolus. *If medical advice indicates that massage is advisable, it is recommended that a lighter massage is given, of a shorter duration initially.*

- thrombosis/embolism

Health and safety note

Always seek medical advice before massaging a client with a history of thrombosis or embolism, as there is a risk that the blood clot could become detached and be carried to another part of the body, where it could obstruct the flow of blood to a vital organ. *If medical advice indicates that massage is advisable, it is recommended that a lighter massage is given, of a shorter duration initially.*

- high blood pressure – clients with high blood pressure should have medical referral prior to massage, even if they are on prescribed medication, due to their susceptibility to form clots

Health and safety note

Clients on antihypertensive medication may be prone to postural hypotension and may feel light-headed and dizzy after treatment. Therapists are advised to carefully monitor a client's reaction and advise clients to get up slowly from the chair following treatment. *If medical advice indicates that massage is advisable, techniques applied are generally soothing and relaxing.*

- low blood pressure

Health and safety note

Care should be taken with a client suffering from low blood pressure when sitting or standing up after massage, due to the fact they may experience dizziness and could fall.

- dysfunction of the nervous system – clients with any dysfunction of the nervous system should be referred to their GP before treatment is given; a light, relaxing massage may be indicated in the case of a client with cerebral palsy, multiple sclerosis or Parkinson's disease, as massage may help to reduce spasms and involuntary movements and reduce rigidity and stiffness

Health and safety note

Always seek medical advice before offering treatment to a client with a nervous dysfunction.

- epilepsy – always refer to the client's GP regarding the type and nature of epilepsy the client may suffer from; caution is advised due to the complexity of this condition and the risk that deep relaxation or overstimulation could provoke a convulsion (although this has never been proven in practice)

Health and safety note

As some types of epilepsy may be triggered by smells, care should be taken with choice of oils or medium.

- diabetes – this is a condition that requires medical advice, as some clients with diabetes may be prone to arteriosclerosis, high blood pressure and oedema; pressure should be carefully monitored and administered, as any loss in sensory nerve function may result in the client being unable to give accurate feedback regarding pressure

Health and safety note

If the client is receiving insulin by injection, care should be taken to avoid massage on recent injection sites. Clients should have their necessary medications with them when they attend for treatment, in the event of an emergency.

- cancer – medical advice should always be sought before massaging a client with a cancerous condition
  There is a risk of certain types of cancer spreading through the lymphatic system; massage is also thought to aid in the metastasis of the cancer. It is unlikely that gentle massage can cause cancer to spread through the stimulation of lymph flow; however, it is important always to obtain advice from the consultant/medical team concerning the type of cancer and the extent of the disease. Once medical advice has been sought, massage may help in relaxing the body and supporting the immune system. It may also be used in palliative care (therapy that eases or reduces pain or other symptoms).

Health and safety note

When massaging a client with cancer, always avoid massage over areas of the body receiving radiation therapy, close to tumour sites and areas of skin cancer. It is usual to avoid massage while clients are actively undergoing chemotherapy or radiotherapy treatment, as they may be too unwell to tolerate treatment. However, in between courses of medical treatment you can offer short, light massage sessions, which will be beneficial in relaxing the client and supporting the immune system.

- recent operations – depending on the nature of the operation and the area/s affected, it may be necessary to seek medical advice before proceeding with treatment

Health and safety note

If a client has recently undergone surgery to the head and neck, Indian head massage should be avoided, as it may interfere with the healing process. Medical advice is often necessary to establish when the area has completely recovered.

- osteoporosis – due to the fact that bones can break easily and vertebrae can collapse with this condition, it is advisable to seek medical advice before giving treatment

Health and safety note

In the case of a client with osteoporosis, care needs to be taken to ensure comfortable client positioning; avoid excessive joint movement and apply a lighter pressure.

Conditions that present as localised contraindications

These include:

- skin disorders – care should be taken as the condition may be worsened. Some skin conditions such as eczema, dermatitis and psoriasis should be treated as a localised contraindication as affected areas may be hypersensitive and the condition may be exacerbated by massage.
- recent scar tissue – massage should only be applied once the tissue is fully healed and can withstand pressure. Gentle frictions may be applied over the healed scar tissue in order to help break down adhesions.
- severe bruising, open cuts or abrasions – these should be treated as localised contraindications, and if presented in the treatment areas they should be avoided.
- undiagnosed lumps, bumps and swellings.

Health and safety note

In the case of an undiagnosed lump or swelling, the client should be referred to their GP for a diagnosis. Massage may increase the susceptibility to damage in the area by virtue of pressure and motion.

Additional cautions

These include:

- allergies – care should be taken to ensure that any oils or products used do not contain items to which the client may be allergic

Health and safety note

In the case of a client with allergies, patch tests should be carried out to avoid adverse reactions.

- asthma – care should be taken to position the client comfortably during treatment

Health and safety note

In the case of a client with asthma, take care to avoid using any massage mediums or substances that a client may be allergic to.

- medication – certain medications may inhibit or distort the client's ability to give feedback regarding pressure, discomfort and pain

Health and safety note

Always check with the client's GP if you are unsure as to the type of medication a client is taking and its effects.

- pregnancy – pregnancy is not strictly a contraindication, unless there are serious complications, in which case treatment should be avoided altogether; however, special care should be taken for a pregnant client, to ensure that they are comfortable during the treatment, and therefore additional supports or alternative positioning may need to be offered

Health and safety note

Therapists should be aware that some women may experience side effects as a result of the pregnancy, such as dizziness and high blood pressure. Pressure and duration of treatment may need to be adjusted according to the individual circumstances.

Total contraindications	**Referral to GP/medical advice**
High temperature or fever	Recent surgery
Infectious/contagious diseases	Severe circulatory disorder/heart condition
Recent haemorrhage	Thrombosis/embolism
Recent head or neck injury	High/low blood pressure
Intoxication	Dysfunction of the nervous system
Migraine	Epilepsy
	Diabetes
	Cancer
	Undiagnosed lumps, bumps or swelling
Localised contraindications	**Special cautions**
Recent scar tissue	Allergies
Bruising, open cuts or abrasions in treatment area	Medication
	Pregnancy

▲ Table 4.2 Summary of contraindications and cautions

Knowledge check 2

1. State six factors to be considered in a client consultation.
2. State four contraindications that would prevent an Indian head massage treatment being carried out.
3. State three conditions that may restrict Indian head massage treatment.
4. State what considerations may need to be taken into account for
   i. a client receiving chemotherapy or radiotherapy treatment
   ii. a client with high blood pressure
   iii. a client with diabetes.

To see the answers to this knowledge check, scan the QR code opposite or visit www.hodderplus.co.uk/indianhead/chapter-4.

Figure 4.1 shows an example of a consultation form that may be used for Indian head massage.

Indian Head Massage Consultation Form

Client Note

The following information is required for your safety and to benefit your health. Whilst Indian head massage is a very safe treatment, there are certain contraindications which may require special care. The following information will be treated in the strictest of confidence. It may however, be necessary for you to consult your GP before any treatment can be given.

Date of initial consultation: 03/05/11 Client ref. No. SW63

PERSONAL DETAILS

Name: Sarath wilson Title: Mr/Mrs/Miss/Ms/Other ______

Address: 23, Ridgestone close, High town park, London, NW12 1MG

Telephone Number~Daytime: 020 875 6987 Evening: 020 522 3612

Telephone Number~Mobile: 11870 123987 Email: S.Wilson25@hotmail.co.uk

Date of Birth: 19/03/72 Occupation: Nail Techenician

MEDICAL DETAILS

Name of Doctor: Johnson Surgery: Street End

Address: Street End Surgery, Jackson place, High town park, London

Telephone Number: 020 555 6688

Do you have/have you ever suffered with any of the following?

(Please give dates and details)

		Dates & Details
Recent head or neck injury?	Y Ⓝ	
Cardiovascular condition?	Y Ⓝ	
Thrombosis or embolism?	Y Ⓝ	
High or low blood pressure?	Y Ⓝ	
Dysfunction of the nervous system?	Y Ⓝ	
Cancer/chemotherapy or radiotherapy?	Y Ⓝ	
Recent haemorrhage?	Y Ⓝ	
Cuts or abrasions in the treatment area?	Y Ⓝ	
Recent operation?	Y Ⓝ	
Diabetes?	Y Ⓝ	
Epilepsy?	Y Ⓝ	
Spastic conditions?	Ⓨ N	Occasional Migraine
Migraine/severe headaches?	Y Ⓝ	
Skin/scalp or hair disorder or infection?	Y Ⓝ	
Do you have any recent scar tissue/bruises/open cuts/large moles lumps/ other swellings?	Y Ⓝ	
Do you suffer with any allergies?	Y Ⓝ	
Any medical condition (not mentioned above)?	Y Ⓝ	

Current Medical Treatment: None

Current Medication (list dosages): None

▲ Figure 4.1 Consultation form

GP referral required: Yes ( ) No (✓)

Genaral State of Health

Do you smoke?
Do you drink alcohol?
How many glasses of water do you drink daily?
How would you describe your diet?
How would you describe your Skin Condition?

	Normal ( )	Dry (✓)	Oily ( )
	Combination ( )	Sensitive ( )	Mature ( )
How would you describe your posture?	Good ( )	Average (✓)	Poor ( )
How would you describe your muscle tone?	Good ( )	Average (✓)	Poor ( )
What is your height and weight?	Height 5′6″	Weight 9st 5	
How would you describe your stress levels?	High (✓)	Medium ( )	Low ( )
How would you describe your sleep patterns?	Good ( )	Average ( )	Poor (✓)

Exercise undertaken/lifestyle: *Mainly socialising with friends*

Do you follow a regular exercise program: Yes ( ) No (✓) Details: ________

Do you have any hobbies/time set aside for relaxation (give details): *Reading in bed*

Have you had an Indian head massage treatment before? Yes ( ) No (✓)
If yes please give brief details of previous treatments and success: ________

Are you currently having any other forms of alternative/complementary treatment? (Please state) *No*

CLIENT DECLARATION

I declare that the information I have given is true and correct and that as far as I am aware, I can undertake treatment with this establishment without any adverse effects. I have been fully informed about contraindications and am therefore willing to proceed.

Client's signature: ________ Date: 3/5/2011
(If applicable) Guardian's signature: ________ Date: 3/5/2011
Therapist's signature: ________ Date: 3/5/2011

(*additional information, treatment adaptions/modifications required*)

▲ Figure 4.1 *Continued*

To access editable and printable versions of this form scan the QR code opposite or visit www.hodderplus.co.uk/indianhead/chapter-4.

Health and safety note

Clients under the age of 16 are considered minors and therefore should not receive an Indian head massage treatment unless accompanied by a parent or guardian, who must sign a consent form.

Formulating a treatment plan for Indian head massage

Once the verbal and non-verbal information has been elicited from the client, the therapist is then in a position to suggest a treatment plan and obtain the client's agreement before proceeding.

A treatment plan for Indian head massage will include the following information:

- the date of the treatment
- feedback from any previous treatment, if applicable
- any updated information on the client's condition since the original consultation
- the treatment objectives (relaxation, sense of well-being, uplifting, improvement in the hair and scalp condition)
- any special considerations/modifications, such as specific areas to be worked on, special needs or requirements
- an outline of the proposed treatment, to include areas for treatment, length and cost of treatment, along with the suggested treatment frequency (this may also be reviewed at the end of the treatment)
- type of oils used (if applicable) and reasons for choice
- the client's agreement.

Treatments should be reviewed at regular intervals in order to monitor progress and elicit client satisfaction. By discussing a treatment plan regularly with a client, their individual needs can be taken into consideration and changes can be made, as required.

Study tip

An important consideration in a client's treatment plan may be the time of day the treatment is undertaken. A client may require the treatment in the morning, to gently awaken the nerves and prepare the body for the day's activities, or may require the appointment later in the day to help remove the stresses of the day and promote sleep.

Figure 4.2 shows an example of a treatment plan, including a record of Indian head massage treatments.

Date	Feedback/update from last treatment	Treatment objective/s	Adaptations required	Proposed treatment plan (inc. frequency)	Oil/ medium to be used	Client's agreement	Outcome	Future treatment recommendations
20th Jan 2011	N/A	Stress relief and relaxation Reduction of muscular tension, particularly in the neck	Additional neck support to assist client comfort Be aware of neck mobility as neck muscles may be sore and stiff	Treatment of all areas (45 mins) concentrating on neck due to tension Relief of sinus congestion with pressure points on face Recommend frequency once a week	Coconut oil for dry scalp condition	[signature]	Client very relaxed and refreshed After care leaflet given	Once a week for 4 weeks and then monthly

▲ Figure 4.2 Treatment plan, including a record of treatments

To access editable and printable versions of this form scan the QR code opposite or visit www.hodderplus.co.uk/indianhead/chapter-4.

Liaising with other health care professionals

As the benefits of Indian head massage become more widely known and validated, there are more opportunities opening up for therapists to work alongside other health care professionals. Therapists therefore need to be aware of professional and medical etiquette when liaising with other professionals.

Health and safety

When referring clients to their GP with a contraindication, it is important to avoid diagnosing medical conditions, as you are not qualified to offer medical advice.

Referral to a health care professional

If a contraindication is established with a client at the time of consultation, treatment cannot usually proceed without reference to the client's GP. In this case, it is helpful to have a pre-prepared referral form on headed notepaper that may be taken by the client to their doctor, or may be posted with a stamped, addressed envelope.

When referring to a client's GP, it is important to note that a doctor's insurance will not cover them for giving permission or consent to holistic therapy treatments. It is therefore essential that therapists make it clear that they are seeking advice about the client's medical condition, in order to decide whether Indian head massage treatment is suitable, and that their proposed treatment is in accordance with medical advice.

In order to raise awareness of Indian head massage among doctors and other health care professionals, it is important for a therapist to include literature on Indian head massage, concerning its methodology, benefits and effects.

Handling referral data from other health care professionals

If a client has been referred to you by another health care professional, it is professional etiquette to reply with a status report on the client's progress. Report writing is an essential part of networking with other professionals, as it helps to raise awareness of the benefits of the treatment and its value in a client's physical and emotional well-being.

A status report should include the following information:

- a general introduction to the client and how they were referred
- a summary of the client's main presenting problems
- an evaluation of the therapist's findings
- the treatment used and an explanation of the techniques involved
- the client's progress
- recommendations for future/continued treatment.

The most important factor in the consultation, besides whether the client is medically suitable for treatment, is their expectations and objectives of the treatment.

Knowledge check 3

1. State three essential factors that need to be recorded on a client's treatment plan.
2. Why is the time of day a consideration in formulating a treatment plan?
3. Explain why it is important to avoid diagnosing medical conditions when referring clients to their GP.

Referral form

Therapist's Name: Carol Spencer

Clinic Address: The Holistic Clinic, 2 Swallow Rd, Netley Abbey, southampton

Date: 12/10/11

F.A.O. Dr James
Stanley Surgery
12 –14 High Street
Liphampton
Hampshire
S012 3AB

Dear Dr James

I am writing with regard to one of your patients Mrs Brown of West end cottage 21 common rd, Fareham, Hampshire.

who has requested Indian head massage treatment (*please see attached information on Indian head massage*).

Your patient has informed me that he/she suffers from high blood pressure.

Please can you advise me, in your medical opinion, if there is any reason why this patient should not receive an Indian head massage?

Thank you for your assistance in this matter

Therapist's name and signature

Doctor's advice note

The proposed treatment of Indian head massage you suggest would be suitable/~~unsuitable for this patient.~~

Doctor's name and signature

Dr. BR James

▲ Figure 4.3 Referral form

To see the answers to this knowledge check, scan the QR code opposite or visit www.hodderplus.co.uk/indianhead/chapter-4.

To access editable and printable versions of this form scan the QR code opposite or visit www.hodderplus.co.uk/indianhead/chapter-4.

Setting professional boundaries

In order to have a healthy and professional relationship with clients, there should be a balance between care and compassion for the client, and keeping a distance from any personal involvement. The setting of boundaries can provide the foundation on which a therapist can build a professional relationship with a client. A therapeutic relationship should always involve distance between a therapist and a client, in order to make it safe for both parties.

There is always a risk of transference in a client–therapist relationship, in which a client begins to personalise the professional relationship and thus steps over the professional boundary. There is also risk of counter-transference, when a therapist has difficulty in maintaining a professional distance from the client's problems and begins to step into a friend/counsellor role. If either of these situations occurs, it is important to realise how potentially damaging this can be for a client and for the therapist, and how it detracts from the healing process.

When to refer a client to another health care provider

While Indian head massage can be very beneficial in relaxing a client and relieving minor stress-related conditions, it is important to realise that all treatments have their limitations.

If a client presents a condition that is beyond the scope of the treatment, such as a serious medical physical or psychological condition, it is essential that a therapist is able to recognise this and refer the client to the professional who can best help them. In this instance, it is useful for therapists to have resources available for clients to access, such as information on:

- other complementary therapies
- counsellors or psychotherapists
- professional therapy organisations that members of the public can contact for details of qualified members
- advice centres
- self-help groups.

Displaying information offers the client the chance to choose for themselves a way of moving forward with their own situation.

Key fact

Holistic therapy treatments such as Indian head massage always tend to work best when there is a combined treatment strategy; this may involve a client receiving regular treatments, making lifestyle adjustments and attending for treatment with another health care professional.

Multiple-choice self-assessment questions

1. **Which of the following is the most essential skill needed for a therapist to carry out an effective consultation for Indian head massage?**
   a Talking
   b Being friendly
   c Showing empathy
   d Listening
2. **What action should be taken if, during a consultation, a client informs you that they have very high blood pressure?**
   a Offer a lighter treatment that is soothing and relaxing.
   b Proceed with a normal treatment, but keep checking that the client does not feel dizzy.
   c Ask the client to seek advice from their GP to see if treatment is advisable.
   d Do not offer a treatment unless the client is taking medication.
3. **Which of the following conditions would indicate that Indian head massage treatment could not be offered?**
   a Recent scar tissue
   b Low blood pressure
   c Acute infectious disease
   d Open cut or abrasion
4. **Which of the following conditions would not require referral to a GP for advice before offering treatment?**
   a Thrombosis/embolism
   b Dysfunction of the nervous system
   c Recent head or neck injury
   d Open cut or abrasion
5. **Which of the following conditions would restrict an Indian head massage treatment?**
   a Conjunctivitis
   b Herpes zoster
   c Recent head or neck injury
   d Sebaceous cyst
6. **In the case of a client with osteoporosis, you would**
   a avoid treatment, as it will be painful for the client
   b ensure comfortable client positioning, avoid excessive joint movement and apply a lighter pressure
   c ensure comfortable client positioning, avoid excessive joint movement and apply a firmer pressure
   d offer a shorter treatment, but use firmer pressure to ensure it is effective.
7. **Why is it important to seek medical advice before treating a client with a history of thrombosis or embolism?**
   a The treatment would be uncomfortable for the client.
   b There is a risk of cross-infection.
   c The client may feel dizzy and faint.
   d It could cause serious or fatal results.
8. **Skin conditions such as eczema, dermatitis and psoriasis should be treated as a localised contraindication, as**
   a affected areas may be infected and may be spread via the massage
   b affected areas may be hypersensitive and the condition may be exacerbated by massage
   c affected areas may be painful
   d affected areas may become more dry as a result of the massage.
9. **Why is it important to avoid using the words 'permission' or 'consent' on a doctor's referral note?**
   a It is unethical.
   b The correct medical terminology must be used for insurance purposes.
   c It is not professional etiquette.
   d A doctor's insurance will not cover them for giving permission or consent to holistic therapy treatments.
10. **An Indian head massage consultation and treatment plan should always contain**
   a the client's date of birth
   b the client's agreement
   c the client's occupation
   d a record of the client's food habits.

To see the answers, scan the QR code opposite or visit www.hodderplus.co.uk/indianhead/chapter-4. To access an interactive version of these multiple-choice self-assessment questions visit www.hodderplus.co.uk/indianhead/chapter-4.

To access an interactive crossword for this chapter visit www.hodderplus.co.uk/indianhead/chapter-4.

5 Indian head massage case studies

Introduction

As part of the development process for therapists studying to become professional practitioners of Indian head massage, it is necessary to carry out a number of case studies to explore the practical efficacy of the techniques and, most importantly, to gain valuable practical experience of the skills learnt. Carrying out several treatments on case studies encourages repetitive practice and can help to increase confidence levels through client feedback.

This chapter is devoted to providing general guidelines on how to approach case studies, along with three examples.

Learning objectives

By the end of this chapter you will:

- know how to present an Indian head massage case study as part of an assessment for a professional qualification.

Indications for treatment

There are many conditions that a client may present that may benefit from Indian head massage. Common conditions that Indian head massage has been known to help with include:

- tension headaches
- eye strain
- muscular tension
- emotional stress
- anxiety and depression
- insomnia and disturbed sleep patterns
- sinusitis
- poor hair condition.

What is a case study?

A case study is a record of a series of treatments carried out on a client that has been evaluated for effectiveness.

Study tip

When considering who to choose for your case studies, it is advisable to choose as wide a range of clients as possible, in order to meet the requirements of a professional award and to prepare yourself for commercial practice.

The essential components of a case study are as follows.

Health and safety note

As part of a case study, a full consultation must be carried out and recorded, including personal, medical and lifestyle details, along with a declaration and the client's signature. (See the example of a consultation form on pages 131–2.)

Client profile

This is a general introduction to the client and will include background information, such as age range, occupation, lifestyle issues, sleep patterns, hobbies and interests, along with their main presenting problems and any factors that may affect them in their daily life.

Consultation form

Before any treatment commences, the client needs to be assessed in order that their individual considerations may be taken into account (health problems or special needs).

Observations

This may include initial and ongoing observations from information elicited at the original consultation and subsequent treatments. Therapists need to be perceptive of non-verbal signs the client may exhibit, such as their posture, facial expressions and breathing rate. These are all factors that will not be evident from the recording paperwork. The noting of these factors will assist the reader or assessor to build a fuller picture of your case study, and will reflect the development of your perceptive skills.

Treatment plan

Once the initial consultation has taken place, a course of treatment may then be recommended. A treatment plan will typically include the following information:

- client's name
- date and time of treatment
- outline of proposed treatment and areas to concentrate on
- treatment timing
- cost
- client expectations
- treatment objectives
- special client considerations
- oils to be used
- recommended treatment frequency.

(See the example of a treatment plan on page 134.)

Record of treatments

It is important that a record is kept of all treatments carried out. This will typically include:

- an assessment of the client's physical condition (noting any areas of tension, physiological responses), as well as psychological responses and body language (client nervous or apprehensive)
- visual assessment of the client (noting posture, non-verbal signs)
- any known reactions, their effects and any advice given
- aftercare advice given
- homecare advice, along with any oils or products suggested for home use
- outcome and general evaluation of the treatment
- recommendations for future treatment and the suggested frequency.

Evaluation

The evaluation is an essential part of a case study, as it is only through feedback and evaluation that a therapist can gauge the effectiveness of the treatments given, and ultimately measure their own professional development.

Factors to consider in evaluating the treatment are:

- Was the course of treatment effective? If so, in what ways?
- What benefits, if any, were derived from the treatments?
- Were there any particular parts of the treatment that the client liked or disliked?
- Were there any contra-actions?
- Is the client keen to continue with regular treatments?

Written testimonial

Once the course of treatment has been completed, it is necessary for the purposes of assessment and authenticity to ask your case studies to complete a written testimonial, which is a handwritten letter to confirm that they have received a course of treatment on the dates concerned, and should outline any benefits they have noticed as a result.

Alternatively, you could ask a client to complete a pre-prepared evaluation form, like the one in Figure 5.1.

Client Evaluation Sheet - Indian Head Massage

Dear Client, we would be grateful if you would kindly answer the following questions about the treatment you have received today. Your comments will be greatly appreciated and are invaluable to the student therapist's progress. All information given is treated with the strictest confidence.

Therapist's Name: Jane Longman Date of Treatment: 17/07/11

Client Care

a) Was the reason for the consultation explained to you? Yes
b) Was a treatment plan discussed with you? Yes
c) Was your comfort and modesty ensured throughout the treatment? Yes

Speed/flow/rhythm of movements

a) Did your massage seem rushed or unhurried? Unhurried
b) Were the movements smooth and flowing? Yes
c) Did the massage seem disjointed in any way? No
d) Did you find any of the movements uncomfortable or irritating? Slightly tender on shoulders.

Pressure

a) Was the massage firm/light/other? Fairly firm
b) Did the pressure used meet with your requirements? Yes, just right.

Outcome

a) How did you feel after the massage? Relaxed.
b) Is this the outcome you expected? What I was hoping for.
c) In general, were you pleased with your treatment? Yes, very pleased.
d) What aftercare advice were you given? Drink plenty of water, relax, and avoid alcohol or smoking.

Do you have any additional comments you would like to make?

Found the massage very helpful.
I enjoyed it because it helped me to relax and release tension in my muscles.

Client's Signature: 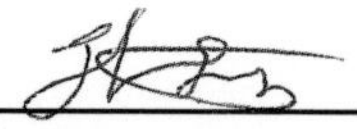 Date: 17/07/11

▲ Figure 5.1 Client evaluation sheet

To access editable and printable versions of this form scan the QR code opposite or visit www.hodderplus.co.uk/indianhead/chapter-5.

Self-evaluation

It is also important for therapists to carry out a self-evaluation, in order to assess their own development. By objectively analysing their own performance, therapists can perfect their skills and commit to continual improvement.

Examples of Indian head massage case studies

Case study 1

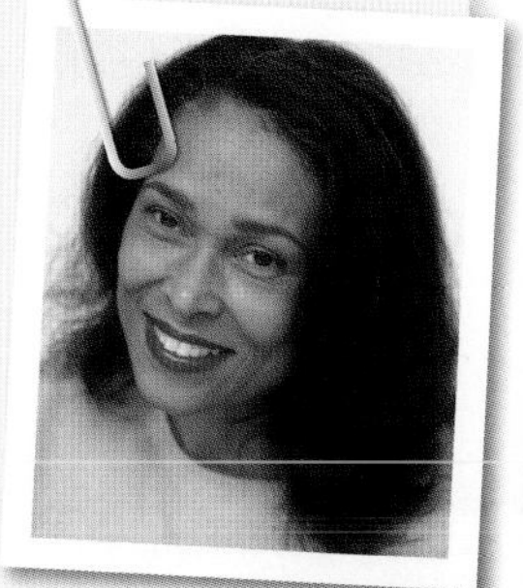

Client profile

Name: Janet

Age: 42 years

Occupation: mature student and homemaker

Background information

Janet is a mature student, with two girls of 17 and 14 years of age. She is currently training to be a counsellor and is on work placement at a local doctor's surgery.

Her life is therefore very busy, looking after her two daughters, completing her studies and looking after their home. Despite her busy schedule, Janet does find some time to relax; she swims, goes for walks and loves reading.

Physically, Janet is fit and healthy, with no medical conditions. However, she does sometimes feel stressed out due to the pressures of her studies and running a home. She finds her neck muscles are often tight, in particular the right trapezius muscle often aches, causing her a degree of discomfort.

Janet's energy and stress levels are average.

Treatment objectives

Janet had never experienced Indian head massage before. The effects and benefits of the treatment were therefore explained to her.

After consultation, it was agreed with Janet that the treatment objectives were to:

- ✓ help relieve muscular tension in the shoulders and neck
- ✓ aid general relaxation and relief of tension
- ✓ help uplift Janet psychologically and aid stress relief.

Treatment plan

It was agreed with Janet that a course of three treatments would be given over a period of two weeks; the first two were given in the first week, and the third the following week.

Coconut oil was to be used on the scalp, as Janet's hair and scalp has a tendency to dryness.

Record of treatments

Treatment 1

On commencement of the first treatment, Janet indicated that she was very tired mentally, as she had just returned from her work placement.

The treatment uncovered a lot of tension in the neck and shoulder area. The neck and shoulders were very stiff. A lot of deep breathing was suggested throughout the treatment to help ease tension. By the time we reached the scalp massage, Janet was almost asleep.

After the treatment, Janet reported that at the start she was aware of all her thoughts and her mind was not still; however, at the end of the treatment she felt calm, extremely relaxed, but at the same time energised.

Janet was advised to drink plenty of water following treatment, to rest, have a light meal and to avoid alcohol or caffeine consumption. She was also encouraged to leave the oil on for a few hours following treatment, before shampooing.

Janet did not have any adverse reactions after the treatment and reported that she felt quite energetic the next day.

Treatment 2

The second treatment was given three days after the first. Janet had been at college all day and was tired, but less tension was noticeable. She relaxed from the beginning and fell asleep. At the conclusion of the treatment, she felt relaxed, calm and contented.

Janet did not report any adverse reactions after her second treatment and reported that she felt relaxed but energetic the next day.

Treatment 3

The third treatment was given a week later. During this treatment, Janet commented on the overall improvement she was experiencing and how the muscular tension had decreased to the point where it no longer caused her discomfort. She reported that she was also feeling more relaxed and energetic.

Outcomes and recommendations

The course of three treatments have proved very beneficial to Janet. During and after each treatment, the improvements have been visibly noticeable. Janet has also commented enthusiastically on how much better she has felt.

Further treatments were recommended to maintain Janet's progress and condition, and it was suggested that treatments be continued once fortnightly as a preventative measure against tension build-up.

Client testimonial

'The experience of the head massage was quite different from anything I had experienced before. I was aware of my tension during the first treatment and found the shoulder and upper arm movements quite strange. However, the pressure was just right and by the second and third treatments I knew what to expect and was much more relaxed. In the second and third treatments I actually fell asleep – something I never realised I could do sitting upright in a chair!

I think I slept better and definitely felt more invigorated in the days afterwards, and less tense.

I really enjoyed and appreciated the experience and shall definitely be continuing with regular treatments.'

Case study 2

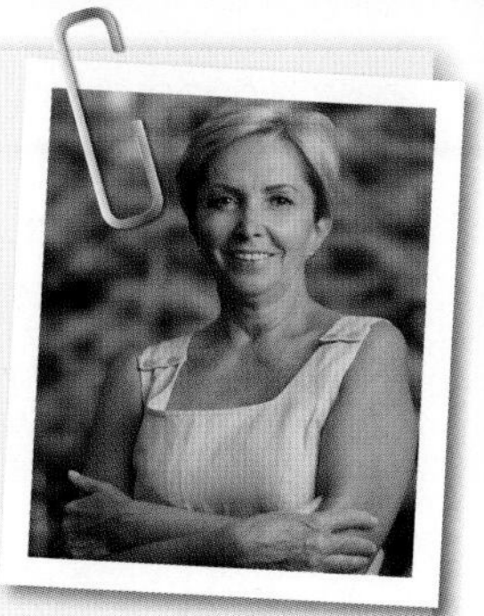

Client profile

Name: Pauline

Age: 59 years

Occupation: retired

Background information

Pauline is a widow with two daughters and four grandchildren, whom she looks after on a regular basis. Although Pauline is retired, she has quite an active social life, playing tennis and swimming, and she enjoys gardening.

Generally, Pauline is in good health and has no major illnesses, but sometimes suffers from sinusitis, headaches and disturbed sleep. She takes HRT and cholesterol tablets, for which she has regular reviews with her GP.

During the consultation, Pauline revealed that she had manipulation on her left shoulder under anaesthetic two years ago. However, Pauline's current condition did not prove to be contraindicated to treatment, although caution was observed when treating the shoulder and upper arm area. She did not present with any other conditions or considerations for treatment.

Generally, Pauline has low levels of stress and medium energy levels, but recently has been experiencing low energy levels. While the benefits were explained to her, Pauline mentioned her dry scalp and thinning hair.

Treatment objectives

After consultation, it was agreed that the treatment objectives were to:

- ✓ aid general relaxation
- ✓ improve congestion in the sinus area
- ✓ improve scalp and hair condition
- ✓ relieve muscular tension
- ✓ improve energy levels.

Treatment plan

It was agreed with Pauline to give a course of three treatments over a four-week period. The first and second treatments would be weekly and the third after a fortnight.

Record of treatments

Treatment 1

Pauline has never had any form of massage treatment before and was quite apprehensive. As a result, she was unable to relax fully during her first treatment. She enjoyed the scalp massage and felt that the pressure points over the sinus area on the face helped to ease congestion. Pauline commented that she felt relaxed at the conclusion of the treatment.

She felt calm and experienced no adverse reactions the next day.

Treatment 2

During this treatment the muscles in Pauline's neck and upper back felt very tight. She explained that this was due to the fact that she had been gardening during the day. Deep breathing was advised to help ease tension during the treatment. Pauline was visibly more relaxed during this session and commented that her neck and upper back felt better.

Pauline reported that she experienced a headache for a couple of days after the second treatment; this she felt was caused by congestion and the sinuses.

Treatment 3

The third treatment was given two weeks later. During the treatment Pauline commented on how the pressure points over the sinus area helped and how the use of oil had helped with the dryness of the scalp and hair. Pauline relaxed really well during this treatment and almost fell asleep.

Aftercare advice was given after each treatment: to drink plenty of water, rest, have a light meal and avoid consumption of alcohol and stimulants. Pauline was also shown some simple massage techniques to use at home with oil for the long-term care of the hair and scalp condition.

Outcomes and recommendations

The course of treatments has been successful for Pauline. She felt relaxed after each treatment and indicated how they have helped with her sinusitis, sleep pattern and hair and scalp condition. She also commented on how her energy levels have improved since treatments commenced.

Pauline has requested that she continue with regular treatments for relaxation and body maintenance. Suggested frequency is once a fortnight.

Client testimonial

'The course of Indian head massage I have received has been a beneficial and new experience for me. Having never received a massage, I was unsure of what to expect and felt quite nervous to start with. Everything was so well explained, and the pressure was perfect for me. Although I felt relaxed after the first treatment, I was able to relax more fully on the second and third, knowing what to expect. I would very much like to continue with regular treatment, as this seems an ideal way to relax. It has certainly helped to improve my sinusitis and headaches, and after each treatment I found I slept more soundly and woke feeling more refreshed.'

Case study 3

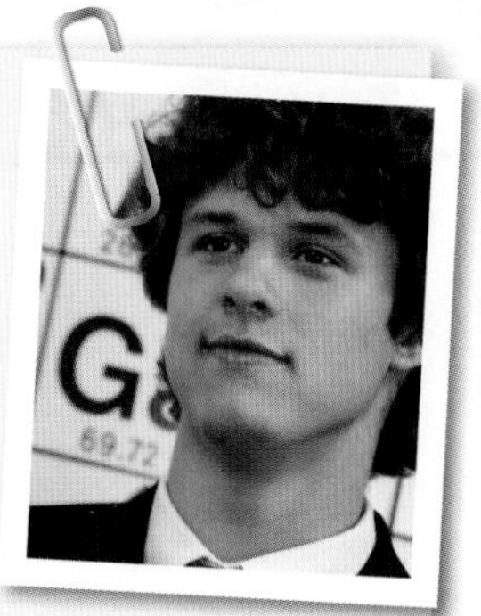

Client profile

Name: Michael

Age: 18 years

Occupation: student

Background information

Michael is completing his A levels in maths and the sciences. He is fit and in good health, but suffers from hay fever, for which he takes antihistamines.

Michael has never experienced Indian head massage before; however, due to exam stress he was keen to try the treatment, for stress relief and relaxation.

Treatment objectives

After consultation, it was agreed with Michael that the treatment objectives were to:

- ✓ help relieve muscular tension
- ✓ help relieve mental fatigue
- ✓ promote psychological uplift
- ✓ aid relaxation and stress relief.

Treatment plan

It was agreed with Michael that, due to his high stress levels at exam time, two treatments would be given in the first week and the third treatment given a week later.

Record of treatments

Treatment 1

During the first treatment, Michael was unable to relax to start with; however, he began to relax with the neck massage and actually fell asleep during the scalp massage. A lot of tension was found in the neck and shoulder muscles. A little more time was devoted to treating the shoulder area and Michael was advised to take plenty of deep breaths throughout the treatment, to help ease tension.

Michael was quite surprised by how relaxed the treatment had made him feel and commented that he could not believe he fell asleep sitting up. He felt calm, relaxed and energetic at the end of the first treatment.

Michael was advised to drink lots of water, rest, eat a light meal following treatment and avoid consumption of alcohol and stimulants.

Treatment 2

The second treatment was carried out after four days. Michael reported that after the first treatment he felt relaxed and a bit tired the next day, but became more energetic as the day went on.

At the commencement of the second treatment, Michael's neck and shoulders felt much looser. During the treatment he relaxed and fell asleep, but during the face massage he was awake and alert. After treatment, he was keen to go to play five-a-side football, but was advised against it and told to rest in order that the energy could be utilised in the body for the healing process. The same aftercare advice was given as that in the first treatment.

Treatment 3

The third treatment was given a week later. Michael reported that he had a slight headache the day after the second treatment, but also felt more calm and relaxed. He commented that he also felt dehydrated and felt better after drinking more water.

During the third treatment, Michael fell asleep soon after the treatment started, but remained awake and energetic during the face massage.

Aftercare advice was specified as in the previous treatments.

The day following the third treatment, Michael reported that he felt quite tired and lethargic in the morning. He also felt dehydrated, but felt better after drinking more water. As the day progressed, he commented on how much more energetic he felt.

Outcomes and recommendations

The series of treatments given has been successful for Michael. He felt he was able to relax, unwind and relieve the mental fatigue he was feeling due to the pressure of his exams. After each treatment Michael felt tired, lethargic and dehydrated, due to toxins being released; however, after drinking more water he felt much better – energetic, calm and relaxed.

Michael is keen to continue treatments for relaxation; suggested frequency would ideally be once a fortnight.

Client testimonial

'I thoroughly enjoyed my head massage sessions. I had never experienced a head massage before and found some of the sensations quite strange for the first time, yet at the same time they were very relaxing. While my back, shoulders and arms were being massaged I felt very lethargic and fell asleep every time these areas of my body were massaged. However, I found that when my neck, scalp and face were massaged I felt very energised and revitalised. The massage always left me feeling energetic and lively, yet calm and relaxed inside. During each massage I was aware that my body was relaxing, my heart rate slowed slightly and I fell asleep very easily as I became used to the movements. I also noticed that during the massage I was unaware of time passing as I was so relaxed.

The days following the massages I sometimes felt quite tired and lethargic. I was also slightly dehydrated, but soon felt better when I increased my intake of water.

I feel the head massage sessions have enabled me to relax and cope with my increased stress levels at this time and therefore I feel I have really benefited from the treatments. I would also like to continue with the treatments regularly to maintain the benefits.'

Knowledge check

1. Suggest a suitable treatment plan for each of the following case study scenarios, including

i. suggested frequency
ii. any modifications/special care needed
iii. suggested oil or medium to be used.

Profile for case study 1

Case study 1 is a client who regularly receives massage treatments, although she has never experienced an Indian head massage before.

- 46 years of age, with a highly stressed job, divorced, with two grown-up children
- has an old whiplash injury, and due to this and work-related stress, frequently experiences headaches and neck/shoulder pain
- skin and scalp condition are very dry and scaly.

Profile for case study 2

Case study 2 is a new client to massage, although she has received beauty treatments before.

- 30 years of age, currently working part-time, married with two children under five years of age
- suffers with backache, the onset of which started after the birth of her second child
- lifestyle is hectic, and with two small children has very little time for herself
- scalp and skin condition is fairly sensitive.

Profile for case study 3

Case study 3 has never experienced any form of massage treatment before.

- 21 years of age, single and studying for a degree at university
- stress levels are high due to workload (both university course work and part-time job)
- has poor sleep patterns and low energy levels (always feeling tired)
- suffers with headaches and sinusitis
- skin and scalp condition is oily.

6 Indian head massage techniques

Introduction

In India, massage has long been adopted as a daily practice in order to help maintain a healthy mind and body throughout the course of life. In the modern day of high stress levels in the western world, massage is a must for relaxing both mind and body, and recharging depleted energy levels. Indian head massage is uniquely different from other types of therapeutic massage practised in the West in that it is applied through the clothes to a client in a seated position, so there is no need for special or sophisticated equipment.

Learning objectives

By the end of this chapter you will be able to:

- understand the massage movements used in Indian head massage, along with their effect
- prepare a treatment area for Indian head massage
- understand the properties and benefits of oils and herbs used in Indian head massage
- carry out a step-by-step Indian head massage treatment to the upper back and shoulders, upper arms, neck, scalp and face
- understand how to adapt an Indian head massage treatment to suit different client needs
- provide aftercare advice.

Massage movements used in Indian head massage

The massage techniques used in Indian head massage are simple, but extremely effective. They consist of a combination of traditional Indian techniques and westernised techniques.

Effleurage

Effleurage is one of the principal techniques used in Indian head massage. It is a stroking or *smoothing* movement that signals the beginning and end of a massage. Effleurage is also used as a linking movement to facilitate the flow from one technique to another.

Effleurage is applied with the whole hand, the fingers or the forearms. Pressure can be superficial or deep, depending on the effects to be achieved. Effleurage can be applied slowly and gently to produce a calming and soothing effect, or more briskly to stimulate the circulation and energise and revitalise the person being massaged. In Indian head massage, a combination of slow, gentle stroking and brisker, energetic effleurage is used.

Effects of effleurage

- Dilates the capillaries and increases the circulation
- Relaxes the client by soothing sensory nerve endings in the skin
- Prepares the area for deeper strokes
- Aids in moving waste out of congested areas
- Soothes tired, aching muscles
- Warms the tissues, making them more extensible.

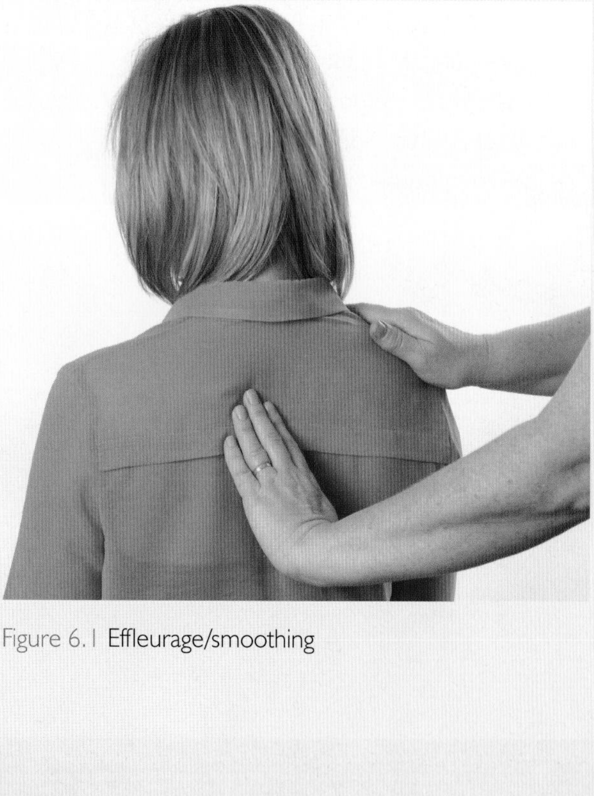

▲ Figure 6.1 Effleurage/smoothing

Petrissage

Petrissage movements are deeper movements using the whole hand, thumbs or fingers. There are many types of petrissage used in Indian head massage – for example, picking up, squeezing and releasing, rolling. Petrissage movements involve the skin and muscular tissue being moved from their position, squeezed with a firm pressure away from the underlying structure and then released.

Effects of petrissage

- Increases the removal of waste products from the tissue and encourages fresh oxygen and nutrients to be delivered to the tissues
- Stretches muscle tissue and fascia
- Reduces adhesions and muscular spasms
- Relaxes muscle tissue and reduces accumulated stress and tension from the muscles.

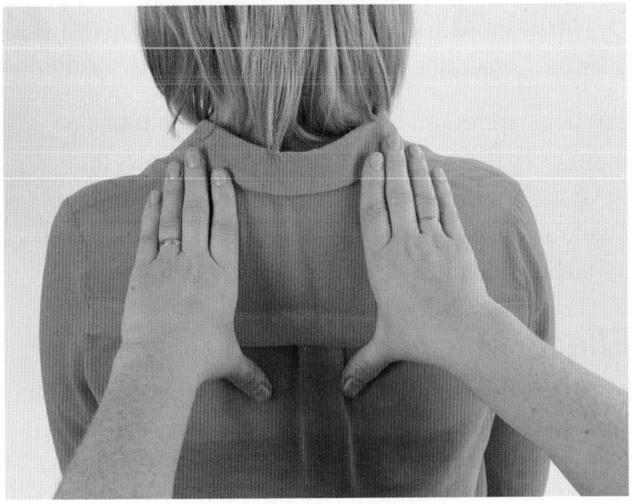

▲ Figure 6.2 Petrissage

Tapotement

These techniques are performed with the fingers and are similar to percussion movements in Swedish massage. They involve a series of light, brisk, springy movements applied with both hands in rapid succession.

The main tapotement movements used in Indian head massage are as follows.

Hacking

This technique involves flicking the hands rhythmically up and down in quick succession, using the ulnar borders of the hands.

Champi

This technique is also known as double hacking. It is performed by holding the hands in a prayer position, and allowing them to relax so that the heels of the hands and the pads of the fingers and thumbs are gently touching. A series of light, rapid striking movements are then performed across areas such as the shoulders.

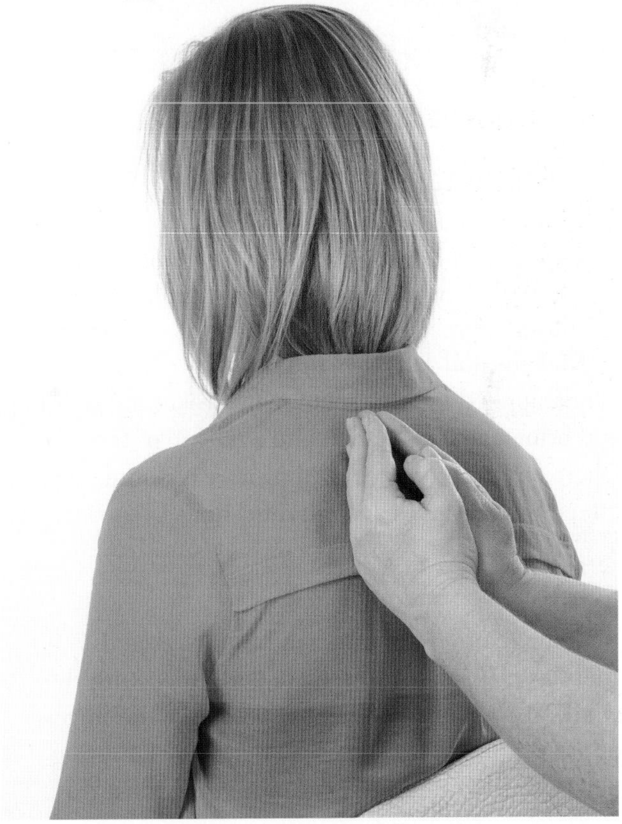

▲ Figure 6.3 Champi/double hacking

Tabla playing (tapping)

Tabla refers to a drum used in the classical and popular music of northern India. It is a light technique that uses the fingertips to tap on the head.

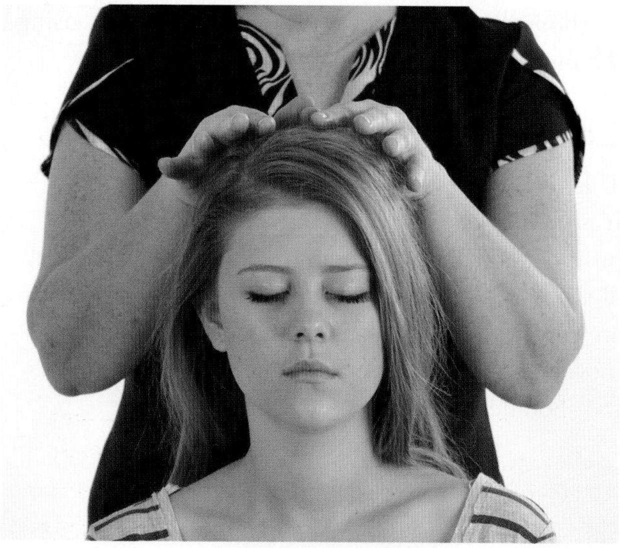

▲ Figure 6.4 Tabla playing

Effects of tapotement

- Stimulates the nerve endings
- Increases the circulation and local blood flow
- Increases muscle tone through stimulation of muscle fibres
- Wakens and refreshes the body.

When applied lightly, tapotement strokes are soothing and bring about relaxation and a release of tension; when applied more deeply they have a stimulating effect on the nerves and are refreshing.

Frictions

A strong feature of the Indian head massage is friction movements, which are performed with the whole of the hand, the heel of the hand, the fingers or the thumbs. They are deeper, more penetrating movements that cause the skin to rub against the underlying structures.

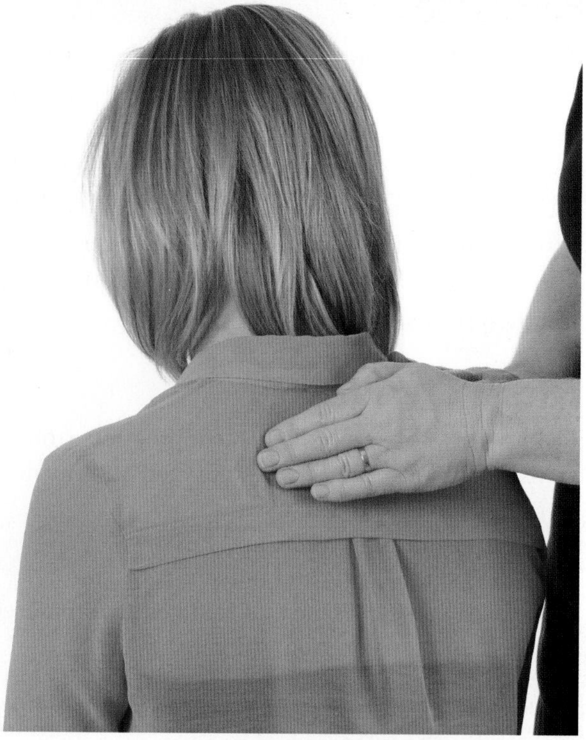

▲ Figure 6.5 Frictions

Frictions are excellent for breaking down tension nodules that have accumulated due to stress and tension. Frictions are particularly useful in Indian head massage for working around the scapulae and on either side of the spine.

Effects of frictions

- Dilate the capillaries and increase the circulation
- Generate heat locally in the area massaged
- Loosen stiffness and tension by relaxing muscles
- Break down and help free adhered tissue in restricted areas.

Vibrations

These are fine, shaking, trembling or oscillating movements that are applied with one or both hands, using either the whole palmar surface of the hand or the fingertips. A fine trembling movement may be achieved by moving the fingers up and down or side to side, while maintaining contact with the skin.

Vibrations may be performed either in a static form or where the hands or fingertips travel over a point while still vibrating. Vibration movements may be fine, deep or vigorous, depending on the effect required.

Effects of vibrations

- Help relieve tension and aid relaxation, creating a sedative effect
- Stimulate and clear nerve pathways, creating a refreshing effect
- Stimulate muscle spindles, thereby creating minute muscle contractions
- Help relieve pain.

Pressure points

Pressure points are vital energy points, similar to acupressure used in Chinese medicine. In Ayurveda it is said that the 'life force' is located in the head. By balancing the energy within these vital points, health at all levels within the body is promoted. The stimulation of pressure points in the head is said to stimulate the hypothalamus, pituitary and other areas of the brain, to encourage healing to be relayed to various parts of the body.

Effects of pressure points

Pressure points are applied with the fingers and the thumbs; their effects are to:

- clear congestion in the nerve pathways
- relieve pressure and pain from tense muscles
- relieve sinus congestion
- encourage lymph drainage
- increase circulation locally to the area
- restore the energy balance to the body.

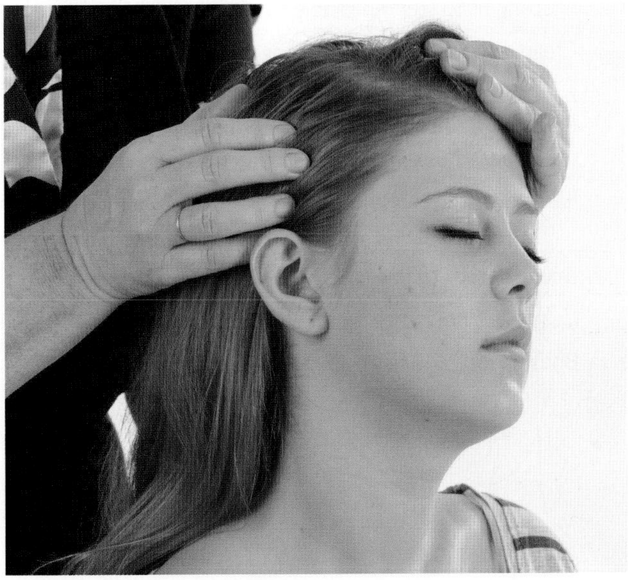

▲ Figure 6.6 Pressure points

Marma points

Marma points are an integral part of Ayurveda and are the subtle pressure points, similar to points used in acupressure, that stimulate the life force or pranic flow. The marmas are anatomical places on the body, mostly composed of flesh and bones.

There are a total of 107 marmas in the body:

- 37 in the head and neck
- 12 in the front of the body
- 22 in the upper limbs
- 14 in the back of the body
- 22 in the lower limbs.

Marma points are naturally sensitive points, measured by finger widths known as *anguli*. The finger width is the finger of the person being treated and not the therapist's own finger. The location of marmas are given in this way because each person is made differently and has a different size and proportion. The location of marmas may vary from one to eight finger widths, and often relate to regions of the body and not a point.

In Indian head massage the marmas may be used to:

- treat the pranas
- treat a specific organ or system of the body
- treat a specific dosha imbalance.

Marma point	Location	Helps with
1. Adhipati	At the crown of the head and the midline (11 finger widths above the eyebrows)	Calming the mind, heightening perception, assisting with spinal alignment and mental clarity
2. Brahma randra	Over the anterior fontanelle	Insomnia, elevation of mood, easing of headaches
3. Shiva andra	Over the posterior fontanelle	Lowering of high blood pressure, relieving dizziness, improving the memory and sense of alertness
4. Vidhura	Behind and slightly below the mastoid process (bony bump behind ear lobe)	Congestion in the ears, relief of tension in the jaw and facial muscles, mental tension and anxiety
5. Krikatika	Either side of spine, where the neck meets the skull	Releasing neck and shoulder tension, relaxing the body, improving posture
6. Simanta	Bony joints at the top of the skull	Whole body relaxation, aids sleep
7. Arshak	On top surface of collar bone, in the L made with the large neck muscles as you turn the head from side to side	Stimulates energy to the liver and spleen, aiding digestion, stabilising blood sugar levels
8. Manya	Side of neck, four finger widths below the ear lobe	Improves circulation to the face, stimulates lymph drainage, helps ease a sore throat or upper chest congestion
9. Sira matrika	Either side of the windpipe on the upper half of the neck	Helps improve circulation and improves the voice
10. Nila	Either side of the windpipe on the lower half of the neck	Helps the voice and helps ease a sore throat
11. Kantha	In the middle of the neck at the level you feel your voice vibrate	Healthy functioning of the thyroid gland and expression of inner feelings, helps regulate the mood
12. Kathanadi	Behind the top of the sternum	Helps sore throats and upper respiratory congestion
13. Hanu	In the middle of the chin	Increases circulation to the face and helps your head connect with your heart feelings
14. Oshta	In the middle of the upper lip	Mental clarity and improves sexual desire
15. Phana	Either side of the nose, just above the flare of your nostrils	Helps clear lung energy, clears the sinuses and helps to balance functioning of right and left sides of the brain, enabling us to feel more able to cope with stress
16. Gandu	Either side of the nose, just above the Phana marma point	Clears the sinuses and brightens the eyes
17. Apanga	In the outer corner of the eye, slightly on the outer surface of the bony orbit of the eye	Relieves puffiness around the eyes and eye strain, clears the upper sinuses
18. Brhuh	Either side of the very top of the nose where you can feel little bumps just above the eyes	Eases eye strain and headaches
19. Avarta	In the middle above each eyebrow	Brings energy to the head, helps you feel more centred
20. Shankha	In the hollow of the temples	Calms and nourishes the brain and the mind
21. Sthapani	Just above the eyebrows, in the centre of the forehead (third eye area)	Brings peace and harmony to the mind

▲ Table 6.1 Marma points relating to the head and neck

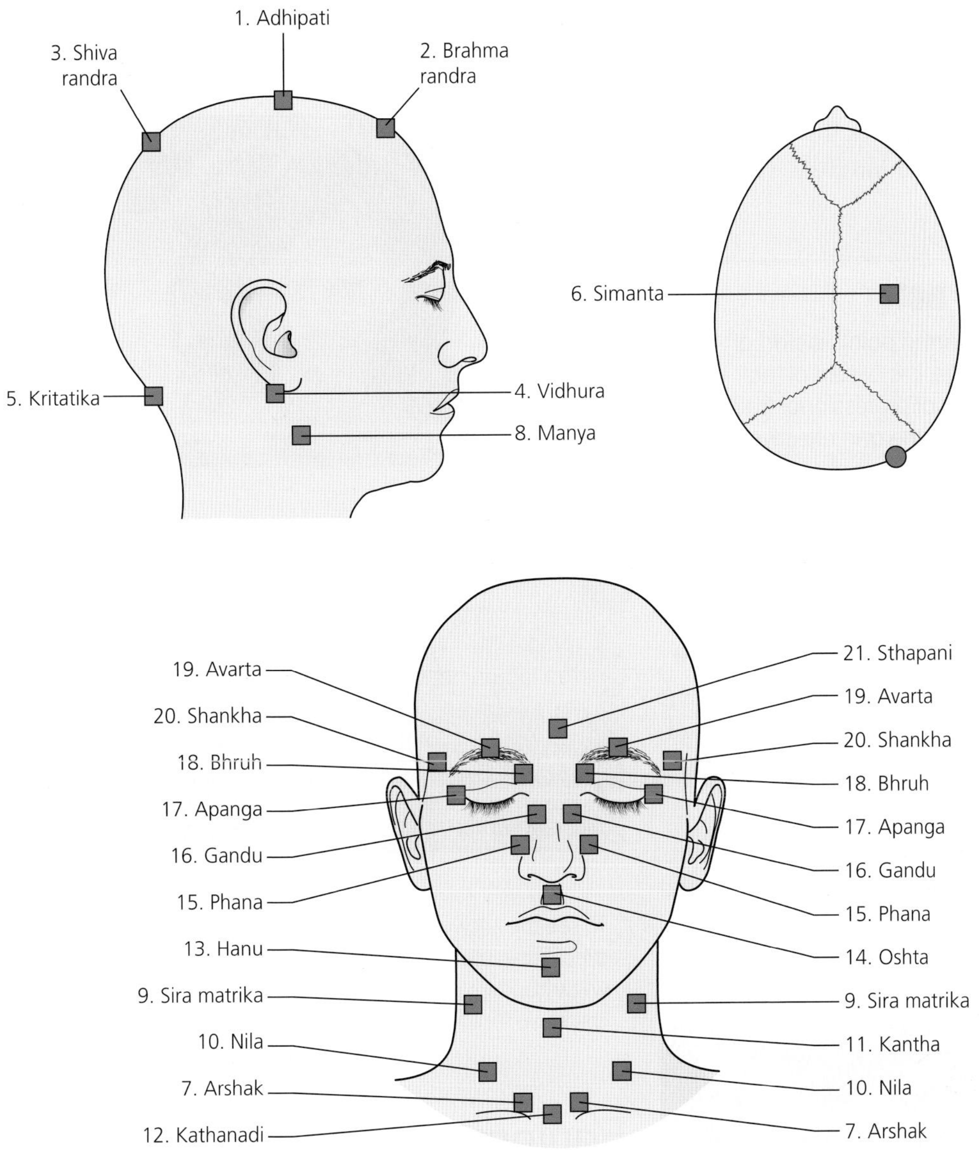

▲ Figure 6.7 Marma points relating to the head and neck

Treatment methods of marma points

Marma points may be treated with pressure, circular massage, heat and oils. Pressure is used on the marmas in the same way as any other form of pressure therapy. The marma is first found and located by the practitioner finding a hard, tender or sensitive point. Pressure is then increasingly applied with conscious breathing, in the knowledge that prana is going out from the fingers and into the client. When enough pressure has been applied, small counterclockwise massage movements may be used to break up the tension from the point.

In general, clockwise movements stimulate or energise a marma point, and counterclockwise movements dispel and liberate blocked or stagnant prana.

The key to using pressure therapy on a marma point is to go slowly and deeply and to work within the comfort zone of the client. It is essential to avoid pushing forcibly through a marma, as this can go against the internal harmony and interfere with the healing process.

Health and safety note

Although the treatment of marma points is part of traditional Ayurvedic massage, it is essential that practitioners undergo additional professional training and study in order to promote safe and effective use of them, as any injury to these subtle energy points may cause danger to life.

Compression

This is a form of petrissage in which the muscles are gently pressed against a surface such as the scalp, top of the shoulders or the upper arms, with the palms of both hands, and then slowly released.

Effects of compression

- increase blood flow locally to the area being treated
- help relieve tension in the muscles and alleviate pain, through gentle compression of the blood vessels and nerves.

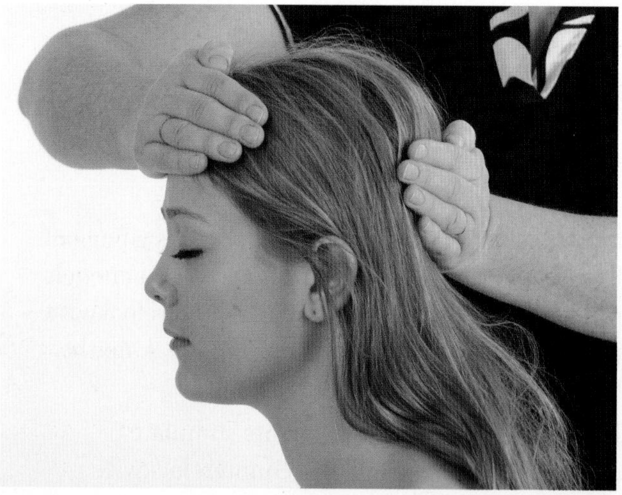

▲ Figure 6.8 Compression

Hair tugging

This is a technique used in the scalp massage where the roots of the hair are lifted in between the fingers of both hands and pulled upwards. Hair tugging stimulates hair growth by stimulating the nerves in the hair root.

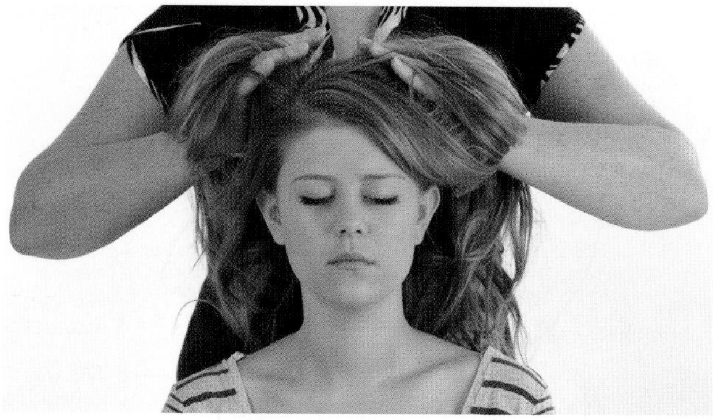

▲ Figure 6.9 Hair tugging

Knowledge check 1

1. Name the five massage techniques carried out in an Indian head massage treatment.
2. State two effects of each of the five movements.
3. What is a marma point?
4. How many marma points are there relating to the head and neck?

To see the answers to this knowledge check, scan the QR code opposite or visit www.hodderplus.co.uk/indianhead/chapter-6.

Equipment and materials for Indian head massage

The beauty of Indian head massage lies in its simplicity. It can be performed in an ordinary chair, without the need to purchase expensive equipment.

The products, tools and equipment needed to carry out an Indian head massage include:

- chair or stool with backrest (ideally one with a relatively low back and without an armrest)

Health and safety note

An important factor for the therapist is the height of the chair. It is therefore preferable to use a chair with an adjustable height and backrest, so that the therapist's working position is comfortable.

- couch – if a client requests to be treated in an inclined position, a couch may also be used during the treatment
- suitable skin cleansing products for cleansing the face to remove facial make-up, if appropriate
- dampened cotton wool and facial tissues
- a variety of oils for optional use on the scalp
- suitable alternative massage medium (light non-allergenic cream)
- a selection of small towels for draping across the shoulders/wrapping up the hair after the scalp oil massage, or for wrapping up the feet
- a dry hand cleanser (the type of hand cleanser most suited to a visiting therapist is a dry, antibacterial cleanser that is easy and practical to use)
- a comb or brush to ensure the hair is unknotted and free from hair products prior to the massage
- a variety of clips to help secure the client's hair out of the way when massaging the upper back, neck and shoulders
- a small footstool/cushion (for the client to rest their feet if desired)
- a mirror for the client
- a magnifying lamp for checking skin and scalp condition
- a covered waste bin with disposable bin liner.

Hair types

An important factor in deciding on the type of oil to use is identifying the client's hair type.

Hair type	Description
Dry	Dry, flaky appearance Scalp may also be dry and flaky May have a coarse appearance, lacking in shine
Oily	Presents with a shiny appearance due to excess sebum May look lank and lifeless
Fine	Fine hair is smaller in diameter than medium or coarse hair Generally limper, but shinier than coarse hair
Thick/dense	Larger in diameter than thin or fine hair May also be coarse
Chemically treated	Hair may be weak and damaged May be dry and brittle due to overprocessing
Coarse	Has a larger diameter and fewer hair follicles, which means the hair produces less oil, therefore it can tend to be dry

▲ Table 6.2 Hair types

Key fact

Indian hair oils

Ayurvedic suppliers will sell oils for use on the skin, hair and scalp, according to the client's dosha profile. For instance, a pitta hair and scalp oil will be rich in cooling Ayurvedic herbs (including sandalwood and blue water lily), while a vata hair and scalp oil will be rich in nourishing Ayurvedic herbs, including Bhringaraj ('lord of the hair'). (See the resources section for suggested suppliers.)

Oils used in Indian head massage

The use of oil is optional when massaging the scalp. Oil that is applied to the head is absorbed into the roots of the hair, which are connected with nerve fibres leading to the brain. Applying oil to the head helps to strengthen the hair and remove dryness; and by relaxing the muscles and nerves of the head, fatigue is eliminated, leaving the recipient feeling refreshed and revitalised. Massaging the head increases the supply of oxygen and glucose to the brain, and improves the circulation of spinal fluid around the brain and the spinal cord.

There are several oils that may be used for Indian head massage. Traditionally, oils such as sesame, coconut, olive, mustard and almond have been used by Indian women as part of their grooming ritual, to keep their hair in good condition.

Note: the oils used in Indian head massage are seasonal, with mustard and olive being a popular choice in the winter due to their warming effects, and sesame and coconut being more popular in the summer months.

Oil	Description	Source	Properties	Hair/skin type	Additional notes
Almond 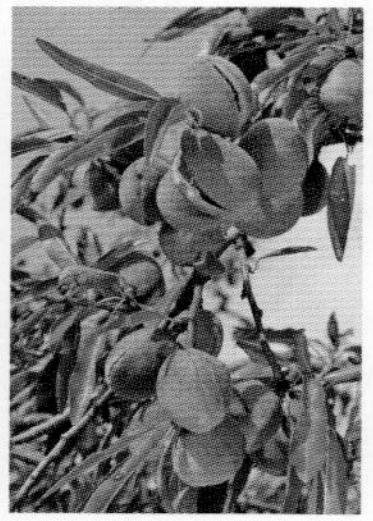 ▲ Figure 6.10 Source of almond oil	A popular oil, full of nutrients, which makes it an excellent hair conditioner	Extracted from the kernels of the sweet almond tree	High in nutrients such as unsaturated fatty acids, protein, vitamins A, B, D and E Helps to soften, moisturise and protect the hair Has warming effects on the body and is therefore useful for stimulating hair growth, as well as helping to reduce muscular pain and tightness	Suitable for all hair/ skin types	Caution: avoid this oil if your client has an allergy to nuts
Coconut 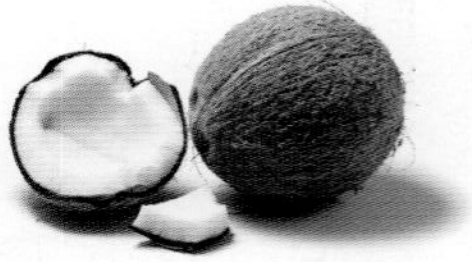 ▲ Figure 6.11 Source of coconut oil	A popular light oil for Indian head massage and is widely used in southern parts of India, especially in the spring	Extracted from the dried flesh of the coconut	Very moisturising and softening on the skin and the hair Also helps to relieve inflammation	Dry, brittle and lifeless hair Dry, dehydrated skins	Caution: take care with hypersensitive skin
Sesame 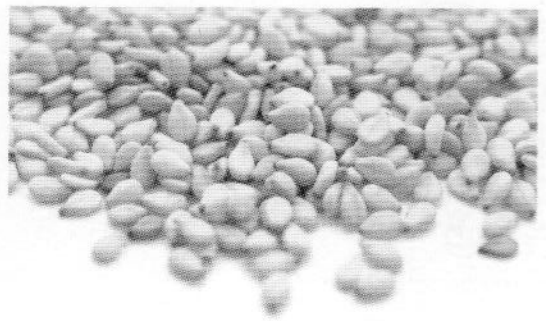 ▲ Figure 6.12 Source of sesame oil	One of the most popular oils used in the western part of India Used as a base oil for all oils used in head massage and is very popular in Ayurveda	Extracted from the sesame seeds	Sesame seeds are high in minerals such as iron, calcium and phosphorus, which help to strengthen, nourish and protect the hair Can also help to improve skin texture, reduce swellings and alleviate muscular pain	All skin types, especially dry skin and hair	It is particularly popular in India during the summer, as it does provide some protection from the rays of the sun

▲ Table 6.3 Oils used in Indian head massage

Oil	Description	Source	Properties	Hair/skin type	Additional notes
Olive 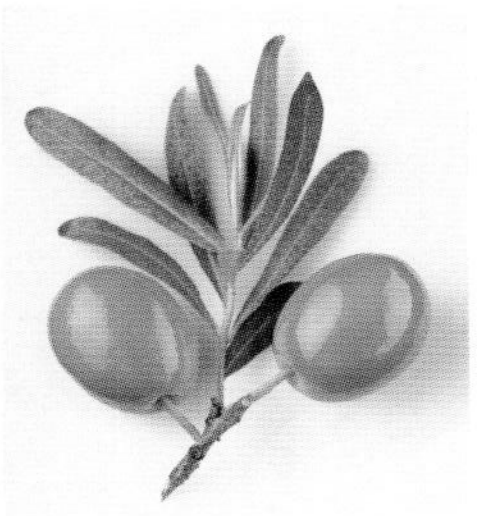 ▲ Figure 6.13 Source of olive oil	Very popular in the western world Of vicious consistency, with a strong smell, it is often mixed with another lighter oil, such as almond	Extracted from the flesh of the olive	Contains high levels of unsaturated fatty acids and has excellent moisturising properties Is soothing and penetrative Has stimulating properties that help to increase heat in the body and is therefore helpful in reducing swellings and alleviating muscular tightness and pain	All skin/hair types, especially dry skin and hair	
Mustard 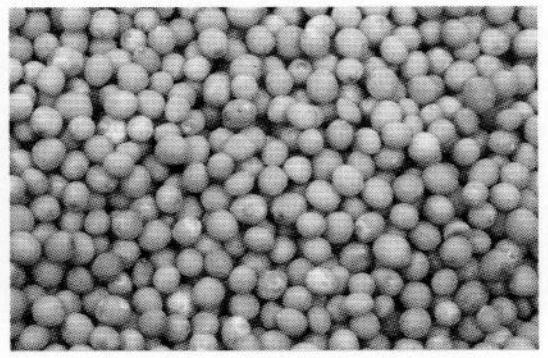 ▲ Figure 6.14 Source of mustard oil	Often found in Indian grocery stores and is one of the most popular oils in north-west India Especially used during the winter months because of the hot, warming sensation it creates Pungent smell and, by increasing body heat, its effects are very warming Popular among wrestlers and bodybuilders in India	Extracted from the crushed seeds of the mustard plant	Well known for its ability to break down congestion and swellings from tense muscles and to relieve pain	For dryness of the scalp, using mustard oil with a small amount of turmeric powder can prove very effective	Caution: this oil may irritate the skin because of its stimulating nature

▲ Table 6.3 *Continued*

In addition to the oils mentioned above, there are other oils that are traditionally used in India for the treatment of hair. These oils are blended with eastern herbs and spices not readily available in the West. These may be imported and sold in traditional Indian supermarkets and health stores.

Key fact

When the body is subjected to stress and illness, the skin and hair are often affected, resulting in dryness and sometimes loss of hair.

With tension, the scalp becomes tight, restricting the flow of the nutrients that promote healthy hair growth.

Using oils on a regular basis can help to encourage healthy, shiny hair, nourish the hair follicles, slow down hair loss and soften and moisturise the hair.

Storage of oils used in Indian head massage

Oils should be stored in airtight bottles, with tops tightly secured, in a cool, dark place in order to maximise their shelf life.

Always check the shelf life of oils with the manufacturer once opened, and dispose of any residual oil safely and hygienically.

Use of essential oils in Indian head massage

Traditionally, essential oils such as sandalwood, jasmine and rosemary have long been used in India as part of Ayurvedic preparations.

Health and safety note

While the properties of essential oils can be extremely beneficial on the hair and the scalp, it is recommended that essential oils are not individually blended by a therapist practising Indian head massage unless they are qualified and insured for the practice of selecting and blending essential oils.

Many essential oils suppliers offer pre-blended preparations for sale, which may be used in Indian head massage. However, caution is advised on safe proportions, due to the fact that when carrying out Indian head massage you are close to the brain and the olfactory response, and the effects of essential oils may be enhanced.

Name of oil	Source	Properties/benefits
Amla 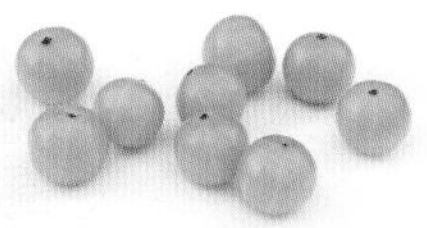 ▲ Figure 6.15 Source of Amla oil	Extracted from the seeds and pulp of the Indian gooseberry Amla is the name given to the fruit of a small leafy tree (*Amlica embillicus*) that grows throughout India and bears an edible fruit (the Indian gooseberry).	In combination with henna, this is an excellent hair tonic. It promotes the growth of healthy and lustrous hair, and has a cooling and nourishing effect.
Brahmi	Extracted from the Brahmi (*Eclipta alba*), which is a small, creeping plant that grows in waterlogged conditions	This is a unique combination of carefully selected exotic herbs blended with pure coconut oil. Brahmi oil is used medicinally in India as a tonic for the nervous system for those suffering from anxiety and emotional exhaustion. Brahmi oil helps the growth of long, lustrous hair and provides relief from dandruff and joint pain. It is also said to help improve the memory and dispel mental fatigue.

▲ Table 6.4 Hair oils

Name of oil	Source	Properties/benefits
Bhringaraj	The oil is extracted from the Bhringaraj, which is an annual herb that is found growing as a weed in marshy land in many parts of the world (most commonly India, China, Thailand and Brazil).	This is a popular oil for daily head and scalp massage in India. As well as helping to promote hair growth, it is said to nourish brain cells, help encourage better sleep and relieve stress and tension. Traditionally, it is used to help strengthen and nourish hair wearied by the stresses of modern life and environment.
Neem oil 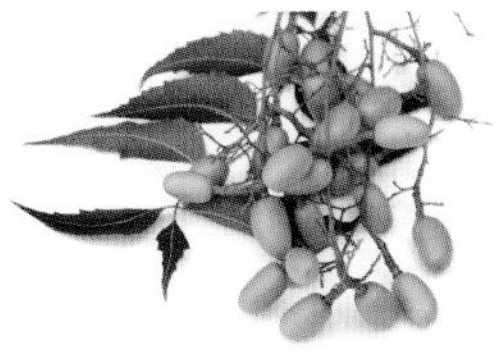 ▲ Figure 6.16 Source of Neem oil	Neem oil is a vegetable oil pressed from the fruits and seeds of the neem (*Azadirachta indica*), an evergreen tree that is grown extensively in the Indian subcontinent.	This oil is native to India and has antiseptic, astringent and antibacterial properties. Early Sanskrit medical writings refer to the attributes of neem. It is particularly effective for relieving itching and irritation, on the scalp and the skin.
Pumpkin seed	Extracted from the seeds of the squash-like fruit	This oil is extremely nourishing for dry and stressed hair, as pumpkin seeds are rich in vitamins A, E, C and K, unsaturated fatty acids and proteins.
Shikakai 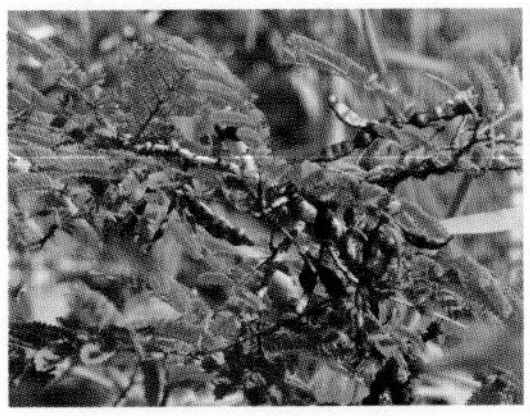 ▲ Figure 6.17 Source of Shikakai oil	Extracted from the fruit pods, leaves and bark of the *Acacia concinna* plant, one of the Ayurvedic medicinal plants. It is dried and ground into a powder, and then made into a paste.	This is an excellent hair rejuvenator and has astringent and antiseptic properties. Is said to help with eczema and dry scalp. It has been traditionally used for hair care in the Indian subcontinent since ancient times.

▲ Table 6.4 *Continued*

Other massage mediums

An alternative to using oil in an Indian head massage would be the use of a non-allergenic massage cream or light skin care cream. Some clients may prefer the use of a lighter skin care cream when massaging the face.

Take care to check ingredients of skin care/massage creams carefully, to ensure they are not likely to sensitise the skin.

Significant points on the head for oil application

There are three important points on the head according to the Ayurvedic tradition:

- The first point can be found by measuring eight finger widths above the eyebrows. This is where it is recommended that oil is poured on to the scalp initially, and then distributed symmetrically down both sides of the head with the fingers.

- The second point is at the crown of the head on the midline – an important therapeutic point – and it is where blood vessels, nerves and lymphatics meet. Oil is traditionally poured on to the crown and then evenly distributed down the sides of the scalp.
- The third point is at the base of the skull and is the point at which the neck meets the skull. Oil is traditionally poured on to this point, with the person's head inclined forwards, and then mixed in either side and towards the ears.

Preparation for an Indian head massage treatment

Preparing the environment

Hygiene/health and safety

The treatment room or area for Indian head massage should always look hygienically clean and tidy, but comfortable and welcoming. Attention should be paid to ensure that there are no trailing wires/obstructions (place all clients' belongings under the couch or hang up), and that tools and equipment are in a safe working position (check height and safety of chair or couch, and so on).

A comfortable and relaxing atmosphere can be aided by giving thought to the following factors.

Lighting

This should be soft and discreet. Try to avoid overhead lights that are glaring.

Ventilation

Ensure the atmosphere is well ventilated and draught-free. The smell of a room is also very important, and with good ventilation, the atmosphere will remain fresh.

Temperature

This should be comfortably warm (about 21–24 degrees Celsius), without being too hot. Do not forget that the body can cool down considerably during the course of a massage.

Decor and colours

Colouring should be chosen carefully, as some colours are warm, while others will feel too cold and clinical. Towels should preferably match the decor and add to the warmth of the room.

Privacy

A treatment room should always be private to ensure client relaxation. If a designated area is being used for Indian head massage, privacy can be effected by creating a semi-private area with a screen.

Atmosphere and noise level

Atmosphere is a very important part of the massage treatment. Relaxation CDs can create a wonderfully relaxing atmosphere, conducive to massage, and will disguise other sounds in the salon.

As Indian head massage is so portable, it is still possible to create the right environment for relaxation by paying attention to sound, lighting and privacy (even if it is only a semi-private area, away from other workplace distractions).

Client preparation

1. Check client is a suitable candidate for treatment by carrying out a consultation.
2. Formulate the client's individual treatment plan, checking if they need any modifications or adaptations (see pages 190–1 for guidelines on adaptations).
3. Seat client comfortably in a chair, ensuring that their legs are uncrossed and feet are placed on the ground. It is usually more comfortable and relaxing for the client to remove their shoes before treatment. Comfort may be assisted further by the use of a cushion, pillow or stool for clients to rest their feet on, and a comforting therapeutic touch is to wrap the feet in a warm towel.
4. Ensure the chair is at a suitable height for you and your client.
5. Drape a towel over the back of the chair and have a clean towel ready for placing over the shoulders for the scalp massage.

6. Ask the client to remove any obtrusive jewellery, such as necklaces, earrings and nose rings, and to remove glasses.
7. Ask the client to brush their hair to remove any residue of hairspray, gel and mousse, and to remove face make-up.
8. If the client's hair is long, it should be tied up with a suitable hair clip. (If your client is wearing a false hairpiece, advise them that it will need to be removed before treatment commences.)
9. Prepare oil for the scalp massage, if required (approximately 2–5 ml, depending on the length of the hair and the condition of the scalp). The client may prefer the oil to be warmed before application to the scalp. If this is desired, place the oil container in a bowl of warmed water or in an oil warmer before treatment.

Therapist preparation

Present a smart and professional appearance by

- wearing professional workwear that is clean, freshly laundered and ironed, and low-heeled, comfortable, enclosed shoes
- tying hair neatly back off the face, with fringe secured
- removing all obtrusive jewellery (including piercings)
- wearing a light day make-up
- observing good personal hygiene (oral and body)
- keeping nails short and well maintained.

Hygiene precautions

- Cleanse hands before and after treatment.
- Check client for any infectious conditions.
- Avoid carrying out treatment if you have any infection that may be transmitted.
- Cover any open cuts or abrasions with a waterproof plaster.
- Pour oil into a separate container for individual client use and dispose of residual oil.
- Where possible, use disposable consumables – for example, spatulas – and pump dispensers to reduce cross-contamination.

Sterilisation and disinfection

Sterilisation is the total destruction of all living micro-organisms in metal tools and equipment. Disinfection is the destruction of most living micro-organisms in non-metal tools, equipment and work areas.

Common methods of sterilisation/disinfection in a salon include:

- radiation – for example, a UV steriliser
- heat – for example, an autoclave
- chemical solutions – Cidex/other manufacturer specific brands (Sterilsafe/Barbicide).

Health and safety note

It is important to always follow manufacturer's instructions and relevant COSHH (Control of Substances Hazardous to Health) guidelines. Refer to pages 234–5 in Chapter 9 for more information on COSHH.

Before carrying out the Indian head massage treatment, ensure that the work environment is clean and hygienic. All work surfaces should be wiped with warm, soapy water and disinfectant. At the end of the service, ensure that any waste is disposed of in a sealed bag and that clean towels are provided for each client.

Professional ethical conduct

As well as presenting a professional image, it is also important for a therapist to:

- have a polite and friendly manner towards clients and colleagues
- respect colleagues and competitors
- be punctual and ready to start work
- take pride in your work
- have a friendly and positive attitude, with approachable facial expressions
- maintain eye contact, with open body language
- avoid gossip
- maintain confidentiality
- maintain loyalty to your clients and employer.

Preparing mentally and physically for treatment

As well as preparing yourself in terms of presentation, it also important for the therapist to prepare mentally and physically for treatment, by adopting breathing exercises before and during treatment, and utilising the correct posture in order to keep healthy.

Breathing techniques

It is important for therapists to be aware of their own breathing during an Indian head massage treatment, and realise that correct breathing can help to increase the effectiveness of the treatment.

Correct breathing helps both the therapist and the client to relax and regain their natural balance, while helping the therapist to maintain concentration and provide the right energy needed for a positive treatment outcome.

Posture and correct body mechanics

Body mechanics involves using correct posture in order to apply Indian head massage techniques with the maximum efficiency and minimal trauma to the therapist. Initially, therapists often find it difficult adjusting from massaging a client on a couch to massaging a client who is seated in a chair. It is therefore essential that correct adjustments are made to body mechanics in order to increase the effectiveness of the massage, help prevent repetitive strain injuries, decrease fatigue and increase comfort for the therapist.

Health and safety note

Failing to apply the correct posture when carrying out an Indian head massage treatment may result in a repetitive strain injury and will affect a therapist's ability to work effectively.

Guidelines for ensuring the correct posture when working include:

- checking the chair height – a chair at the correct height will enable a therapist to use body weight effectively to develop pressure
- wearing low-heeled shoes with good support
- keeping the back straight by tilting the pelvis forwards
- using body weight effectively, by lunging in order to create pressure needed
- keeping the shoulders and upper back relaxed (avoiding raising shoulders to ears)
- keeping feet firmly placed on the ground
- bending knees slightly and keeping knees soft, taking care to avoid locking them straight
- keeping wrists as straight as possible
- avoiding joint hyperextension
- keeping the body in correct alignment by maintaining head erect over neck and shoulders
- keeping head-forward posture to a minimum and avoiding spending too much time looking down
- taking breaks between clients to stretch the neck, shake out the arms and relax
- varying the massage techniques used and varying hand and foot placements
- having regular treatments in order to keep your body working at an optimum level.

Knowledge check 2

1. How should the treatment environment for Indian head massage be prepared to ensure the client receives the maximum benefit from the service?
2. In preparing equipment for treatment, what is the most important factor to ensure comfort and correct posture for the therapist?
3. What is the most important factor in deciding on the type of oil to use in the treatment?
4. State three factors to consider when preparing a client for Indian head massage.
5. How should a therapist be presented when carrying out an Indian head massage. State six factors.
6. State three hygienic precautions to take when carrying out an Indian head massage treatment.

To see the answers to this knowledge check, scan the QR code opposite or visit www.hodderplus.co.uk/indianhead/chapter-6.

Indian head massage techniques

An Indian head massage treatment typically consists of massage to the upper back and shoulders, upper arms, neck, scalp and face. Treatment is traditionally applied through the clothes, with the use of oil being optional on the scalp.

Due to the fact that Indian head massage has been taught within families for generations and has now also been westernised, it should be noted that techniques may vary in their content and application.

The shoulders

The shoulders are the place where most people hold a considerable amount of tension. When the body is in a state of tension, the shoulders are lifted towards the ears and often remain this way, causing the muscles to go into spasm. This restricts the blood flow to the head, neck and shoulders, and causes the neck and shoulders to become stiff and inflexible. Sitting with hunched shoulders can reduce chest capacity and thus impair breathing.

> **Key fact**
>
> Indian head massage can help to counterbalance the effects of stress; by relaxing the shoulders, they will drop and allow the energy to flow more freely to the area, encouraging deeper and easier breathing and improved joint flexibility.

Upper back and shoulder massage

1. **Starting position** with hands over the top of the client's shoulders

   Therapist's stance: standing behind the client in a relaxed posture

Practical tips on technique

- Commence by holding your hands lightly on your client's shoulders.
- Ask your client to take three deep breaths, with the emphasis on breathing in and out slowly and deeply. This helps both client and therapist to relax and prepare themselves for treatment.

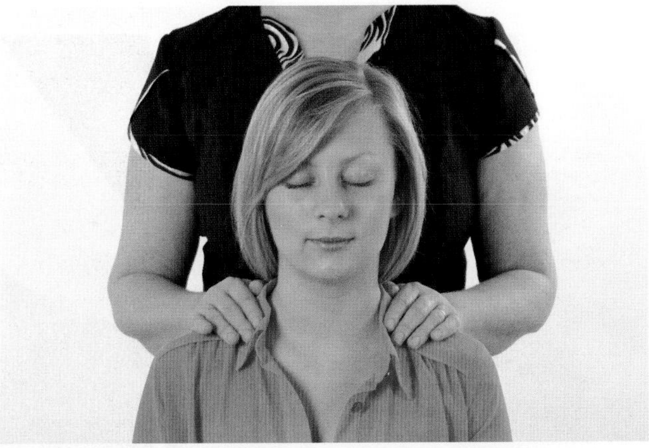

▲ Figure 6.18 Starting position

2. **Holding position** over the top of the head

   Therapist's stance: standing behind the client in a relaxed posture

Practical tips on technique

- Hold your hands lightly on either side of the head for about a minute, waiting for a feeling of relaxation and calm.
- You are now ready to commence the massage.

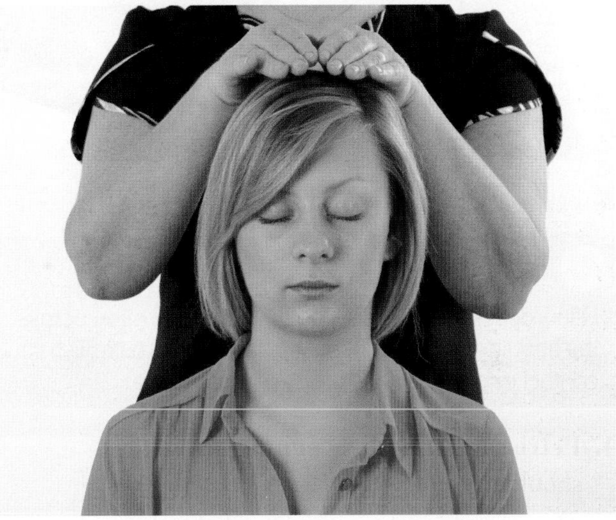

▲ Figure 6.19 Holding position

> **Key fact**
>
> The holding position helps to create a feeling of stillness and calm before commencing the massage.

3. **Effleurage/smoothing** across the shoulders and upper back

   Therapist's stance: standing behind the client in a walk standing position. The walk standing posture is used to lunge forward and increase the pressure and effectiveness of the techniques.

Practical tips on technique

- Use one hand to support one side of the upper back.
- Use the palmar surface of the other hand to stroke up either side of the spine, across the top of the shoulder and around the lateral border of the scapula to return to the starting position.
- The stroke upwards should be deeper than the stroke downwards.
- Repeat three times one side and then repeat the other side, gradually increasing in pressure with each stroke.

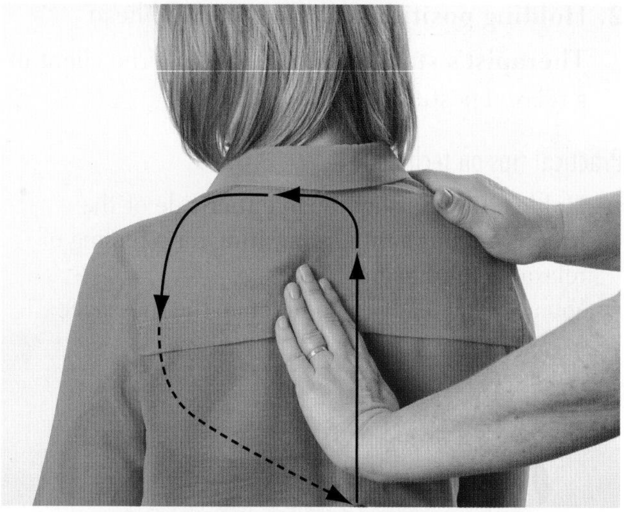

▲ Figure 6.20 Effleurage/smoothing

Key fact

Effleurage/smoothing is the first communication across the shoulders and enables the therapist to establish contact and feel for any areas of tension.

4. **Petrissage/thumb sweeping** across the shoulders

   Therapist's stance: standing behind the client in a walk standing position. The therapist uses the walk standing posture to lunge forward and increase the pressure and effectiveness of the techniques.

Practical tips on technique

- With fingers resting on the top of the client's shoulders, reach down the upper back with your thumbs and place them as far as they can go either side of the spine, across the lower border of the trapezius muscle.
- Now draw the thumbs up and across the trapezius muscle, fanning out towards the little finger.
- Repeat three times, gradually increasing in pressure.
- Now draw the thumbs up towards the middle finger and repeat three times.
- Then draw the thumbs up towards the index finger and repeat three times.

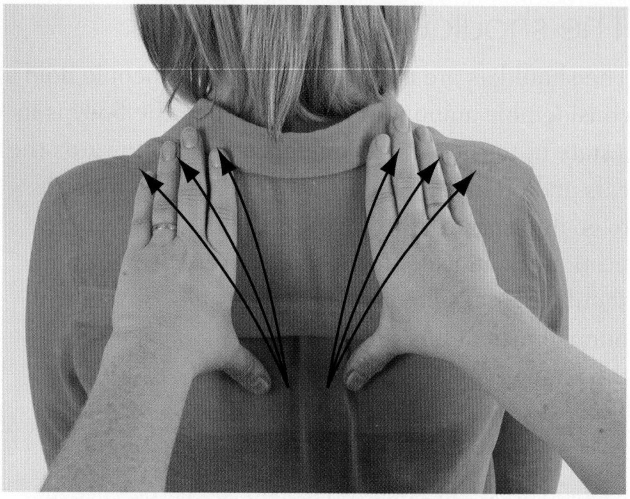

▲ Figure 6.21 Petrissage/thumb sweeping

Key fact

Petrissage/thumb sweeping is a deeper technique that helps to unlock tension and free fibrous adhesions from the trapezius muscle.

5. **Frictions with the heel of the hand** rubbing around the scapulae

   Therapist's stance: standing to the side so that you are facing your client's shoulder from the side

Practical tips on technique

- Support one side of the back with one hand.
- Use the heel of your other hand to rub lightly and briskly (in a side-to-side motion) across the top of the scapula, in between the scapula and below the scapula in the characteristic 'C' shape.
- Repeat three times each side.

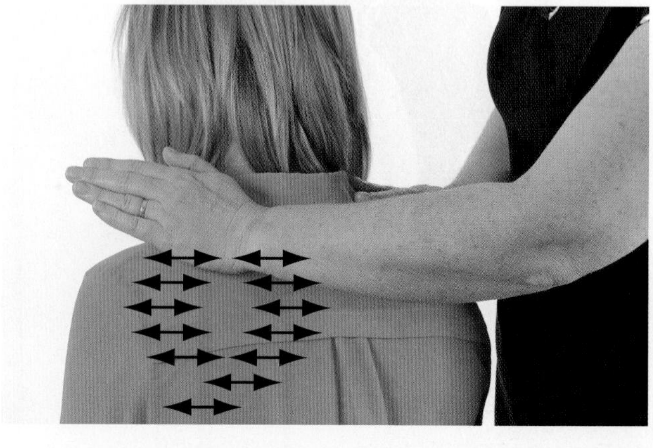

▲ Figure 6.22 Frictions with the heel of the hand

> **Key fact**
> Frictions help to create a considerable amount of heat in the tissues, which helps to break down fibrous adhesions and restrictions around the scapulae.

6. **Frictions with the finger** rubbing round the scapulae

   Therapist's stance: standing to the side so that you are facing the client's shoulder from the side

Practical tips on technique

- Support one side of the back with one hand.
- Join the fingers of the other hand and place fingertips so that they face away from the spine.
- Rub vigorously backwards and forwards across the top of the scapula, in between and below the scapulae in the characteristic 'C' shape.
- Repeat three times each side.

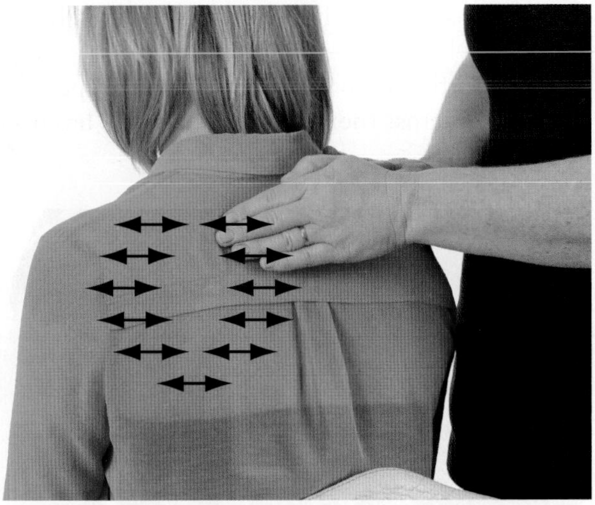

▲ Figure 6.23 Frictions with the fingers

> **Key fact**
> This technique is similar to the previous technique in helping to free restrictions and tension from around the scapulae.

7. **Effleurage/smoothing** (as step 3)
8. **Pressures** with the knuckles either side of the spine

   Therapist's stance: standing behind the client in a walk standing position

Practical tips on technique

- Place the middle knuckles of the forefinger *and* middle finger on either side of the spine at the top of the shoulders.
- Ask the client to take a deep breath in, and *as they breathe out* apply pressure inwards and then slowly release back towards you.
- Continue working down either side of the spine, approximately 2.5 cm at a time until you reach the mid-spine.
- Make a light sweep back up to the top of the shoulders. Repeat twice.

> **Key fact**
> Pressures stimulate the nerve endings either side of the spine, releasing blockages in the nerves and easing tension.

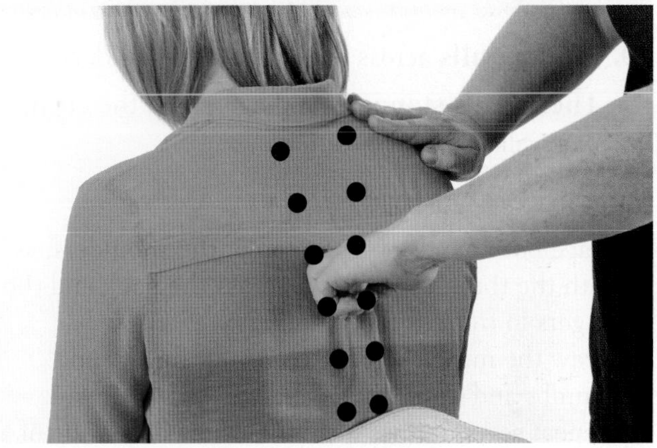

▲ Figure 6.24 Pressures with the knuckles

9. **Thumb rushes** over the shoulders

   Therapist's stance: standing behind the client in a walk standing position

Practical tips on technique

- Place the palms of the hands around the cap of the shoulder (deltoid muscle), with thumbs resting above shoulder blades.
- Starting from the outer edge of the shoulder, use the pads of the thumbs to push in one long sweep from the trapezius muscle (back of the shoulders) over to the pectoralis major muscle (front of the chest).
- Slowly release and then move further in towards the neck and repeat.
- Repeat the movement until the whole of the top of the shoulders has been covered.

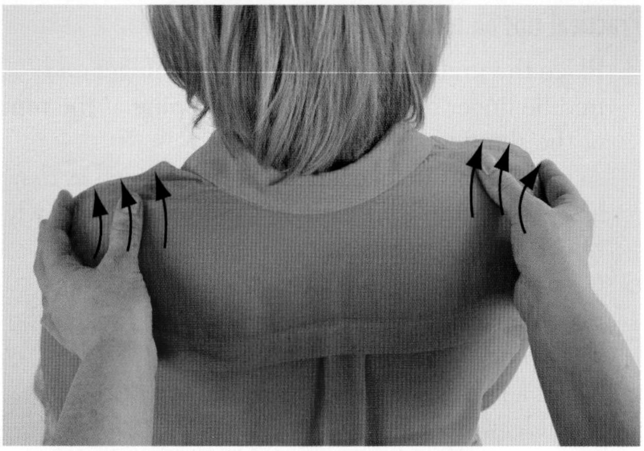

▲ Figure 6.25 Thumb pushes over the shoulders

> **Key fact**
>
> The thumb pushing technique loosens tension in the muscles across the top of the shoulders by squeezing the toxins from the muscle and mobilising the tissues.

10. Finger pulls across the top of the shoulders

Therapist's stance: standing behind the client in a walk standing position

Practical tips on technique

- Place both hands over the top of the shoulders, with the thumbs anchored across the back and the fingers in front of the shoulders.
- Draw the muscles in between your fingers and thumbs and lift upwards and back towards you.
- Repeat several times until the whole of the top of the shoulder has been thoroughly covered.

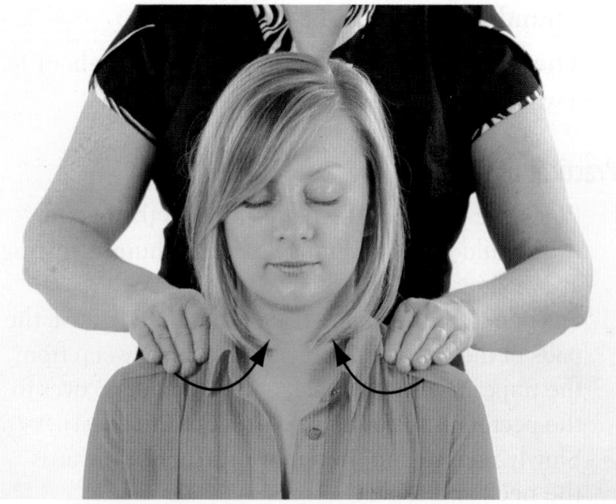

▲ Figure 6.26 Finger pulls

> **Key fact**
>
> The finger pulls technique helps to squeeze the toxins from the muscle fibres and encourages fresh oxygen and nutrients into the muscles. It also helps to soften and loosen the muscles, thereby easing tension.

11. Squeezing and releasing across the top of the shoulders

Therapist's stance: standing behind the client in a walk standing position

Practical tips on technique

- Place palms of both hands on the top of the shoulders, with the heel of the hand lying on the trapezius muscle and fingers resting on the front of the shoulder.
- Lift and squeeze the muscles in an upwards motion, heel of the hands and fingers clasping them tightly in the palm of the hands.
- Squeeze using medium pressure and hold for a few seconds before releasing.
- Move further in towards the neck and repeat until the area across the top of the shoulders has been covered.

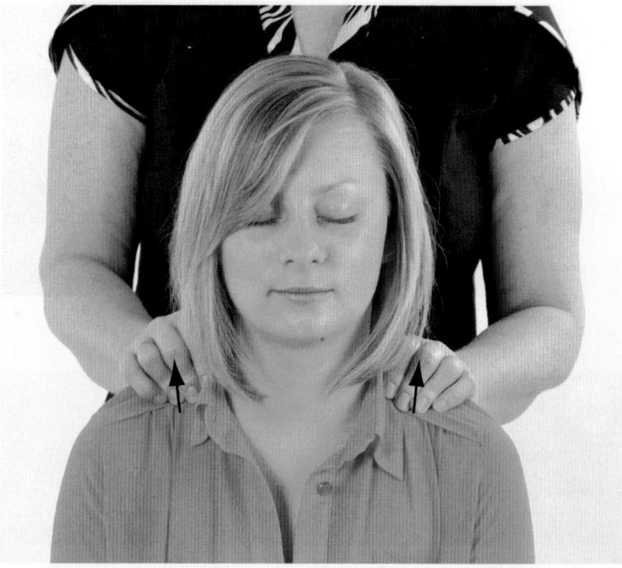

▲ Figure 6.27 Squeezing and releasing across the top of the shoulders

Key fact

The squeeze and release technique helps to squeeze and release toxins from the muscles, as well as softening and loosening tight muscle fibres.

12. Heel pushes across the tops of the shoulders

Therapist's stance: standing behind the client in a walk standing position

Practical tips on technique

- Place palms of both hands on the top of the shoulders, with the heel of the hand lying on the trapezius muscle and fingers resting on the front of the shoulder.
- Lift up and squeeze the muscles in an upwards motion and then roll the hands forwards across to the front of the shoulders, slowly releasing the muscle from your hands as you go.
- Repeat several times until the whole of the top of the shoulders has been covered.

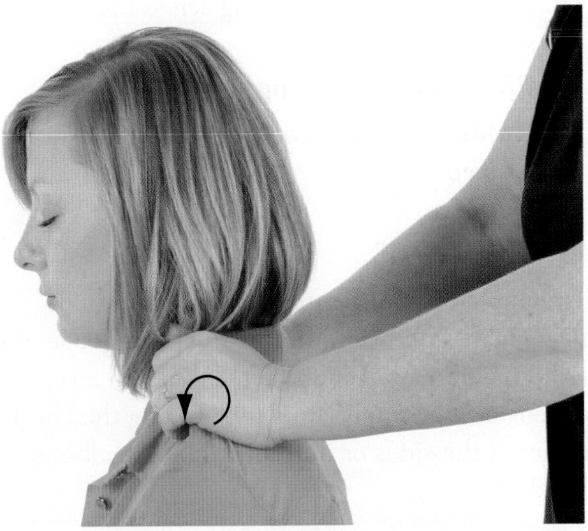

▲ Figure 6.28 Heel pushes

Key fact

The heel pushes technique helps to mobilise and loosen the muscles across the top of the shoulders, encouraging the client to release tension.

13. Smoothing with the forearms

Therapist's stance: standing behind the client in a walk standing position

Practical tips on technique

- Place the inside of the forearms across the top of the client's shoulders and gently apply pressure downwards.
- Glide the forearms across the top of the shoulders, rotating them as you proceed to the outer edge of the shoulder and down the upper arms to just above the elbow.
- Release and then brush the forearms back up the arms and on to the top of the shoulders.
- Repeat three times.

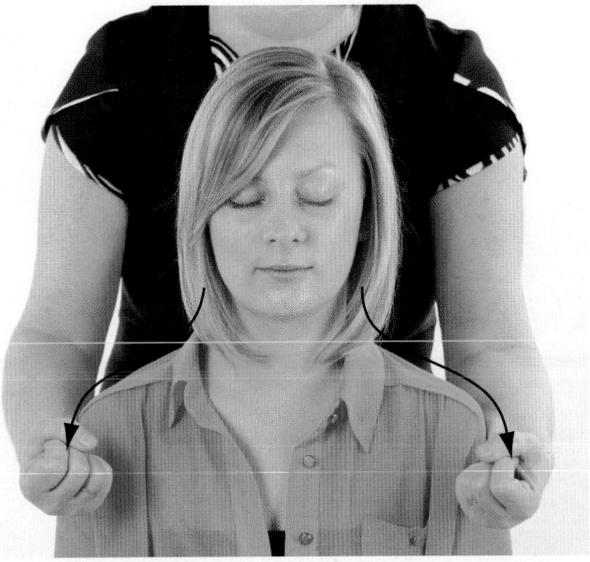

▲ Figure 6.29 Smoothing with the forearms

Key fact

The smoothing with the forearms technique stretches and releases the muscles across the top of the shoulders and helps to encourage the drainage of toxins from the tissues. It also encourages the shoulders to release tension.

14. Chopping across the shoulders and upper back

Therapist's stance: behind the client, kneeling down or standing up with the knees bent, depending on preference and client height

Practical tips on technique

- Place the palms of both hands across the upper back, with fingers together and fingertips pointing upwards.

- Perform light, brisk, chopping movements by quickly moving the index fingers of both hands together, picking up and squeezing the tissue between the index fingers of both hands before releasing them.
- Work across the whole of the upper back and shoulders.

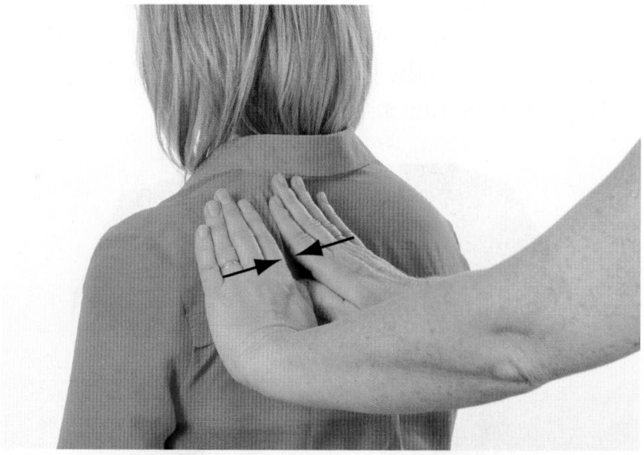

▲ Figure 6.30 Chopping

> **Key fact**
>
> The chopping technique helps to loosen the muscles across the upper back and shoulders, and stimulates the blood circulation and nerve endings, giving a refreshing feeling.

15. **Champi/double hacking** across the shoulders and upper back

    Therapist's stance: standing behind the client in a walk standing position

Practical tips on technique

- Hold your hands in a praying position, leaving the heels of the hands and the fingertips loosely in contact.
- Relax the hands and wrists.
- Using the tips of both fingers joined like a cage, lightly strike the surface and then spring off again.
- Start on one side of the spine of the upper back, around the shoulders and then back down again.
- Repeat the other side.

Note: take care to ensure that hacking is NOT performed directly over the spine.

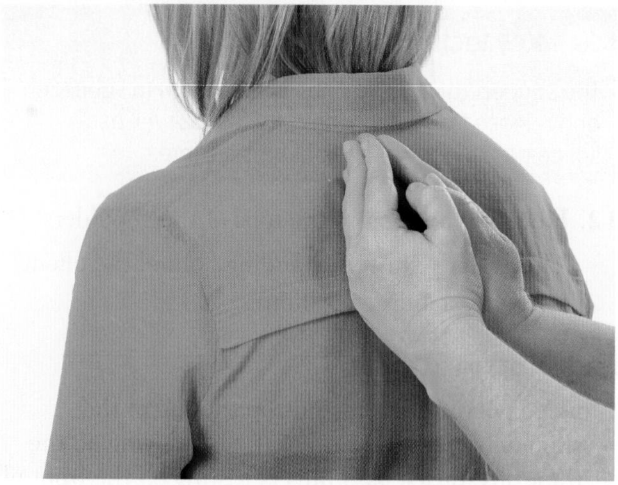

▲ Figure 6.31 Champi/double hacking

> **Key fact**
>
> Champi, or double hacking, stimulates the nerve endings and blood circulation, giving a refreshing and revitalising feeling.

16. **Squeezing and releasing** across the tops of the shoulders (as step 11)
17. **Effleurage/smoothing** (as step 3)
18. **Holding position** over the tops of the shoulders (as step 1)

Upper arms

The upper arms are important for upper body movement, and when the shoulders are tense, they tighten and restrict movement. When in a state of tension, the upper arms tend to hug the chest, either at the sides or in front, while the elbows bend up.

> **Key fact**
>
> Indian head massage can help to reduce tension and tightness in the upper arm muscles, to help improve flexibility of the arms and shoulders.

1. **Squeezing and releasing** to the upper arms

   Therapist's stance: to the side of the client, standing behind the upper arms

Practical tips on technique

- Place the palms of both hands (one above the other) around the upper arm (thumbs resting towards the back of the upper arm and fingertips resting towards the front).
- Starting at the top, gently squeeze and release the upper arm muscles by pressing the fingers towards the thumbs and then slowly releasing.
- Continue working down the upper arm towards the elbow.
- Stroke lightly back up to the top of the upper arm and repeat three times.
- Lightly brush across the top of the client's shoulders to repeat the movement on the client's other arm.

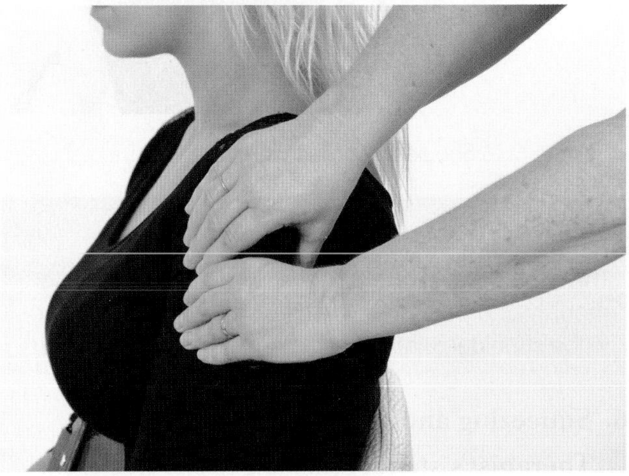

▲ Figure 6.32 Squeezing and releasing to the upper arms

> **Key fact**
>
> The squeezing and releasing technique helps to loosen tension in the upper arms.

2. **Compression** of the upper arms

   Therapist's stance: to the side of the client, standing behind the upper arms

Practical tips on technique

- Stand to face your client's upper arm.
- With fingers facing towards the floor, place one palm on the front of the upper arm and one on the back.
- Starting from the top of the upper arms, use the palms of both hands to compress towards one another gently, squeezing the muscles of the upper arms.
- Slowly release and then continue working down the upper arm until you reach the elbow.
- Brush lightly back up to the top and repeat twice.

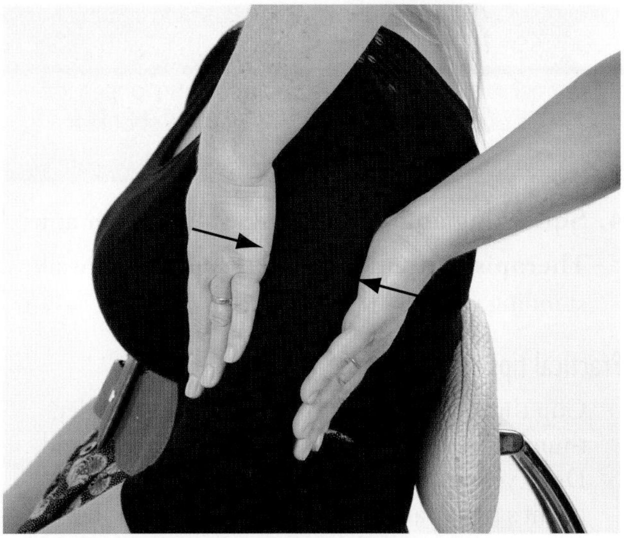

▲ Figure 6.33 Compression of upper arms

> **Key fact**
>
> The compression technique helps to encourage lymphatic drainage by squeezing toxins from the tissues of the upper arms.

3. **Heel rolls** embracing the upper arms

   Therapist's stance: behind the client in a walk standing position

Practical tips on technique

- Place your hands facing forwards on top of the deltoid muscles, heels of the hands behind.
- Roll the heels of your hands over the muscles of the upper arm until they reach your fingertips.
- Repeat at the middle of the upper arm and just above elbow.

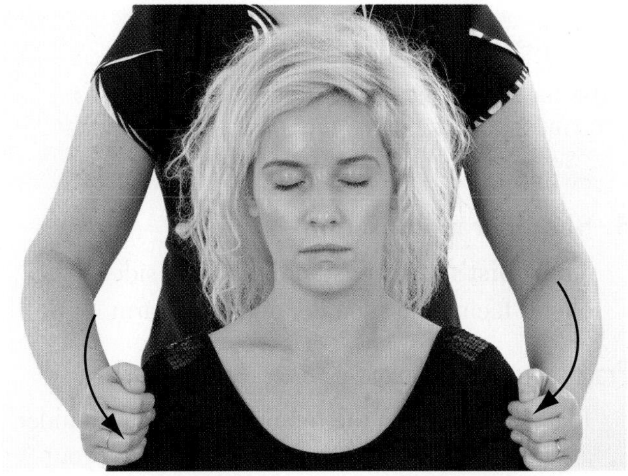

▲ Figure 6.34 Heel rolls

> **Key fact**
> The heel rolls technique helps to relax and loosen the muscles of the upper arms and top of the shoulder (biceps, triceps and deltoid muscles).

4. Squeezing and kneading down the upper arms

Therapist's stance: behind the client in a walk standing position

Practical tips on technique

- Cup the hands around the cap of the shoulder, thumbs pointing forwards and fingertips behind.
- Draw your hands from under the back of the client's upper arm and squeeze up and round towards the front of the upper arms.
- Repeat this movement down to the elbows and then sweep back up to the cap of the shoulder and repeat.

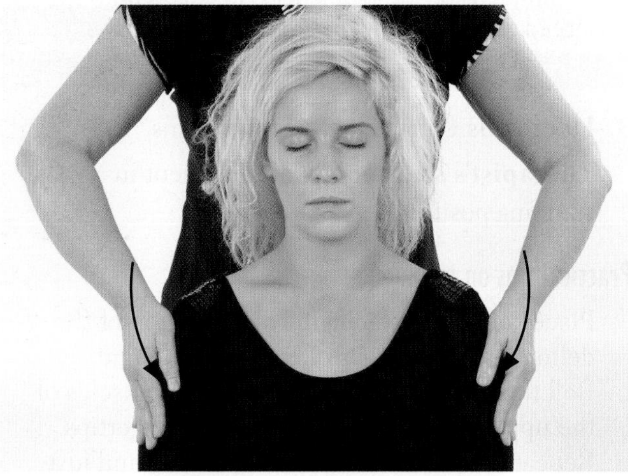

▲ Figure 6.35 Squeezing and kneading down the upper arms

> **Key fact**
> The squeezing and kneading technique mobilises the muscles of the upper arm and helps to release tension.

5. Shoulder mobilisation

Therapist's stance: standing to one side of the client, facing the shoulder and upper arm

Practical tips on technique

- Place one hand on the top of the client's shoulder and one hand under the elbow, supporting your client's hand in the crook of your elbow.
- Gently mobilise the shoulder in a clockwise and anticlockwise direction, taking the shoulder through its full range of movement.
- Repeat on the other side.

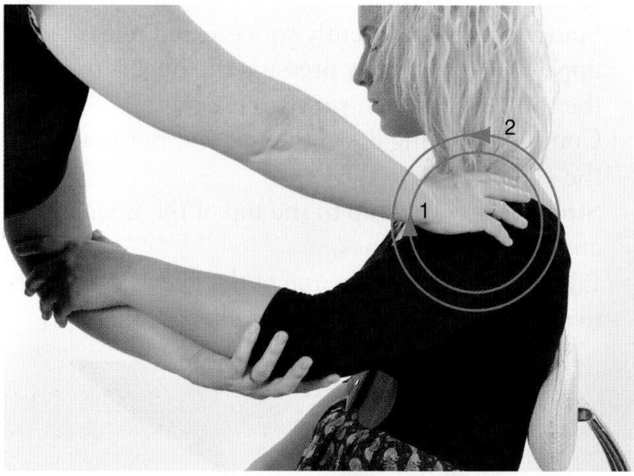

▲ Figure 6.36 Shoulder mobilisation

> **Key fact**
> The shoulder mobilisation technique encourages joint mobility and helps to release tension and restrictions in the shoulder joint.

6. Squeezing and kneading to the forearms

Therapist's stance: standing to one side of the client, facing the shoulder and upper arm

Practical tips on technique

- Support the weight of the client's forearm with one hand, and with the other hand gently use a squeeze and release action down the forearm to just above the wrist.
- Repeat three times.

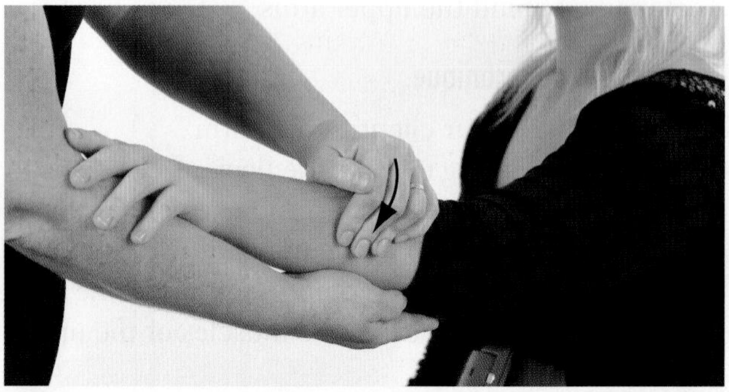

▲ Figure 6.37 Squeezing and kneading to the forearms

> **Key fact**
> The squeezing and kneading technique mobilises the muscles of the forearm and helps to release tension.

7. **Squeezing and kneading** to the fingers

   Therapist's stance: standing to one side of the client, facing the shoulder and upper arm

Practical tips on technique

- Support the client's wrist from underneath with one hand.
- Take each finger between your thumb and fingers and use the squeeze and release technique from the bottom of the finger to the tips, ending on the thumb. End with a gentle traction to each digit.

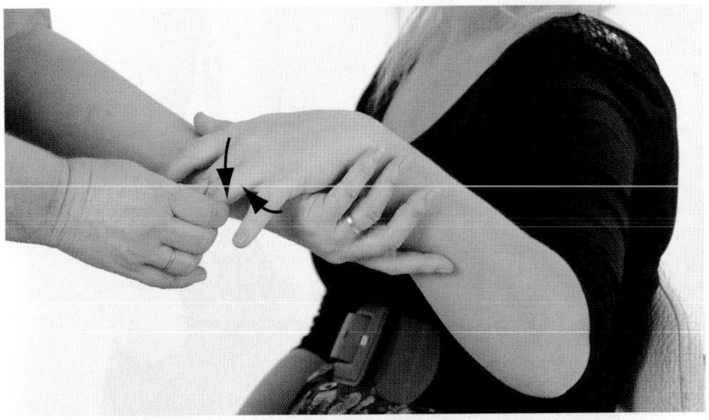

▲ Figure 6.38 Squeeze and knead fingers

> **Key fact**
> The squeezing and kneading technique to the fingers helps to mobilise the fingers and release tension from the hand.

8. **Circular pressure massage** to the pressure point between the thumb and index finger

   Therapist's stance: standing to one side of the client, facing the shoulder and upper arm

Practical tips on technique

- While supporting the client's wrist from underneath with one hand, use the thumb and the index finger to apply gentle circular pressure massage to the area on the top of the hand, between the thumb and finger.
- Apply the circular pressure massage in a clockwise direction, followed by an anticlockwise direction, to slowly release any stagnant energy.

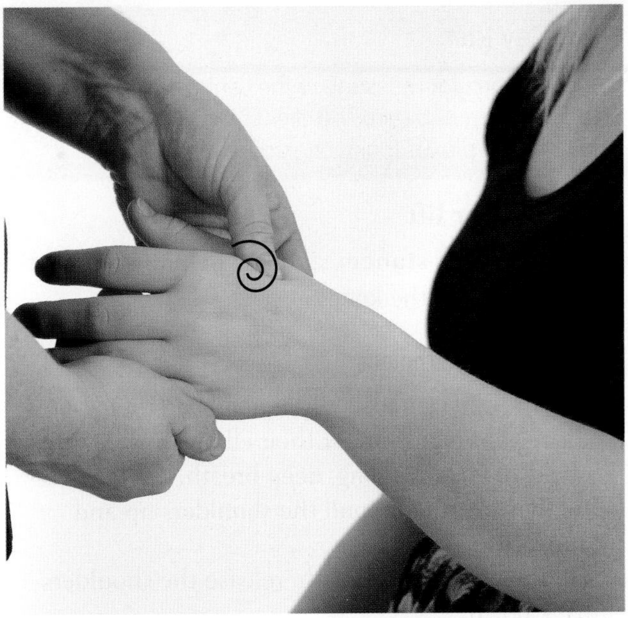

▲ Figure 6.39 Circular pressure massage between thumb and index finger

> **Key fact**
> Applying pressure to the pressure point between the thumb and index finger can help to relieve tension and headaches.

9. **Circular pressure massage** to the pressure point in the centre of the palm

   Therapist's stance: standing to one side of the client, facing the shoulder and upper arm

Practical tips on technique

- Turn the client's hand over to reveal the palm.
- Use the thumb to apply circular pressure massage, as above, to the centre of the palm.

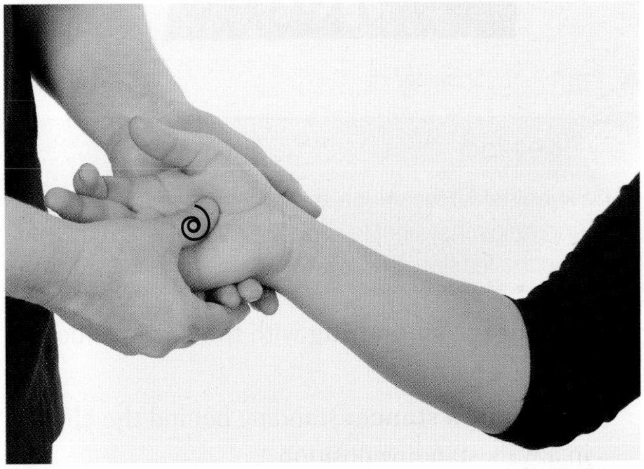

▲ Figure 6.40 Circular pressure massage on palm

> **Key fact**
>
> Applying circular massage to the centre of the palm helps to calm and relax the client as you are working on the solar plexus (palm chakra).

10. Shoulder lift

Therapist's stance: standing behind the client and bending the knees

Practical tips on technique

- Ask the client to place their hands on their lap.
- Place your hands under their elbows and ask the client to take in a long, deep breath.
- As they breathe in, pull the shoulders up and outwards.
- On the client's out breath, release the shoulders back down.
- Repeat twice.

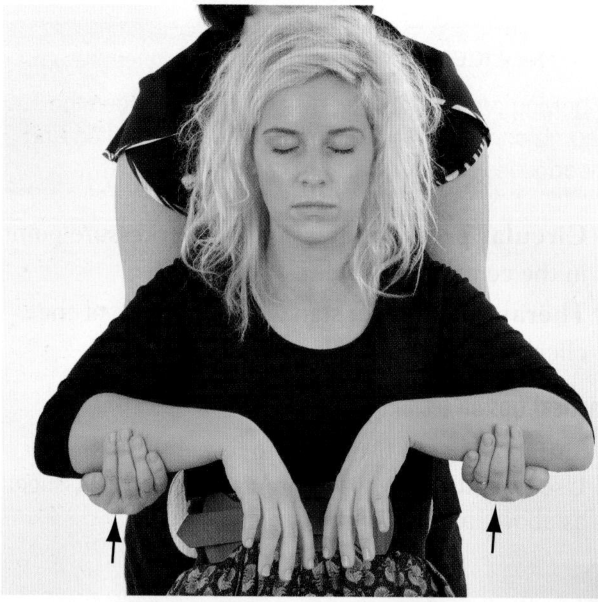

▲ Figure 6.41 Shoulder lift

> **Key fact**
>
> The shoulder lift technique symbolises letting tension go and helps the client to drop their shoulders and release the tension.

11. Effleurage/smoothing with the forearms down the upper arms

Therapist's stance: standing behind the client in a walk standing position

Practical tips on technique

- Using the inside of the forearms, apply gentle pressure on both sides across the top of the shoulders.
- Glide the forearms across the top of the shoulders, rotating them as you proceed to the outer edge of the shoulder and down the upper arms to just above the elbow.
- Release and then brush the forearms back up the arms.
- Repeat three times.

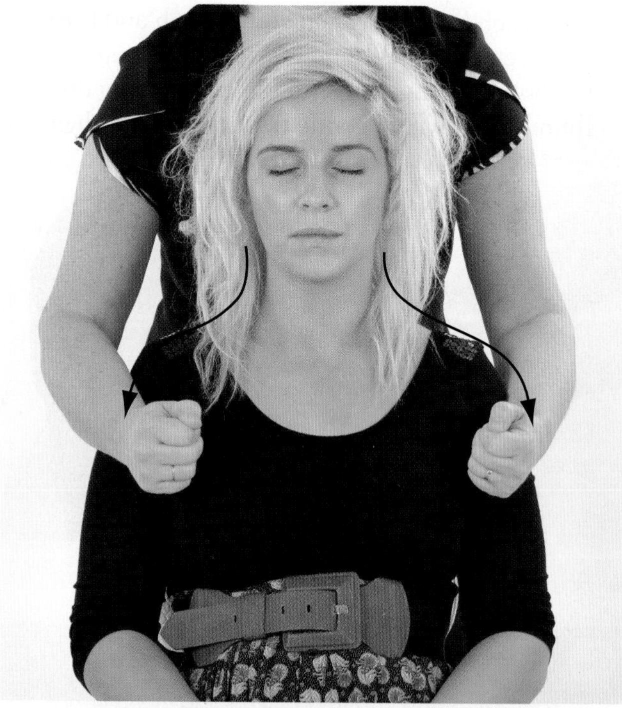

▲ Figure 6.42 Effleurage/smoothing with forearms

The neck

When the body is balanced, the neck is designed to allow the head to move in a variety of directions. When the body is out of balance and under stress, the head tends to come forwards and the chin juts out. This throws the body out of alignment, as the neck muscles tense and take the weight of the head. The neck muscles are then in a permanent state of contraction and can cause the neck to become stiff and tight. The tension then reduces mobility of the neck and shoulders.

Health and safety note

During the neck massage it is important to fully support the client's head to avoid neck strain.

Key fact

Working on the neck with Indian head massage helps to open up the energy flow from the spine to the whole head and can help to reduce tension and improve posture by realigning the muscles, thereby increasing mobility and allowing the head to move more freely.

Neck massage

1. **Rocking** the head backwards and forwards

   Therapist's stance: standing to the side of the client

Practical tips on technique

- Place one hand on the client's forehead and one hand at the back of their neck.
- Ask the client to drop the head slightly forwards so you can support its weight.
- Gently rock the head forwards and backwards, taking care to avoid hyperextending the neck.

Helpful tip: if the neck appears tight, ask the client to breathe deeply three times to relax, after which the head should move more freely and with less resistance.

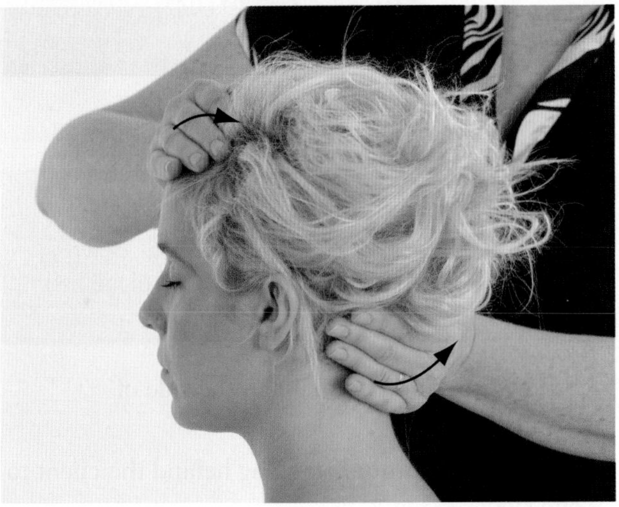

▲ Figure 6.43 Rocking the head backwards and forwards

Key fact

Gently rocking the head back and forth helps the therapist to assess how much tension there is in the neck and can help the client to relax their neck muscles.

2. **Squeeze and release** the muscles at the back of the neck

   Therapist's stance: standing to the side of the client

Practical tips on technique

- Place one hand on the client's forehead.
- Ask the client to tip their head back slightly.
- Spread your thumbs and fingers of the other hand on either side of the base of the neck (forming a V shape).
- Using firm contact with the skin, slide your hand in to squeeze and lift the muscles of the back of the neck and then release by pulling the hand backwards.
- Start from the bottom of the neck and gradually work upwards until you reach the base of the skull.

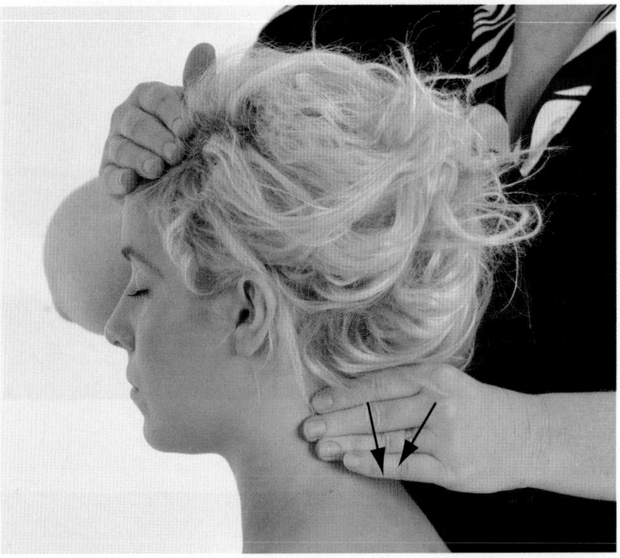

▲ Figure 6.44 Squeeze and release muscles at the back of the neck

Key fact

The squeeze and release technique helps to release tension that builds up in the back of the neck and the skull.

3. Finger frictions to the top of the shoulders and up the side of the neck

Therapist's stance: standing behind the client to one side

Practical tips on technique

- Tilt the client's head gently to one side.
- Support the client's head by using your forearm to cup around the side of their head, so that it rests comfortably in your forearm.

Helpful tip: with this technique you may find it useful to use a support between the client's head and your arm.

- Perform frictions using the pads of the fingers in a side-to-side motion, across the top of the shoulder and up the side of the neck to behind the ear.
- Repeat three times.
- Repeat techniques to the other side of the neck.

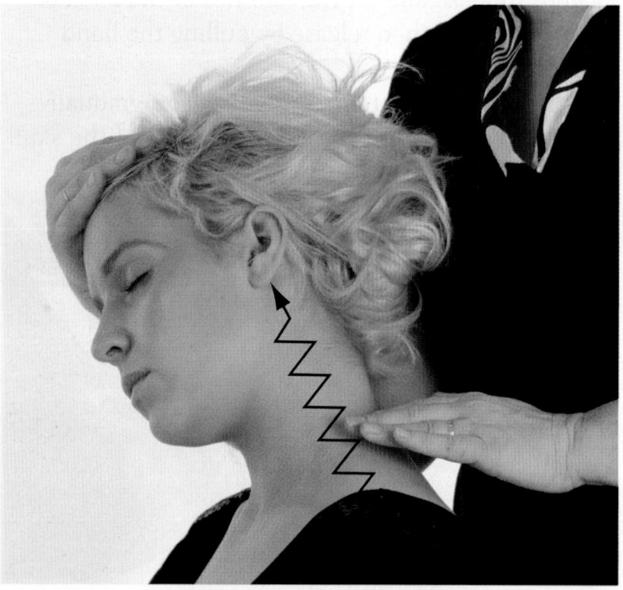

▲ Figure 6.45 Finger frictions to shoulders

> **Key fact**
>
> This technique helps increase the blood and lymph supply to the neck. It also builds up heat in the muscles from the frictions and helps to relieve tightness in the muscles at the side of the neck.

4. Thumb pushes to the side of the neck

Therapist's stance: standing behind the client to one side

Practical tips on technique

- Retain the same support for the client's head as in step 3.
- Use the thumb to push deeply into the muscles of the neck by pushing forwards horizontally, across from the back of the neck to the side of the neck, just below the ears.
- Repeat to the other side of the neck.

> **Health and safety note**
>
> Caution is necessary during this technique in order to avoid applying pressure to the carotid arteries at the side of the neck and to respiratory structures such as the trachea at the front of the neck.

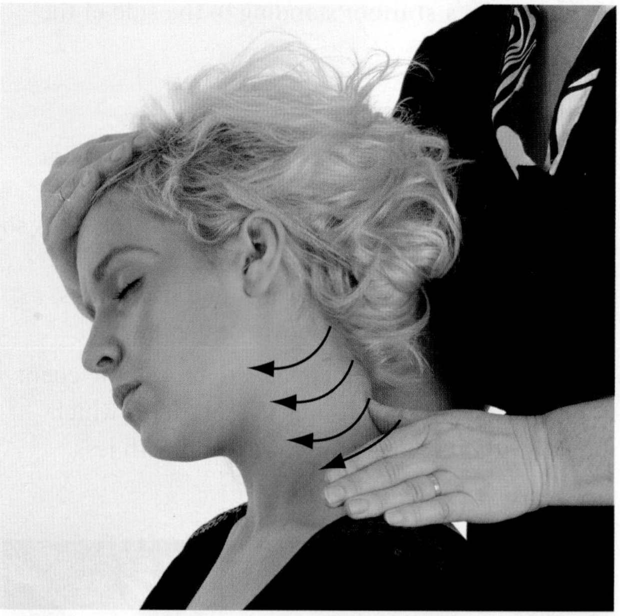

▲ Figure 6.46 Thumb pushes to the side of the neck

> **Key fact**
>
> The thumb pushes technique helps to break down fibrous adhesions that restrict movements of the head and neck.

5. Squeezing and releasing at the side of the neck

Therapist's stance: standing behind the client to one side

Practical tips on technique

- Retain the same support for the head as in step 4.
- Form a V shape between the thumb and the forefinger (thumb is anchored at the back).
- Squeeze and release the muscles at the side of the neck by lifting the tissue and pulling the forefinger back towards the thumb.
- Start from the side of the neck and work from the bottom upwards to behind the ears.
- Repeat to the other side of the neck.

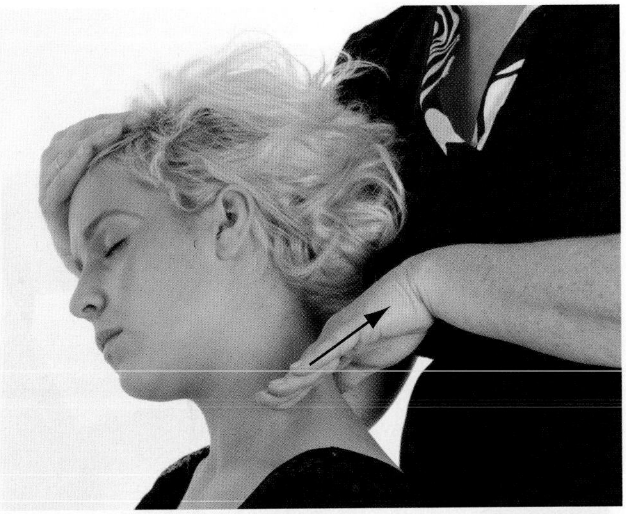

▲ Figure 6.47 Squeezing and releasing at the side of the neck

Key fact

The squeeze and release technique to the side of the neck helps to squeeze the toxins from the muscles and encourages lymph drainage to the neck.

6. **Finger frictions** to the base of the skull

   Therapist's stance: standing to one side of the client

Practical tips on technique

- Support the client's forehead with one hand.
- Use your other hand to perform frictions up and down the back of the neck with the pads of the fingers.
- Work from the base of the neck to the base of the skull.
- Repeat until the back of the neck and the base of the skull has been covered.

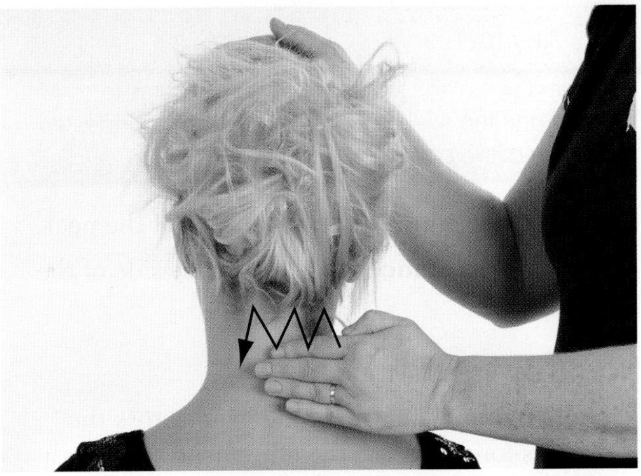

▲ Figure 6.48 Finger frictions to base of skull

Key fact

The finger frictions technique helps to encourage heat to release tight, congested muscles at the back of the neck and the base of the skull, where tension builds up.

7. **Heel of the hand frictions** to the base of the skull

   Therapist's stance: standing to one side of the client

Practical tips on technique

- Retaining the supporting hand on the forehead, use the heel of the other hand to apply friction at the base of the skull.
- Mould the heel of the hand to the base of the skull and use a side-to-side motion to friction briskly across the base of the skull.
- Repeat until the whole area of the base of the skull has been covered.

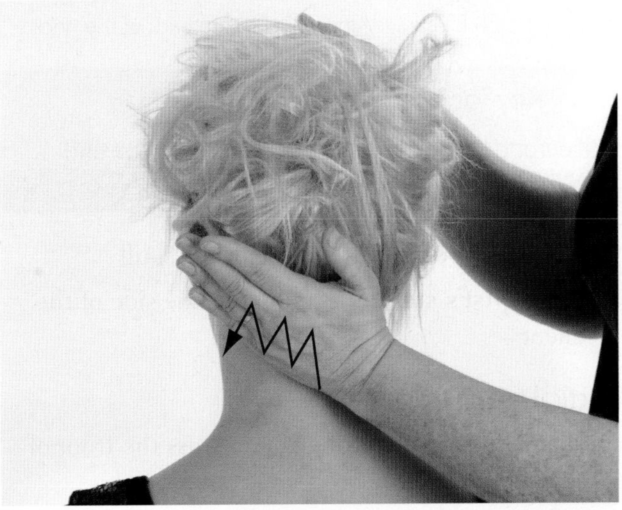

▲ Figure 6.49 Heel of the hand frictions to base of skull

> **Key fact**
> The heel of the hand frictions technique helps to encourage the release of toxins from tight, congested muscles at the base of the skull.

8. **Effleurage/smoothing** to the back of the neck

   Therapist's stance: standing to one side of the client

Practical tips on technique

- Still retaining the supporting hand across the client's forehead, use the other hand to smooth the base of the skull and neck in a circular motion.
- Repeat several times.

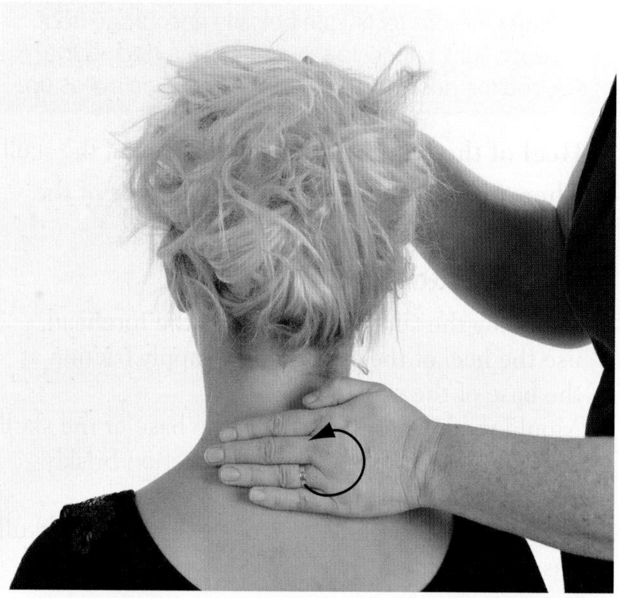

▲ Figure 6.50 Effleurage/smoothing to the back of the neck

> **Key fact**
> Effleurage/smoothing technique helps to relax and soothe the neck muscles.

9. **Pressure points** at the base of the skull

   Therapist's stance: standing to one side of the client

Practical tips on technique

- Maintain the supporting hand across the front of the client's head.
- Use the tip of the middle finger to gently press into the pressure point in the centre of the base of the skull for a few seconds, while at the same time gently rocking the head backwards.
- Pause for a second and then move the head forwards to release.
- Using the thumb and middle finger, press on the points approximately 2.5 cm either side of the central point and rock the head gently backwards.
- Pause and then move the head forwards to release.

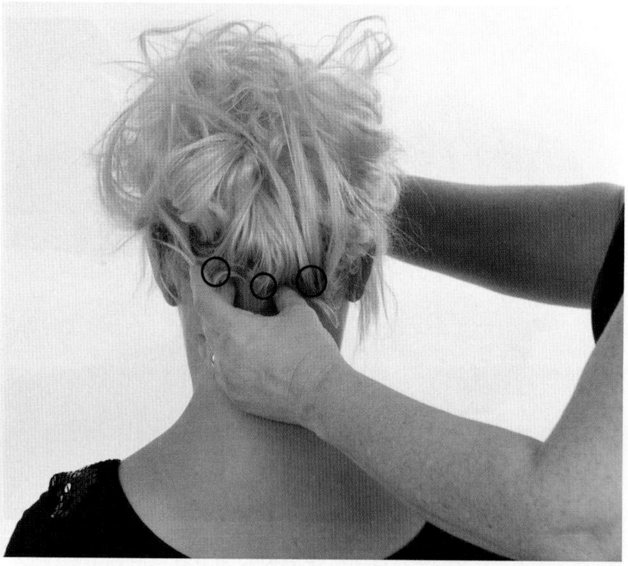

▲ Figure 6.51 Pressure points at the base of the skull

> **Key fact**
> The pressure points technique helps to relieve pressure from congested nerves and muscles relating to the head and neck.

10. **Gentle stretching** to the side of the neck

    Therapist's stance: standing behind the client to one side

Practical tips on technique

- Tilt the client's head gently to one side.
- Support the client's head by using your forearm to cup around the side of their head, so that it rests comfortably in the forearm.
- Place your other forearm on top of the client's shoulder.
- Ask the client to take a deep breath in, and as they breathe out gently press down on the top of the shoulder and hold for a few seconds before sweeping down and over the top of the upper arm.

- Repeat twice.
- Then repeat the technique on the other side of the neck.

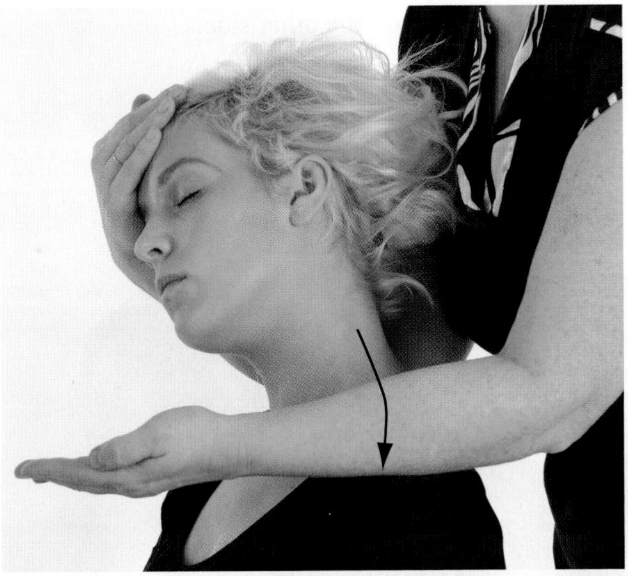

▲ Figure 6.52 Gentle stretching to the side of the neck

> **Key fact**
>
> This technique creates a gentle stretch up the side of the neck.

11. Smoothing with the whole hand at the base of the skull (as step 8)

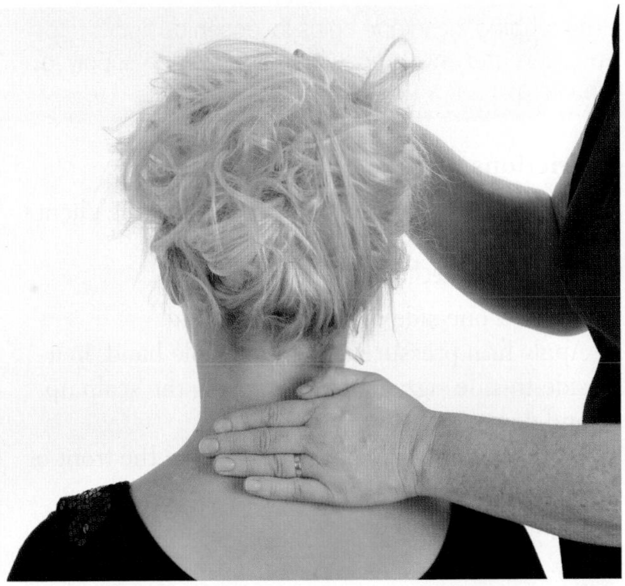

▲ Figure 6.53 Smoothing with the whole hand

The scalp

The scalp muscles tighten when under stress, restricting the blood flow and leading to headaches, eye strain and neck and shoulder tension.

> **Key fact**
>
> Indian head massage helps to counterbalance stress in the head by improving the circulation and the condition of the hair. Regular head massage also helps to relax the muscles and nerve fibres of the scalp, thereby relieving tension and fatigue.

Scalp massage

To watch a video demonstration of scalp massage scan the QR code opposite or visit www.hodderplus.co.uk/indianhead/chapter-6.

1. Rubbing to the side of the scalp, around the ears

Therapist's stance: standing behind the client

Practical tips on technique

- Support one side of the client's head with one hand.
- Use the fleshy part of the palm of the other hand to carry out a light rubbing movement with side-to-side motion, across the temporalis muscle above, in front of and behind the ears.
- Work backwards and forwards three times.
- Repeat to other side.

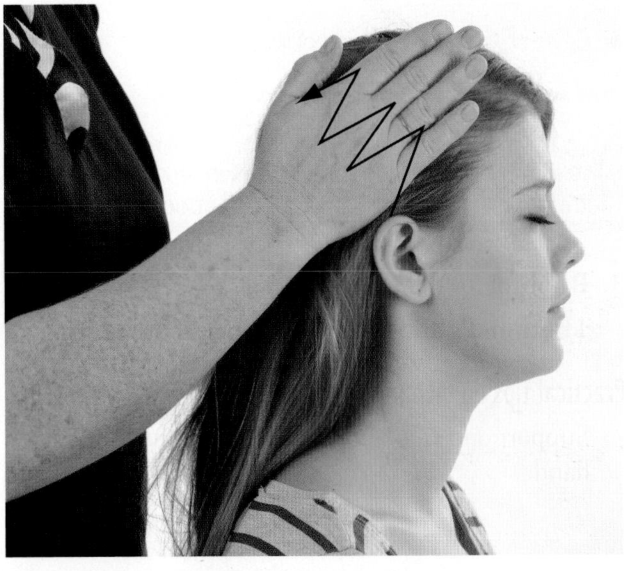

▲ Figure 6.54 Rubbing to side of scalp, around the ears

> **Key fact**
> The rubbing technique helps to lightly increase the circulation of blood to the scalp.

2. **Frictions** to the side of the scalp, around the ears

   Therapist's stance: standing behind the client

Practical tips on technique

- Support one side of the client's head with one hand.
- Use the pad of the fingers of the other hand to perform frictions briskly to the same area as in step 1 (in front of, above and behind the ears).
- Repeat on the other side of the scalp.

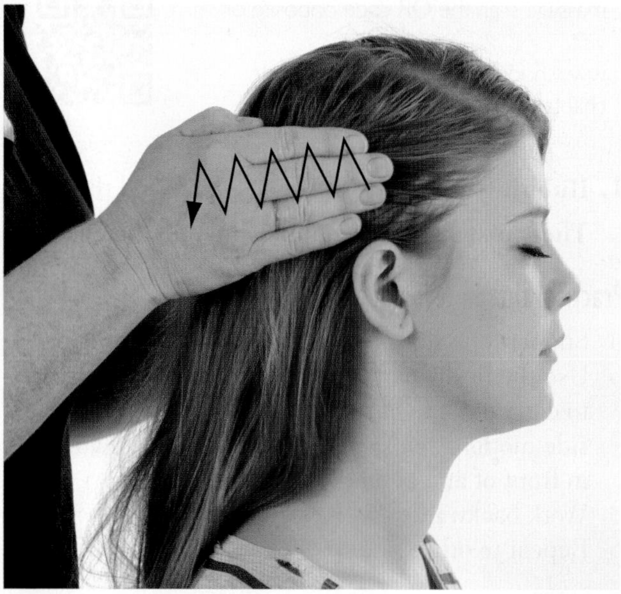

▲ Figure 6.55 Frictions to side of scalp

> **Key fact**
> The frictions technique helps to loosen tension from the temporalis muscle that can cause headaches.

3. **Rubbing** to the whole of the scalp

   Therapist's stance: standing behind the client

Practical tips on technique

- Support one side of the client's head with one hand.
- Use the soft, fleshy part of the other hand to carry out a rubbing motion, using a broad zigzag motion from side to side.
- Work over one side of the head from front to back and then repeat on the other side.

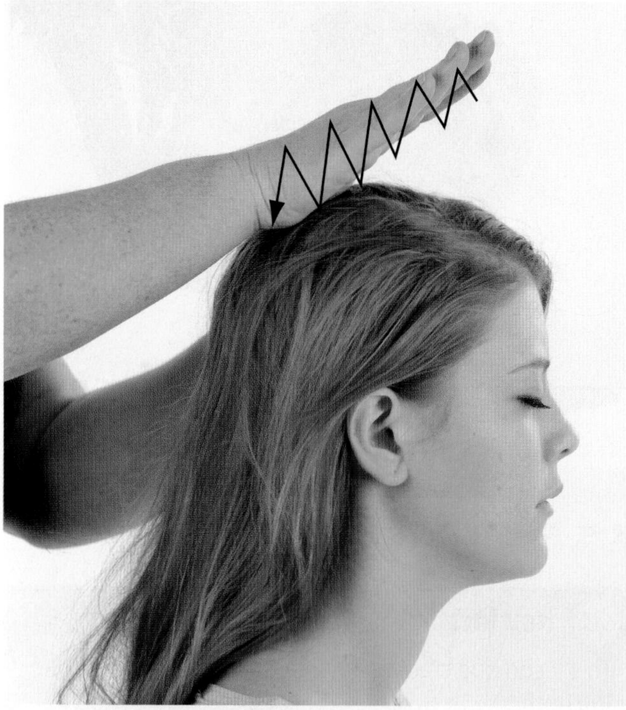

▲ Figure 6.56 Rubbing to the whole scalp

> **Key fact**
> The rubbing technique helps to loosen up tight scalp muscles and encourages blood and lymph supply to the scalp.

4. **Frictions** with the whole of the hand

   Therapist's stance: standing behind the client

Practical tips on technique

- Support one side of the client's head.
- Apply firm pressure using the whole hand, in a side-to-side zigzag motion, moving the scalp up and down.
- Work over one side of the scalp from the front of the scalp to the back.
- Repeat to the other side.

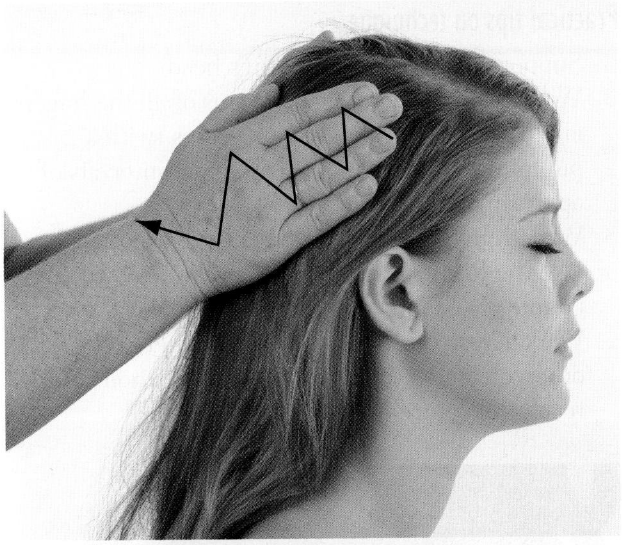

▲ Figure 6.57 Frictions with whole hand

5. **Ruffling** through the hair

Therapist's stance: standing behind the client

Practical tips on technique

- Support one side of the client's head with one hand.
- Separate the fingers of the other hand and use the tips of the fingers to perform a light, wave-like movement from side to side through the hair.
- Work from the front of the scalp towards the back.
- Repeat three times.

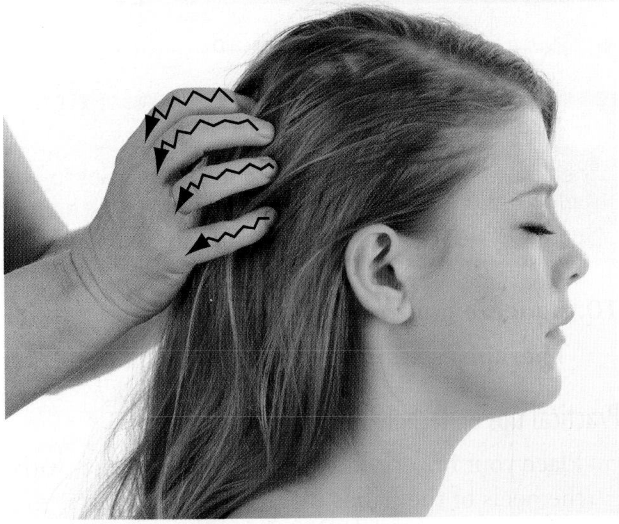

▲ Figure 6.58 Ruffling through hair

> **Key fact**
>
> This ruffling technique has a very soothing and soporific effect on the nerves if performed slowly, and is more stimulating and invigorating if performed more vigorously.

6. **Hair tugging**

Therapist's stance: standing behind the client

Practical tips on technique

- Draw the fingers of both hands through the client's hair, from root to tip, in an upwards direction.
- Release the hair from your fingers, repeating several times.
- Gather the hair between your fingers and give the hair a tug to stimulate its growth.

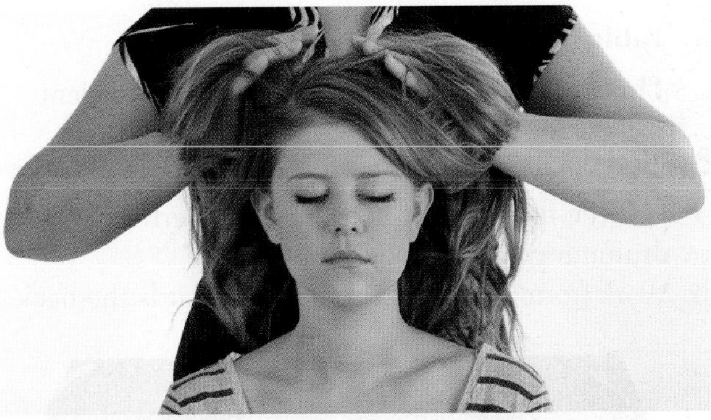

▲ Figure 6.59 Hair tugging

> **Key fact**
>
> The hair tugging technique helps to stimulate the circulation to the scalp and bring fresh blood and lymph to the surface.

7. **Effleurage/smoothing** through the hair

Therapist's stance: standing behind the client

Practical tips on technique

- With alternate hands, stroke through the client's hair using the fingertips.
- Work repetitively from the front of the scalp towards the back several times.
- If the client requires more stimulation to the scalp, use the nails of both hands to comb through the hair from front to back.

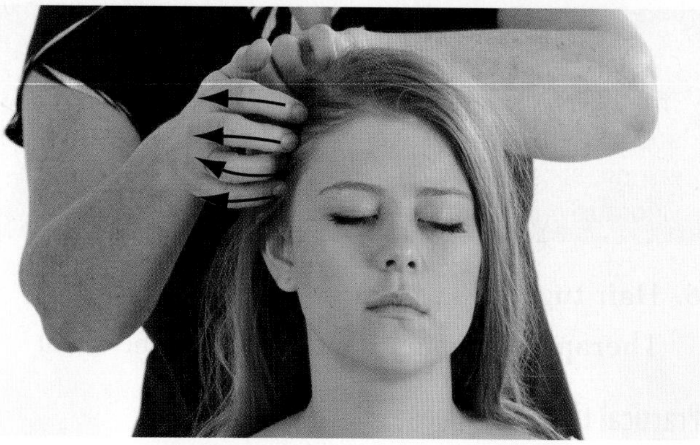

▲ Figure 6.60 Effleurage/smoothing through hair

> **Key fact**
> The effleurage/smoothing technique has a very calming and soothing effect on the client.

8. Tabla playing over the scalp

Therapist's stance: standing behind the client

Practical tips on technique

- Use the fingertips of both hands to perform a light drumming over the client's head.
- Work from the front of the head towards the back.

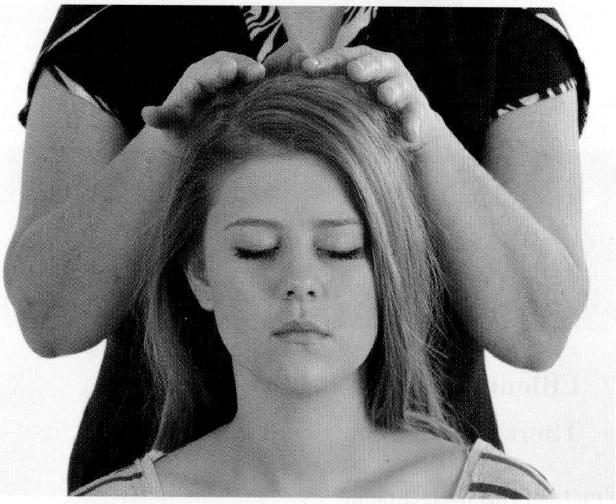

▲ Figure 6.61 Tabla playing

> **Key fact**
> The tabla playing technique is very stimulating and energising to the scalp.

9. Pressure points over the scalp

Therapist's stance: standing behind the client

Practical tips on technique

- Support one side of the client's head.
- With the other hand, use the tips of all the fingers and the thumb to perform pressures (with a pumping action) across the scalp, at intervals of approximately 2.5 cm.
- Work from the hairline towards the back of the head.
- Use the fingers and thumb to press in slowly for a couple of seconds and then release.
- Work across from one side of the head to the other, changing the supporting hand when you reach the centre of the scalp.

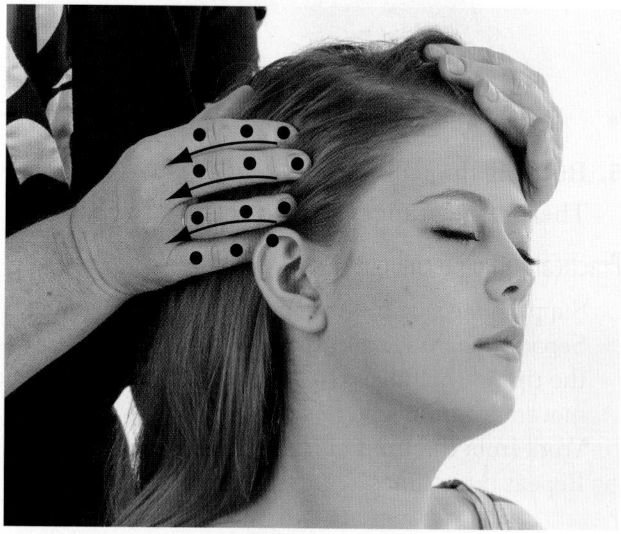

▲ Figure 6.62 Pressure points over scalp

> **Key fact**
> The pressure point technique over the scalp helps to release blockages from the nerves relating to the head and neck and has a stimulating effect on the head.

10. Squeeze and release the scalp muscles

Therapist's stance: standing behind the client

Practical tips on technique

- Place your fingers on top of the client's head, with the heels of the hands placed behind the ears.
- Using the heels of the hands, squeeze inwards with medium pressure.
- Hold, then lift and release upwards.
- Repeat the movement with the heels of the hands above the ears.
- Repeat the movement with the hands placed in front of the ears.

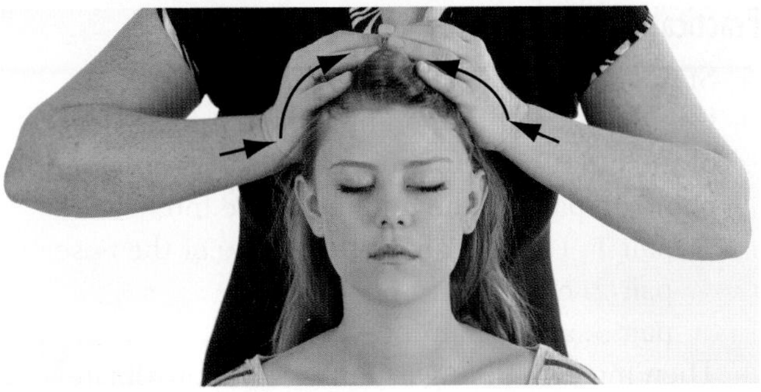

▲ Figure 6.63 Squeeze and release the scalp muscles

Key fact

The squeeze and release technique to the scalp muscles helps to relieve headaches and eye strain.

11. Circular frictions using the heels of the hands across the temples

Therapist's stance: standing behind the client

Practical tips on technique

- Support the client's head against you.
- Use the heels of both hands to make circular movements against the temples.
- Lift upwards and back towards you.
- Repeat several times.

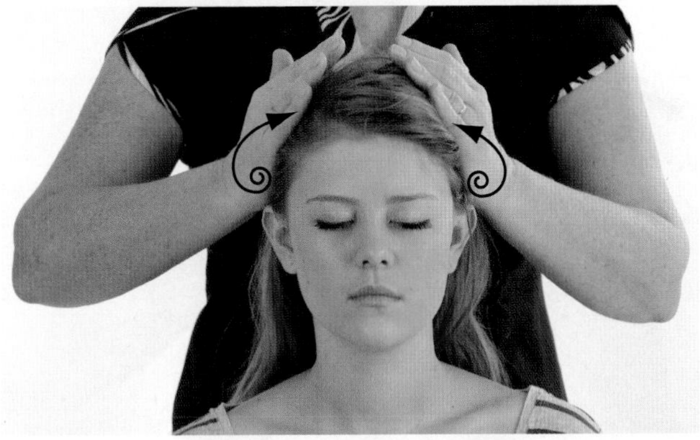

▲ Figure 6.64 Circular frictions using the heels of the hands across the temples

Key fact

Applying circular frictions to the temples is also very effective at helping to relieve tension headaches and eye strain.

12. Compression to the head

Therapist's stance: standing to the side of the client

Practical tips on technique

- Place one hand around the front of the client's head and one around the back.
- Squeeze inwards with the palms of the hands and then release.
- Repeat three times.

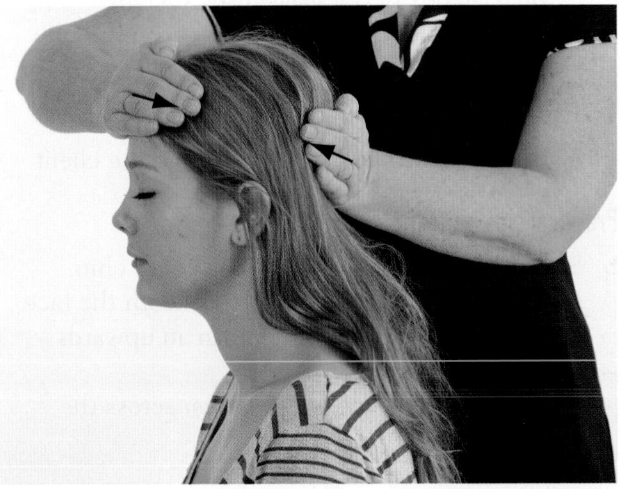

▲ Figure 6.65 Compression to the head

Key fact

This technique is very effective at helping to release tension headaches.

13. Effleurage/smoothing through the hair (as step 7)

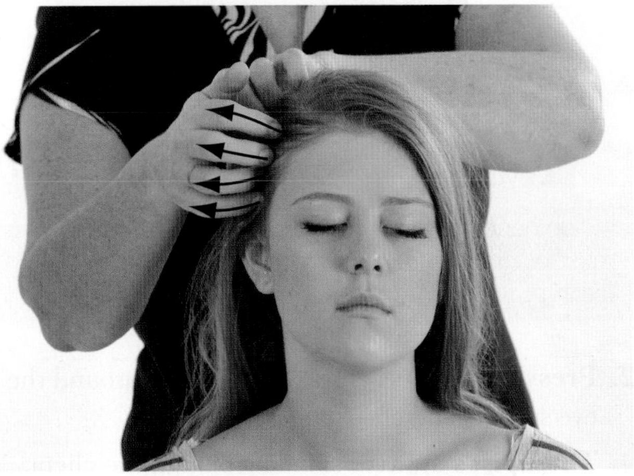

▲ Figure 6.66 Effleurage/smoothing through the hair

The face

The face is an area of the body that cannot help but show tension. When feeling tense, the jaw tends to clamps tight, teeth grind together and the lips tighten.

Before commencing the face massage, you may wish to use a dry hand cleanser to cleanse your hands of any oil or sebum that may be left on the hands from the scalp massage.

For the face massage, the client's head needs to be tilted back slightly to rest against the therapist's upper thorax. Ensure that the client's neck is comfortable and offer a neck support or cushion.

1. **Effleurage/smoothing** across the face

   Therapist's stance: standing behind the client

Practical tips on technique

- Start with the fingers across the client's chin.
- Use the fingers of both hands to smooth the face, with gentle flowing movements in an upwards direction.
- Work across the chin and jaw, then across the cheeks and forehead.
- Repeat three times.

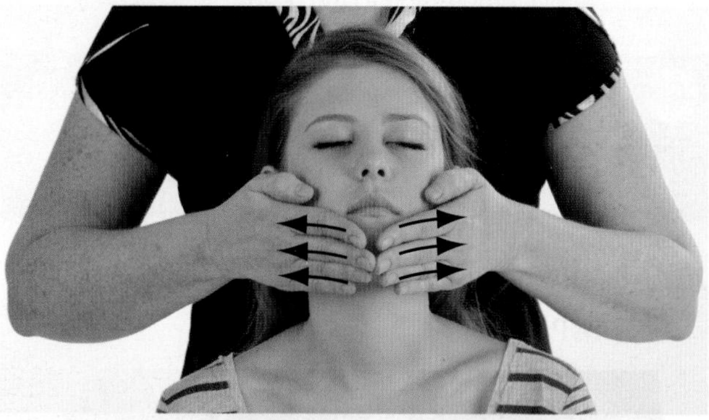

▲ Figure 6.67 Effleurage/smoothing across the face

> **Key fact**
>
> Indian head massage can help to relax the facial muscles and melt away tension, leaving the client feeling calm and refreshed.

2. **Pressure points** across the forehead, around the eye sockets and cheekbones

   Therapist's stance: standing behind the client

Practical tips on technique

- Support the client's head with one hand.
- Use the pads of the forefinger and middle finger of the other hand to press the following pressure points in pairs at the midline of the forehead:
  - pair 1: 1.25 cm above the bridge of the nose
  - pair 2: halfway up the forehead
  - pair 3: at the hairline.
- Then move both fingers outwards approximately 1.25 cm and repeat.
- Then press points on the ridge of bone all round the eyes – outwards along the top and inwards along the bottom.
- Now move to points on either side of the nose and across the curve of the cheekbones, and drain the sinuses by curving forefingers under the cheekbones and holding for a few seconds.

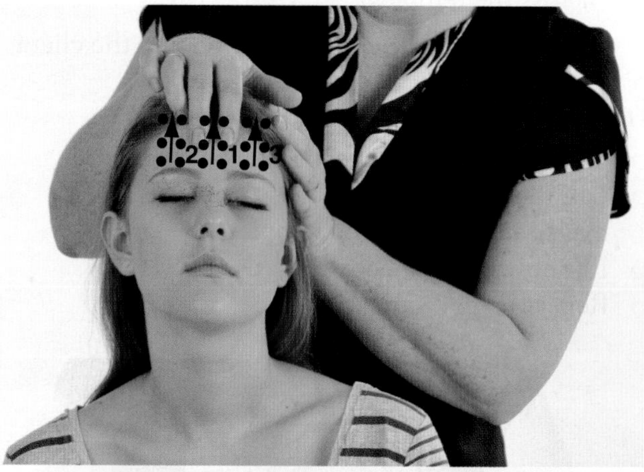

▲ Figure 6.68 Pressure points across the forehead

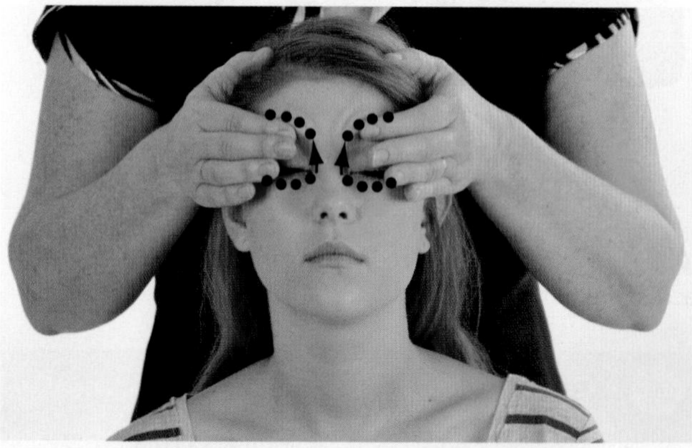

▲ Figure 6.69 Pressure points around the eye sockets

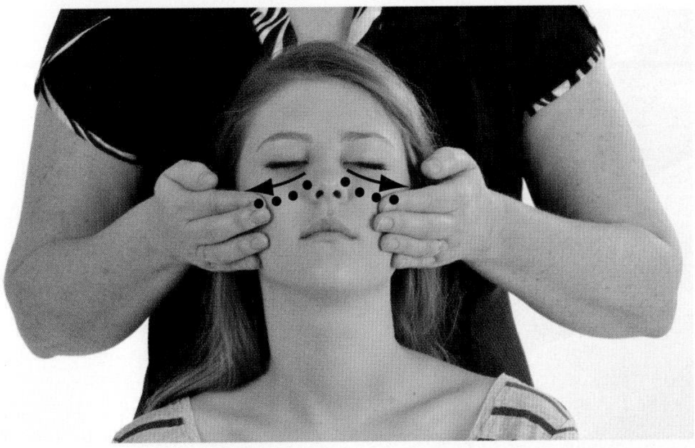

▲ Figure 6.70 Pressure points on the cheekbones

> **Key fact**
> Using this pressure point technique on the face helps to relieve sinus congestion and encourage lymphatic drainage from the head.

3. **Circular temple frictions** with the tips of the fingers

   Therapist's stance: standing behind the client

Practical tips on technique

- Support the client's head against you.
- Use the pads of the fingers to perform circular frictions to the temples.
- Work slowly and deeply over the area several times.

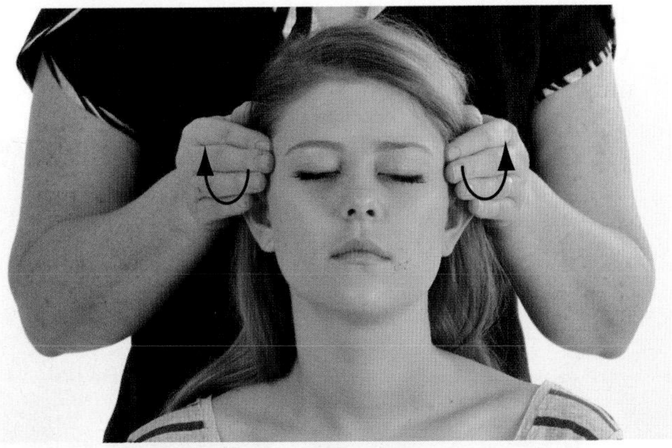

▲ Figure 6.71 Circular temple frictions with the tips of the fingers

> **Key fact**
> This technique helps to relieve tension in facial muscles, helps to relieve headaches and eye strain, and helps to relax the eyes.

4. **Squeezing and twiddling** the ear lobes

   Therapist's stance: standing behind client

Practical tips on technique

- Place your fingers behind the client's ear lobes and the thumbs in front.
- Squeeze the ear lobes between thumb and forefinger.
- Hold for a few seconds and then slowly release.
- Twiddle the ears by rolling the thumb and the forefinger across the ear lobe in a brisk manner.
- Repeat several times.

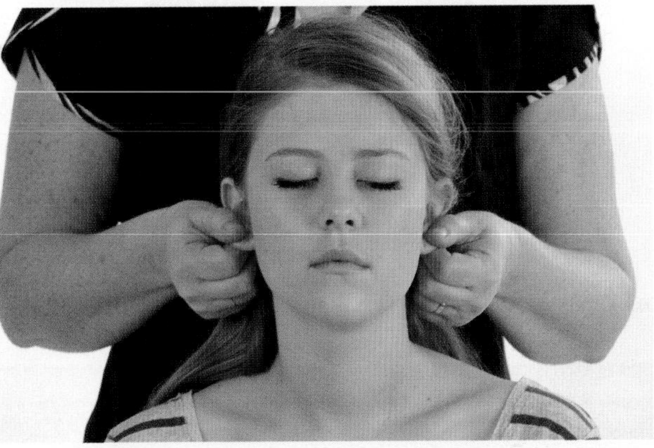

▲ Figure 6.72 Squeeze and twiddle the ear lobes

> **Key fact**
> The squeezing and twiddling technique applied to the ears stimulates the nerve endings to the whole of the body and creates an energising feeling.

5. **Effleurage/smoothing** (as step 1)
6. **Relaxing** the facial muscles

   Therapist's stance: standing behind the client

Practical tips on technique

- Gently place both of your hands so that they cover the lower part of the jaw and cheeks.
- Relax the hands and keep them still and relaxed for a few seconds.

- Gradually move the hands up the face, stopping to place the hands so that the tips of the middle fingers meet at the bridge of the nose.
- Continue up the face, stopping to place the hands so that they cover the eyes.
- Continue up the face to finally place hands over the top of the forehead.

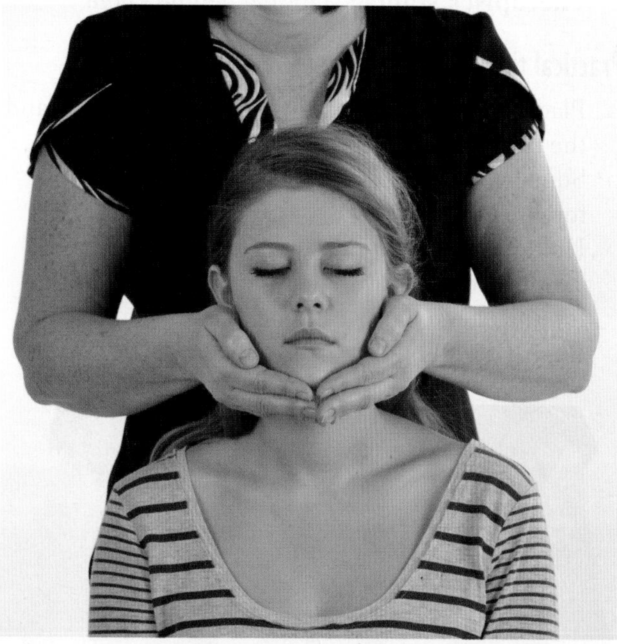

▲ Figure 6.73 Relaxing facial muscles

> **Key fact**
> This technique relaxes the facial muscles and the eyes, and creates a feeling of stillness and calm.

7. **Higher chakra balancing**

   Therapist's stance: standing to the side of the client

Practical tips on technique

- Place one hand lightly over the client's crown chakra (top of the head) and cup the other hand over the throat chakra (without touching the throat).
- Hold your hands there for a short while, breathing deeply and slowly to concentrate.
- Retaining the hand over the crown chakra, move the other hand up to place it lightly over the third eye and hold there for a few moments.
- Then place both hands over the crown.

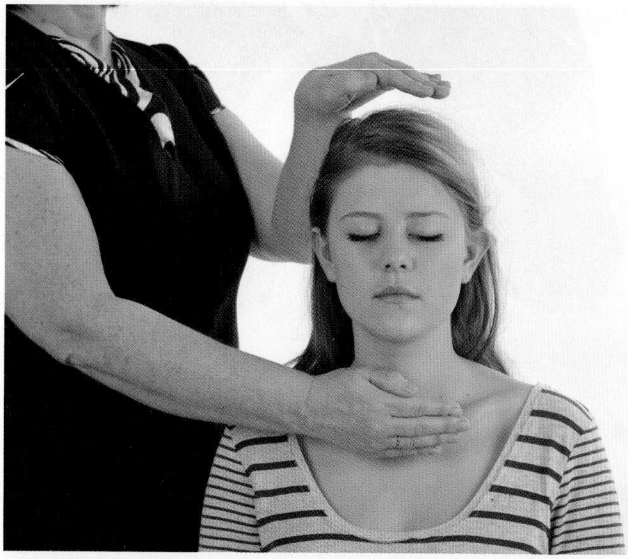

▲ Figure 6.74 Higher chakra balancing

> **Key fact**
> Chakra balancing helps to realign the client's energy and is very soothing and calming, helping to bring about a sense of peace and harmony.

8. **Squeeze and release** to the back of the neck

   Therapist's stance: standing to the side of the client

Practical tips on technique

- Place one hand over the third eye area of the client's forehead.
- Spread the thumbs and fingers of your other hand on either side of the base of the neck (forming a V shape) and gently squeeze and release the muscles at the back of the neck.

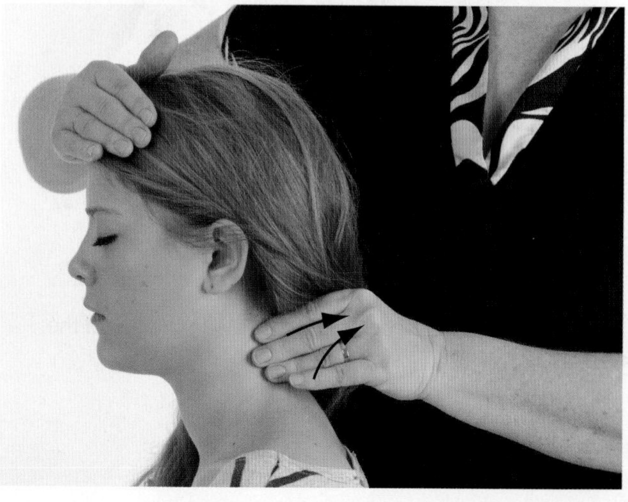

▲ Figure 6.75 Squeeze and release to the back of the neck

9. **Effleurage/smoothing** across the upper back as in step 3 upper back and shoulders.

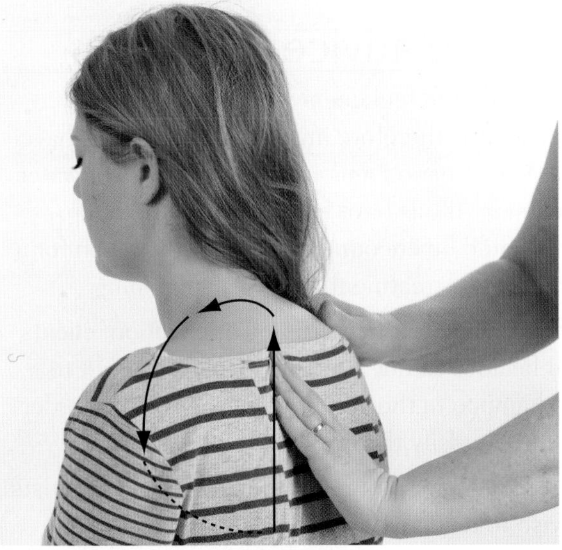

▲ Figure 6.76 Effleurage/smoothing across the upper back

Key fact

The use of effleurage/smoothing at the end of the massage helps to ground the client and brings them back from a deep state of relaxation.

10. Slowly leave the client's aura

After squeezing the top of the client's shoulders, take a step back from the client's aura and gently shake your hands.

Wash your hands.

Full routine quick reference guide

Upper back and shoulders

1. **Starting position** with hands over the top of the client's shoulders
2. **Holding position** over the top of the head
3. **Effleurage/smoothing** across the shoulders and upper back
4. **Petrissage/thumb sweeping** across the shoulders
5. **Frictions with the heel of the hand** rubbing around the scapulae
6. **Frictions with the finger** rubbing around the scapulae
7. **Effleurage/smoothing** (as step 3)
8. **Pressures** with the knuckles either side of the spine
9. **Thumb pushes** over the shoulders
10. **Finger pulls** across the top of the shoulders
11. **Squeezing and releasing** across the tops of the shoulders
12. **Heel pushes** across the tops of the shoulders
13. **Smoothing** with the forearms
14. **Chopping** across the shoulders and upper back
15. **Champi/double hacking** across the shoulders and upper back
16. **Squeezing and releasing** across the tops of the shoulders (as step 11)
17. **Effleurage/smoothing** (as step 3)
18. **Holding position** over the tops of the shoulders (as step 1).

Upper arms

1. **Squeezing and releasing** the upper arms
2. **Compression** of the upper arms
3. **Heel rolls** embracing the upper arms
4. **Squeezing and kneading** down the upper arms
5. **Shoulder mobilisation**
6. **Squeezing and kneading** to the forearms
7. **Squeezing and kneading** to the fingers
8. **Circular pressure massage** to the pressure point between the thumb and index finger
9. **Circular pressure massage** to the pressure point in the centre of the palm
10. **Shoulder lift**
11. **Effleurage/smoothing** with the forearms down the upper arms.

The neck

1. **Rocking** the head backwards and forwards
2. **Squeezing and releasing** the muscles at the back of the neck
3. **Finger frictions** to the tops of the shoulders and up the side of the neck
4. **Thumb pushes** to the side of the neck
5. **Squeezing and releasing** at the side of the neck
6. **Finger frictions** to the base of the skull

7. **Heel of the hand frictions** to the base of the skull
8. **Effleurage/smoothing** to the back of the neck
9. **Pressure points** at the base of the skull
10. **Gentle stretching** to the side of the neck
11. **Smoothing with the whole hand** at the base of the skull (as step 8).

The scalp

1. **Rubbing** to the side of the scalp, around the ears
2. **Frictions** to the side of the scalp, around the ears
3. **Rubbing** to the whole of the scalp
4. **Frictions** with the whole of the hand
5. **Ruffling** through the hair
6. **Hair tugging**
7. **Effleurage/smoothing** through the hair
8. **Tabla playing** over the scalp
9. **Pressure points** over the scalp
10. **Squeeze and release** the scalp muscles
11. **Circular frictions using the heels of the hands** across the temples
12. **Compression** to the head
13. **Effleurage/smoothing** through the hair (as step 7)

The face

1. **Effleurage/smoothing** across the face
2. **Pressure points** across the forehead, around the eye sockets and cheekbones
3. **Circular temple frictions** with the tips of the fingers
4. **Squeezing and twiddling** the ear lobes
5. **Effleurage/smoothing** (as step 1)
6. **Relaxing** the facial muscles
7. **Higher chakra balancing**
8. **Squeeze and release** to the back of the neck

To access a printable version of the full routine quick reference guide scan the QR code opposite or visit www.hodderplus.co.uk/indianhead/chapter-6.

9. **Effleurage/smoothing** across the upper back
10. **Slowly leave the client's aura**

Aftercare advice

Clients will often feel deeply relaxed following treatment. It is therefore important that clients have a suitable rest period and are offered a glass of water before rising. If oils have been used on the scalp, clients should be encouraged to leave the oil on for a few hours after treatment, before shampooing.

When washing their hair after oil application, clients should be advised not to wet their hair first, but to apply shampoo to the scalp before the water in order to help to emulsify the oil.

As part of a client's home care programme, therapists may wish to teach clients simple self-massage techniques with oils, particularly if the client requires an improvement to their hair condition.

In order to aid the healing process and to get the maximum benefit from their treatments, clients are advised to

- increase their intake of water following treatment, to assist the body's detoxification process
- have a suitable rest period after the treatment
- avoid eating a heavy meal after the treatment; try to keep the diet light while the body is using its energy for healing
- avoid smoking
- cut down on the consumption of stimulants such as tea, coffee, alcohol and drugs
- take time out to relax and practise stress-relieving techniques, such as yoga or meditation, if appropriate
- participate in regular, manageable exercise
- practise the correct breathing techniques to create a feeling of calm
- use oils and simple head massage techniques at home for long-term hair care.

Contra-actions/reactions to Indian head massage

A client's reaction to Indian head massage may vary according to their physical and emotional condition. If the body has been under a considerable amount of stress, it is not unusual for there to be some kind of reaction as the body adjusts itself back to balance. This is often referred to as a 'healing crisis'.

Clients should be made aware of the fact that some of these reactions may occur and be reassured that if they do occur, they will only be temporary.

Below are some of the healing reactions that may occur following an Indian head massage treatment:

- a feeling of tiredness and lethargy due to the release of toxins
- a headache due to the release of toxins
- thirst due to temporary dehydration
- a feeling of dizziness or nausea
- an aching and soreness in the muscles due to the release of toxins and the nerve fibres responding to the massage
- a heightened emotional state – depression, weepiness or laughter
- increased urination
- increased secretions of mucous from the nose and mouth
- cold-like symptoms
- a disturbed sleep pattern (restlessness).
- If the client feels nauseous or dizzy, stop the treatment, check the room for ventilation, offer the client a glass of water and stay with the client until they feel better. If the symptoms persist, advise the client to seek medical advice.
- If the client has a skin reaction, remove the product immediately and apply a soothing compress. Advise the client to seek medical advice if the symptoms continue.

Health and safety note

If a client experiences a contra-action during the treatment, such as feeling nauseous or dizzy, or a skin reaction, it is important to discontinue the treatment and provide the appropriate action and advice.

- If the client complains of a headache following treatment, advise them to drink water, rest and get some fresh air.

Many clients will report positive reactions following an Indian head massage. These include:

- relief from stress and muscular tension
- an increased feeling of awareness; clients often experience a feeling of calm, peace and tranquillity due to the rebalancing of the chakras
- improved sleep pattern (deep and restful)
- a feeling of alertness and clarity in mental thought
- increased energy levels
- elevation of mood
- pain relief
- increased joint mobility.

Information to record following a treatment

Important information to be recorded after the treatment includes:

- an assessment of the client's physical condition (noting any areas of tension, physiological responses) as well as psychological responses
- visual assessment of the client (noting posture, non-verbal signs)
- any known reactions, their effects and any advice given
- aftercare advice
- home care advice, along with any oils or products suggested for home use
- outcome and general evaluation of the treatment
- recommendations for future treatment and the suggested frequency.

Frequency of treatment

In India, head massage is often part of a daily schedule. In the western world, as part of a stress management programme, Indian head massage should ideally be carried out once or even twice a week for maximum benefit. It is advisable to offer clients a course of treatments (between four and six initially) and to recommend the client takes the treatments close together initially.

Frequency of treatment may vary due to a client's resources, namely time and money, and clients should be encouraged to attend for treatments as frequently as their schedule and financial resources allow.

Benefits of regular Indian head massage treatments

In order to maximise the benefits of Indian head massage, it is important for clients to receive regular treatment.

Benefits of regular treatment include:

- improvement in hair condition
- reduction in stress levels
- increased energy levels
- a general sense of well-being
- improved sleep patterns
- improvement in circulation.

Adaptations to an Indian head massage treatment

Indian head massage, like any other massage technique, should always be adapted and varied to suit the differences in

- the physical characteristics of clients, such as their body size
- variations in muscle tone and skin elasticity
- variations in age, bone density and tissue elasticity
- hair type, in terms of both length and thickness
- clients' individual preferences, in terms of pressure, treatment objectives and duration
- the environment in which the massage is undertaken.

Therapists are likely to encounter many clients who may require a degree of adaptation due to their physical and health-related situations.

Study tip

The best approach to massage is to see every client's situation as a different challenge and view their individual needs as part of the treatment plan. When adapting a massage it is not the massage movements themselves that change; the difference is the way in which the therapist modifies or adjusts the pressure, speed, duration and frequency of the massage.

Pregnant clients

It is advisable to avoid carrying out Indian head massage in the first trimester until the pregnancy is established. The first trimester can be an unsettling time and some clients may experience nausea and sickness.

Once past the first trimester, and provided the pregnancy has no complications, Indian head massage can often be a popular choice due to the fact that pregnant clients can sit comfortably in a chair for treatment, and no special positioning is required.

Health and safety note

Care should be taken when massaging a pregnant client due to the fact that some clients may experience a feeling of dizziness. Care should also be taken, and if necessary, GP referral sought, for those clients who experience high blood pressure during their pregnancy.

Clients with disabilities

The first consideration for the therapist is to establish the nature of the client's disability and, if necessary, research the condition beforehand to be prepared. It is important for a therapist to enquire tactfully about the limitations of the condition and not to assume anything; just because a client has a disability it is does not mean they are paralysed.

If a client is in a wheelchair, then due to the portability of Indian head massage they may be treated quite easily while sitting in their wheelchair. If the client is in a wheelchair it is advisable for the therapist to sit or kneel when carrying out the consultation, in order that they may talk to the client at eye level. It is essential to take care not to appear patronising to clients with disabilities, and you should not discriminate against them because of their disability.

Mature or elderly clients

There are several considerations to be borne in mind with an elderly client.

- Take care to ensure the client is warm enough throughout the treatment.
- Many elderly people experience a sudden drop in blood pressure, so if you are helping the client up, do it gently and carefully to avoid the risk of loss of balance and falls.
- Avoid deep massage by decreasing the amount of pressure used due to decreased reaction time, possible insensitivity to pain and thinning of skin and blood vessels.
- There may be loss of hearing and vision.
- There will be a decrease in muscle tone, bones will not be as strong and flexible, and joints may be worn.
- Skin may appear pale, wrinkled, thinner, looser and more fragile.
- The circulation may not be as efficient, especially if the client is inactive.

It is best to make the treatment sessions shorter, as the client may tire easily. You should also take care when applying pressure and avoid extreme joint mobilisation, due to loss of bone integrity.

Large-framed clients

Clients with a large frame may find Indian head massage more comfortable due to positioning and the fact that no undressing is required.

Pressure should be applied carefully to areas with dense areas of adipose tissue in order to avoid tissue damage and client discomfort.

> **Health and safety note**
>
> It may be tempting for the massage therapist to consider that areas of fatty tissue are insensitive and apply too firm a pressure. Adipose tissue is in fact highly vascular, making it very susceptible to bruising and damage.

General pointers are to consider pressure and monitor client feedback and use body mechanics correctly.

The therapist may also need to adjust the chair height to suit the size of the client.

Small-framed clients

> **Health and safety note**
>
> Care needs to be taken with thin clients to avoid deep massage or pressure over bony areas, which may cause discomfort.

Stimulating techniques such as hacking should be avoided over unprotected areas, and pressure applied should be carefully monitored in line with client feedback. It is important for the therapist to avoid assuming that because the client is thin they require a light massage.

Male/female clients

In general terms, the male body presents more muscle bulk than the female body, and therefore an adaptation of technique is often required. Male clients will generally require a firmer pressure, and the therapist should take care to apply the correct body mechanics and posture in order to be able to carry out the techniques effectively and to the client's satisfaction.

Always remember to check the client's preference with regard to pressure and take any individual requirements into account for both male and female clients.

Adaptations for differences in muscle tone

Muscle tone may vary due to physical characteristics of the client and the level of physical activity they participate in.

Good muscle tone may be recognised by the muscles appearing firm and rounded. A variety of movements may be used in order to keep muscles in good tone, including deeper effleurage, petrissage/kneading and tapotement.

A degree of adaptation of technique may be needed in order to be able to manipulate muscles with good tone (deeper effleurage to relax the fascia and tendons).

Poor muscle tone may be recognised by the muscles appearing loose and flattened rather than rounded. Poor muscle tone may be due to lack of use through lack of regular exercise.

Care should be taken when massaging a client with poor muscle tone to ensure that muscles are not compressed too hard against the underlying bone and that they are not overstretched.

Adaptations for clients with long/thick hair

When carrying out an Indian head massage on a client with long or thick hair, the first consideration is that generally more oil will be needed, and in some cases it may be necessary to section off the hair for the oil application. When establishing contact with the head/scalp, it is best to slide the fingers from the hair root upwards above the ears. When dealing with thick hair, which has a tendency to be coarse, it is best to use a softening and moisturising oil such as coconut.

Adaptations for clients without hair

Clients with little or no hair will require a slightly different approach when massaging the scalp. Any techniques involving manipulation or tugging of the hair will obviously be omitted and less oil will be required. However, it is still important to work over the scalp, as regardless of whether the client has hair or not, the scalp muscles are still liable to develop tension due to their attachments.

Multiple-choice self-assessment questions

1. **How should the treatment area be prepared for Indian head massage treatment?**
   - a Clean, tidy, soft lighting, relaxing music and well ventilated.
   - b Clean, tidy, bright lighting, relaxing music and well ventilated.
   - c Clean, tidy, soft lighting, stimulating music and well ventilated.
   - d Clean, tidy, soft lighting, relaxing music and poorly ventilated.

2. **Which of the following statements is *false* in relation to Indian head massage techniques?**
   - a Effleurage is a stroking or smoothing movement that signals the beginning and end of the massage.
   - b Petrissage movements are deeper, using the whole hand, thumb or fingers.
   - c Tapotement movements are heavy and applied with both hands in a slow motion.
   - d Friction movements are a strong feature of Indian head massage, and are performed with the whole of the hand, the heel of the hand, the fingers or thumbs.

3. **Friction movements are used in Indian head massage to**
   - a prepare the area for deeper strokes
   - b stimulate and clear nerve pathways
   - c break down tension nodules caused by stress and tension
   - d restore energy balance to the body.

4. **A form of tapotement used in Indian head massage called double hacking is also known traditionally as**
   - a tabla playing
   - b tapping
   - c cupping
   - d champi.

5. **Which of the following will assist in ensuring good posture while carrying out an Indian head massage?**
   - a Keeping the wrists bent.
   - b Ensuring that the chair is at the correct height for use.
   - c Lifting the feet off the ground.
   - d Wearing high-heeled shoes with good support.

6. **Which of the following statements is *false*?**
   - a Marma points are naturally sensitive points measured by finger widths.
   - b Marma points are subtle pressure points that stimulate the life force.
   - c In Indian head massage the marmas may be used to treat a client's internal illness.
   - d The marmas are anatomical places on the body, mostly composed of flesh and bones.

7. **How many marma points are located in the head and neck area?**
   - a 107
   - b 27
   - c 37
   - d 57

8. **The marma point located on the top of the head/crown in known as the**
   - a apanga marma point
   - b adhipati marma point
   - c avarta marma point
   - d none of the above.

9. **Which of the following oils is most suitable for a client with dry, brittle and lifeless hair?**
   - a Sesame
   - b Mustard
   - c Olive
   - d Coconut

10. **How can an Indian head massage be adapted to suit a male client?**
    - a Using a lighter pressure
    - b Using a firmer pressure
    - c Using more oil
    - d Using less oil

11. **Which of the following adaptations is most suitable for a mature/older client?**
    - a Check client comfort and warmth throughout, decrease pressure and avoid deep massage.
    - b Check client comfort and warmth throughout, increase pressure and avoid use of oils.
    - c Check client comfort and warmth throughout, decrease pressure and avoid use of oils.
    - d Check client comfort and warmth throughout, increase pressure and use stimulating oils.

12. In Indian head massage the idea of working on the higher chakras is to

a enable the client to breathe more easily
b de-stress the client
c restore a sense of balance and harmony to the client's energy
d open up a client's spiritual potential.

13. Which of the following may be considered a contra-action to Indian head massage?

a Improved sleep pattern
b Feeling of alertness
c Headache and nausea
d Increased energy levels

14. If a client felt nauseous or dizzy during treatment, what action would you take?

a Stop the treatment immediately, check ventilation in the room and offer the client a glass of water.
b Carry on with the treatment, but ask the client frequently if they are okay.
c Inform the client that their reaction is a normal part of the healing process.
d Shorten the treatment timing and inform the client to go home and rest afterwards.

15. Aftercare advice following Indian head massage includes:

a having a suitable rest period, avoiding stimulants, increasing intake of water and eating a light meal
b having a suitable rest period, avoiding stimulants, increasing intake of water and eating a heavy meal
c having a suitable rest period, increasing intake of water and stimulants and eating a heavy meal
d having a suitable rest period, decreasing intake of water and stimulants and eating a light meal.

16. How would you best respond to a client complaining of a headache after massage?

a Advise them to rest for a longer period of time.
b Advise them to drink water, rest and get some fresh air.
c Advise them to take a painkiller.
d Advise them it will pass in the next few hours.

To see the answers, scan the QR code opposite or visit www.hodderplus.co.uk/indianhead/chapter-6. To access an interactive version of these multiple-choice self-assessment questions visit www.hodderplus.co.uk/indianhead/chapter-6.

To access an interactive crossword for this chapter visit www.hodderplus.co.uk/indianhead/chapter-6.

7 Chakra balancing in Indian head massage

Introduction

Traditional Indian head massage treatments involve balancing of the chakras. There are seven major chakras: the base, sacral, solar plexus, heart, throat, third eye and crown chakras.

In Indian head massage we work on balancing the higher chakras: the throat chakra, the third eye and the crown chakra.

Learning objectives

By the end of this chapter you will understand:

- the relevance of chakras to an Indian head massage treatment
- how to balance the chakras.

Chakras

Everything that happens to us on an emotional level has an energetic impact on the subtle body, which in turn has an impact on the physical body.

Chakras are non-physical energy centres located about 2.5 cm away from the physical body.

The energy field of each chakra extends beyond the visible body of matter into the subtle body or aura.

It is important to remember that chakras do not have a physical form; any illustration of the chakras is merely a visual aid to the imagination and not a literal physical reality. Chakras are a way of describing the flow of subtle energy and are often said to be related to an endocrine gland, which the chakra is thought to influence.

With stress, the chakras can lose their ability to synchronise with each other and become unbalanced. If negative energy becomes stored in a chakra, it can accumulate and the function of the chakra becomes impaired. Ultimately, this can lead to energy blocks, where the chakras virtually cease to function, and creates an imbalance as other chakras attempt to compensate for the blocked centre, creating additional strain for the energy system.

The effects of an accumulation of negative energy in the chakras can manifest itself as an emotional or physical condition. Often we are only aware of a change in the physical body, as our attention is drawn to a physical body in the form of pain or disease; this may not always be linked to being a symptom of a cause within the subtle body.

Key fact

Chakras are the focal points for the energies of the subtle bodies and are the key to restoring balance. By placing hands along the axis of the chakras, energy can be aligned and harmony restored. By working with the subtle energy of the chakras, energy may be strengthened, decreased or balanced, as needed by the body at the time of the treatment.

The seven major chakras

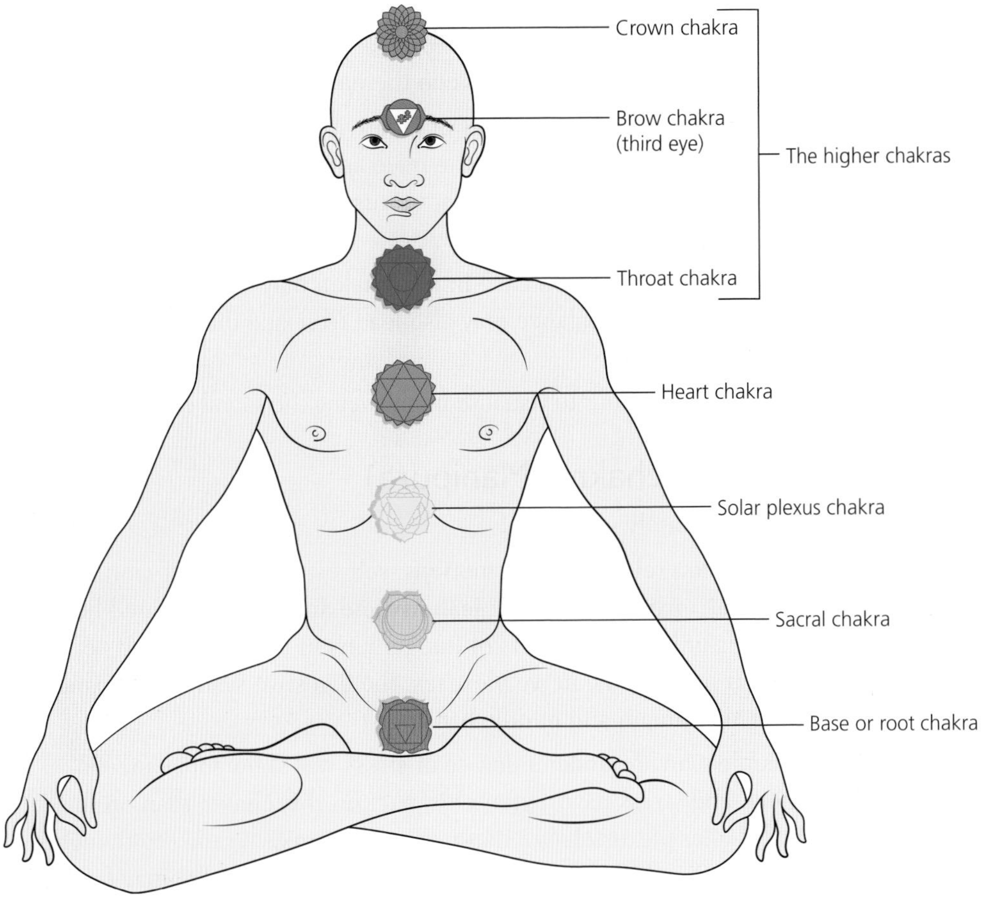

▲ Figure 7.1 Seven major chakras

The base or root chakra (Muladhara)

Location: at the base of the spine

Relevance: it is the foundation chakra and is linked with nature and planet Earth. It is concerned with all issues of a physical nature: the body, the senses, sensuality, a person's sex, survival, aggression and self-defence. At a physical level, it is linked to the endocrine system through the adrenal glands. Its energies also affect the lower parts of the pelvis, hips, legs and feet.

Imbalance: if this chakra is unbalanced it can make a person feel as if they are ungrounded and unfocused. They may feel weak, lack confidence and feel unable to achieve their goals.

Colour association: the colour to visualise in balancing the base chakra is red.

The sacral chakra (Swadhistana)

Location: at the level of the sacrum between the naval and the base chakra

Relevance: it is concerned with all issues of creativity and sexuality. At the physical level, it is linked to the testes in the male and the ovaries in the female. Its energies also affect the urogenital organs, uterus, kidneys, lower digestive organs and lower back.

Imbalance: a person with an imbalance in this chakra may bury their emotions and be overly sensitive. An imbalance may also lead to sexual difficulties and energy blocks with creativity.

Colour association: the colour to visualise in balancing the sacral chakra is orange.

The solar plexus chakra (Manipura)

Location: at approximately waist level

Relevance: this chakra relates to our emotions, self-esteem and self-worth. Feelings such as fear, anxiety, insecurity, jealousy and anger are generated here. At a physical level, it is linked to the islets of Langerhans in the pancreas. Its energies also affect the solar and splenic nerve plexuses, the digestive system, the pancreas, liver, gall bladder, diaphragm and middle back.

Imbalance: people who are under a degree of stress will show imbalance in this chakra; shock and stress have a greater impact on this chakra than on the others. It is in the solar plexus chakra that negative energies relating to thoughts and feelings are processed. People with an imbalance in this chakra may feel depressed, insecure, lacking in confidence and may worry what others think.

Colour association: the colour to visualise in balancing the solar plexus chakra is yellow.

The heart chakra (Anahata)

Location: in the centre of the chest

Relevance: this chakra is concerned with love and the heart. It deals with all issues concerned with love and affection. At a physical level it is linked to the thymus gland. Its energies also affect the cardiac and pulmonary nerve plexuses, the heart, lungs, bronchial tubes, chest, upper back and arms. It is also the point of connection between the upper and lower chakras.

Imbalance: if the energy does not flow freely between the solar plexus and the heart, or between the heart and the throat, it can lead to some form of imbalance, due to the energy withdrawal into the body. A person with an imbalance in this chakra may feel sorry for themselves, be afraid of letting go, feel unworthy of love or terrified of rejection.

Colour association: the colour to visualise in balancing the heart chakra is green.

The throat chakra (Vishuddha)

Location: at the base of the neck

Relevance: this chakra is concerned with communication and expression, it also deals with the issue of truth and true expression of the soul. At a physical level, it is linked to the thyroid and parathyroid glands. Its energies also affect the pharyngeal nerve plexus, the organs of the throat, neck, nose, mouth, teeth and ears.

Imbalance: if this chakra is out of balance it may result in the inability to express our emotions; these unexpressed feelings can lead to frustration and tension. A person with an imbalance in this chakra may feel unable to relax.

Colour association: the colour to visualise in balancing the throat chakra is blue.

The brow chakra (Ajna)

Location: in the middle of the forehead over the third eye area

Relevance: commonly known as the 'third eye', the brow chakra is the storehouse of memories and imagination and is associated with intellect, understanding and intuition. At a physical level, it is linked to the hypothalamus and pituitary gland. Its energies also affect the nerves of the head, brain, eyes and face.

Imbalance: if this chakra is not functioning correctly it can lead to headaches and nightmares. A person with an imbalance in this chakra may be oversensitive to the feelings of others, be afraid of success, be non-assertive and undisciplined.

Colour association: the colour to visualise in balancing the brow chakra is indigo.

The crown chakra (Sahasrara)

Location: on top of the head

Relevance: this chakra is the centre of our spirituality and is concerned with thinking and decision-making. At a physical level it is linked to the pineal gland. Its energies also affect the brain and the rest of the body.

Imbalance: an imbalance in this chakra may be reflected in those who are unwilling or afraid to open up to their own spiritual potential. An imbalance may also show as being unable to make decisions.

Colour association: the colour to visualise in balancing the crown chakra is violet.

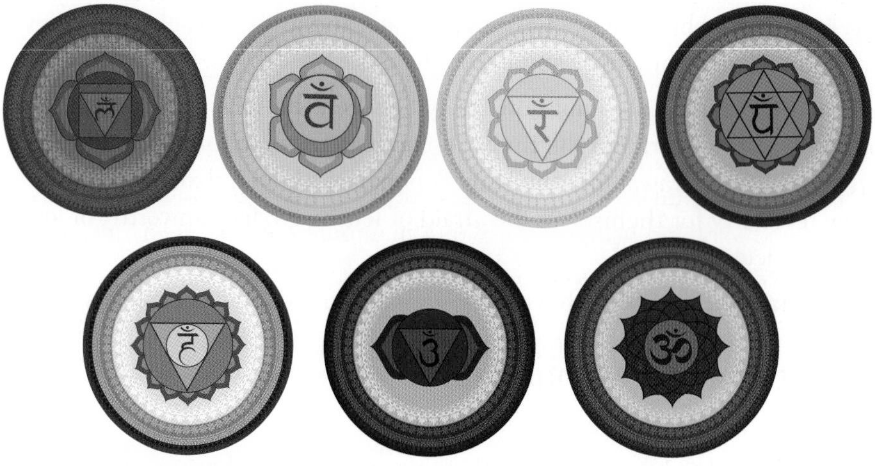

▲ Figure 7.2 The chakra symbols

Keeping chakras healthy

Chakras are like the power stations of our body, bringing it to life and keeping it healthy. Each chakra is associated with different parts of us and they need to spin totally in balance for us to feel good.

In a healthy, fully functioning person, the chakras should all be close to the same size and spinning in the same direction. They should be fully functional, clean and translucent, with no blockages. When they malfunction, unwanted physical and emotional problems may result.

The chakras absorb energy that comes from our thoughts, feelings and outside environment and feed this to our bodies. The body is affected by the quality of the energy that passes through the chakras. For instance, if we have negative feelings, we will be filtering negative energy through our chakras and into the body. Over time, this can make the body ill. Our chakras also absorb energy from the environment. Other people's negative emotions or a room full of clutter will produce an unhealthy energy that we absorb.

Knowledge check

1. What is a chakra?
2. Where are chakras located in relation to the body?
3. List the seven major chakras and where they are located.

To see the answers to this knowledge check, scan the QR code below or visit www.hodderplus.co.uk/indianhead/chapter-7.

Chakra balancing

We cannot avoid coming into contact with negative energy or feeling down sometimes, but we can help to change our feelings from negative to positive and to protect ourselves from harmful energy in the environment. Keeping our chakras in tip-top condition is the key – in other words, keeping them spinning in balance.

Study tip

Chakra balancing is a bit like spring-cleaning the chakras and fine-tuning them. No one is immune; it is therefore important to balance and cleanse the chakras regularly. This is particularly important for therapists, as they are exposed to a considerable amount of emotional energy from their clients, and in order to help their clients effectively their chakras need to be in balance to facilitate the right healing energies.

The technique of balancing or clearing your chakras is based on meditation, and is a relaxation and energy technique recognised for its rejuvenating and healing power. We know that chakras are non-physical centres; therefore you need a non-physical method to stimulate them. This is achieved by focusing your awareness in the area of a chakra and using your mind to manipulate it. You need a localised, mental opening effect in a chakra to stimulate it with your imaginary hands. By moving your point of awareness to the site of a chakra and causing a mental opening effect with your hands, you are directly stimulating the chakra.

There are many different methods of chakra balancing; it is a question of finding one that is effective for you. Some people use coloured crystals, as the energy vibrations of colours aid balancing; some use essential oils for their healing vibrations. Visualisation is powerful, as thought is energy. Affirmations made while chakra balancing create positive feelings. There are many specific exercises associated with each chakra and different books give suggestions for different exercises; find one that you feel intuitively attracted to and go with that (see the Further reading section on pages 287–9, and see also the chakra balancing exercise detailed below).

Whichever methods are used or combined, chakra balancing offers very positive results, improving your health and making you feel good about yourself.

The relevance of chakras to Indian head massage

An important part of Indian head massage treatment is the eastern tradition of balancing of the higher chakras (the throat chakra, the brow chakra, or third eye, and the crown chakra).

With stress and tension the chakras lose their ability to synchronise with one another and become unbalanced.

By placing the hands along the axis of the higher chakras, energy can be realigned and a sense of balance and harmony can be restored.

Activity

Chakra balancing exercise

First, it is important to do some relaxation and breathing exercises, meditate or do whatever you usually do to get centred. This method will only work effectively if you are in a peaceful and centred state.

Once centred, start to visualise your chakras. Do not worry if you feel you cannot see them perfectly in your mind. As you do this regularly, seeing them will become gradually clearer.

Start with the first charka (the root chakra). Visualise it in your mind. Use the colour (red) and see it as an orb. Look at it closely in your mind. Does it look clean and spotless, or do you see any spots?

If you feel you cannot see it, imagine whether it has spots or not. Your imagination is the key to everything spiritual and it is highly accurate in telling you what is there.

Now imagine a golden beam of light shining on your first chakra, removing any impurities or blockages and opening the chakra up to positive energy. Now try to feel the light shining on your chakra. It may be difficult to perceive it at first, but with practice you will soon feel a tingling sensation where your chakra is.

This golden beam is the light of universal energy, the power that flows through everything and gives it life. Allow your intuition to tell you when the light has done the job and burned away the dark spots and blockages. In most cases, under a minute is all the time that is necessary. With practice it will become more obvious.

Now work your way up the chakras, going through the same procedure and concentrating on each one individually: to the second chakra (sacral), visualising the colour orange, followed by the third chakra (solar plexus), visualising the colour yellow, to the fourth chakra (heart), visualising the colour green, to the fifth chakra (throat), visualising the colour blue, to the sixth chakra (third eye), visualising the colour indigo, working your way up to the seventh chakra (crown), visualising the colour violet. This whole procedure should take less than ten minutes.

Once you have purified your crown chakra, look at all seven chakras at once in your mind's eye, as a stack. Perceive whether they are all the same size or whether there are a few larger or smaller ones. Concentrate your energy to help balance them all to the same size and get all of the vortexes spinning in the same direction. Hold the image in your mind and 'imagine' them shifting to the same size, with the vortexes spinning in the same direction.

Chakra sensations

The sensations you will feel in your chakras can vary from a gentle warmth, a localised pressure or bubbling, a localised dizziness, a tingling, a gentle pulsing, to a heavier throbbing, or a combination of some or all of the above. The heavier the thrumming, the more active the chakra. If you place your hand on a chakra when it is active, you will actually feel the flesh pulsing.

You may feel a slight internal contracting, however, a feeling that is not muscular, while you are stimulating your chakras. This is the glands and nerve ganglia linked to the chakras contracting in response to the stimulation. This internal contracting is normal.

Note: you may feel a stronger sensation in some chakras and little or none in others. Concentrate on the lowest ones with the least sensation. This will help to balance the energy flow in the chakra systems.

Key fact

The base or root chakra is the master chakra and is the most important one to activate. This chakra is the doorway for the Kundalini energy. Unless this is opened sufficiently, the energy cannot flow into the other chakras.

Multiple-choice self-assessment questions

1. **Chakras are**
   a physical energy centres located about 2.5 cm away from the physical body
   b non-physical energy centres located about 2.5 cm away from the physical body
   c an energy field surrounding the physical body
   d an energy field surrounding the non-physical body.

2. **Which of the following statements is true in relation to chakras?**
   a Chakras do have a physical form.
   b With stress, chakras can become unbalanced.
   c There are six major chakras in the body.
   d Chakras relate to the flow of physical energy.

3. **The base chakra is associated with the colour**
   a indigo
   b violet
   c blue
   d red.

4. **The throat chakra is associated with**
   a creativity and sexuality
   b emotions and self-worth
   c communication and expression
   d memories and imagination.

5. **The colour to visualise in balancing the heart chakra is**
   a green
   b yellow
   c red
   d brown.

6. **Vishuddha is the name associated with which chakra?**
   a Throat
   b Brow
   c Sacral
   d Solar plexus

To see the answers, scan the QR code opposite or visit www.hodderplus.co.uk/indianhead/chapter-7. To access an interactive version of these multiple-choice self-assessment questions visit www.hodderplus.co.uk/indianhead/chapter-7.

To access an interactive crossword for this chapter visit www.hodderplus.co.uk/indianhead/chapter-7.

8 Stress management

Introduction

Stress is a common feature of modern life and is therefore something everyone experiences. Nobody is born knowing how to handle stress, and as there is no immunity from it, the best way to protect the body from the harmful effects of stress is to learn how to manage it.

Stress undermines the state of physical and emotional well-being; learning how to manage stress effectively can therefore help to maintain good health and vitality. It is now acknowledged that many medical conditions are stress-related, so more importance is being placed on being able to handle stress in order to improve health.

The increasing pressures of modern life have influenced the growth in popularity of holistic therapies such as Indian head massage, as the stress relief and relaxation provided by these treatments can be a major factor in helping clients to manage their stress themselves.

Learning objectives

By the end of this chapter, you will be able to relate the following to your work in Indian head massage:

- definition of stress
- different types of stress and how they affect the body
- recognising stress
- strategies to help clients to take control of and manage their own stress
- Indian head massage as a counterbalance to stress.

By the very nature of their work, holistic therapists are exposed to a considerable amount of emotional energy when dealing with clients. It is therefore important for them to be able to use stress management techniques in order to help both their clients and themselves.

Indian head massage can be a very effective treatment in counterbalancing some of the negative effects of stress. However, for long-term stress relief, clients often need to consider many other factors in their lives. This chapter considers the basic tools of stress management, from identifying the symptoms and causes to employing strategies for coping with stress.

Definition of stress

There is no conclusive definition of 'stress'. It is a difficult term to define, as stress means different things to different people. However, it can be said that stress is the adaptive response to the demands or pressures placed on an individual, and can involve any interference that disturbs a person's emotional and physical well-being. The stress becomes unacceptable when the pressures are beyond the control of the individual, and the results of the stress can then be harmful to others. Stress is therefore the imbalance between the demands of everyday life and the individual's ability to cope with them.

Stress can be positive in that it can act as a stimulus and increase levels of alertness, but it can also be negative when too much stress affects the ability to function effectively. It is the depth and number of stressors at any time that causes stress to become beyond control, which then requires the body to make adjustments to re-establish a normal balance.

Types of stress

Survival stress

This type of stress is when the body reacts to meet the demands of a physically or emotionally threatening situation. The reaction is mediated by the release of adrenaline and produces the so-called 'fight or flight' reaction.

This type of stress is positive in that it enables the body and mind to react quickly and effectively. It is only when the effects of adrenaline are long-term that it can lead to negative stress.

Internally generated stress

This type of stress is often caused by the view of or reaction to a situation, rather than the situation itself. Anxiety and worry can lead to negative thought processes and often leads to a feeling that circumstances are out of control.

There is a relationship between personality and stress, in particular with anxious and obsessional personalities. What may be stressful for one person may be enjoyable and exciting for another.

Work/lifestyle-related stress

Many stresses that are experienced may relate to work or lifestyle. In this context, stress may come from one or more of the following:

- having too much or too little work
- time pressures and deadlines
- demands of a job with limited resources
- insufficient working or living space
- disorganised working conditions
- limited time, to the detriment of leisure and family life
- pollution
- financial problems
- relationship problems
- ill health
- family situations, such as a birth, death, marriage or divorce.

Negative stress

This type of stress is caused by the inability to manage long-term stress.

How to recognise stress

Recognising stress can be very difficult. It is important to realise that as stress levels increase, the ability to recognise stress usually decreases. Stress can manifest itself in different ways, and symptoms may be presented in a number of different ways. These are discussed below.

Short-term physical stress signals

These are symptoms of survival stress, as the body adapts to situations that are perceived as a threat. Effects of short-term physical stress include an increased heartbeat, rapid breathing, increased sweating, tense muscles, dry mouth, frequency of urination and feeling of nausea.

While the effects of short-term physical stress may help you survive in a threatening situation, negative stress can result when the adrenaline is not put to this use. The effects of excess adrenaline can lead to anxiety, frustration, negative thinking, reduction in self-confidence and distraction, and may cause difficult situations to be seen as a threat rather than a challenge.

Long-term stress signals

Common complaints relating to long-term stress are back pain, headaches, aches and pains, excessive tiredness, digestive problems, frequent colds, skin eruptions and exacerbation of asthma. Stress and pressure can also lead to the following:

Internal stress signals

When the body is subjected to long-term stress, the mind becomes unable to think clearly and rationally about situations and problems. This can lead to feelings of anxiety, worry, confusion, feeling out of control or overwhelmed, restlessness, frustration, irritability, hostility, impatience and helplessness, and can also lead to depression and mood changes.

People who suffer from long-term stress may generally feel more lethargic, find difficulty sleeping, change their eating habits, rely more on medication, drink and smoke more frequently and have a reduced sex drive.

Behavioural stress signals

When people are under pressure this can be exhibited in some of the following ways: talking too fast, twitching and fiddling, being irritable, defensive, aggressive, irritated, critical and overreacting emotionally to situations. They may also find that they start becoming more forgetful, make more mistakes, are unable to concentrate, are unrealistic in their judgement and become unreasonably negative. Pressure may cause some people to neglect their personal appearance and spend increasing amounts of time absent from work.

If the body is subjected to excessive short-term stress, it may lead to ineffective performance, which should be treated as a warning sign; stress management strategies can be adopted to avoid the problem in the future. The effects of long-term stress, however, can be much more severe, as it can lead to extreme fatigue, exhaustion, burnout or even breakdown.

Summary of signs and symptoms of stress

Behavioural changes

People who suffer from stress may:

- be argumentative
- be less friendly
- become withdrawn
- avoid friends and relatives
- lose creativity
- work longer and harder and achieve less
- be reluctant to do their own job properly
- procrastinate.

Change of feelings

People who experience stress may:

- lose their sense of humour
- have a sense of being a failure
- lack self-esteem and have a cynical and bitter attitude
- experience irritability with conflict at home and work
- feel apathetic.

Change of thinking

Stress can cause people to:

- be rigid in their thinking, with resistance to change
- be suspicious
- have poor concentration
- feel like leaving a job or a relationship.

Physical changes

People who are stressed may:

- feel tired all the time
- experience sleep problems (usually poor sleep)
- be increasingly absent from work because of prolonged minor illnesses
- have aches and pains
- suffer backache
- experience headaches and migraine
- have indigestion
- hyperventilate
- have palpitations.

Mental health

The effects of stress can cause feelings of:

- anxiety
- depression
- fear of rejection.

Cognitive distortion

Individuals suffering from stress may view themselves in a distorted way:

- **jumping to conclusions**: even in the absence of proof, stressed individuals may jump to conclusions. They may assume that other people see them in a certain way, or they may anticipate that things will turn out badly and act as if their predictions are facts.
- **all or none**: this is the feeling that, if you fail in one way, you see yourself as a total failure. There is then the tendency to overgeneralise and see this single failure as proof of your life's failure.
- **mental filter**: this is when people pick out negative events and dwell on them to the exclusion of everything else. Eventually, the positive aspects of life become rejected and ignored.

Effects of stress on the body

When the body is placed under physical or psychological stress, it increases the production of certain hormones, such as cortisol and adrenaline. These hormones produce marked changes in the heart rate, blood pressure levels, metabolism and physical activity. While this physical action can help a person to function more effectively when under pressure for short periods of time, it can also be extremely damaging and debilitating in the long term.

Dr Hans Selye called the body's response to stress the 'general adaptation syndrome', which he suggested be divided into three stages:

- alarm
- resistance
- exhaustion.

Alarm stage

The alarm stage is the body's initial reaction to the perceived stressor. This involves the so-called fight or flight syndrome, which involves the sympathetic nervous system and the release of the hormones adrenaline and cortisol.

The effects on the body are to effect an alert response and include:

- increased heart rate
- increased breathing rate
- increased diversion of blood to the muscles and brain
- increase in perspiration
- increased release of glucose from the liver
- inhibited digestion.

The alarm stage allows the body to cope and respond, and when the threat is over the body returns to a state of balance through repair and rest (parasympathetic system). However, problems can start to occur when the restoration of balance does not happen because the body is not allowed to rest sufficiently, or due to perceived or real encounters with repeated stressful situations. Repeated alarm reactions can lead to symptoms such as breathlessness, a dry mouth, aching, a clenched jaw or fists, dizziness, palpitations and sweating.

Resistance stage

The resistance stage, which, through the secretion of the circulating hormones, allows the body to continue fighting long after the effects of the alarm reaction have dissipated. This eventually leads to symptoms of disease as the body's energy resources are drained without adequate recuperation and repair. Symptoms associated with the resistance stage include colds and flu, anxiety and depression, high blood pressure, chest pains, tiredness, insomnia, indigestion, headaches and migraine.

Exhaustion stage

The third stage is the exhaustion stage, which takes place if the stress response continues without relief and can result in organs becoming more and more compromised until the adaptation becomes degenerative.

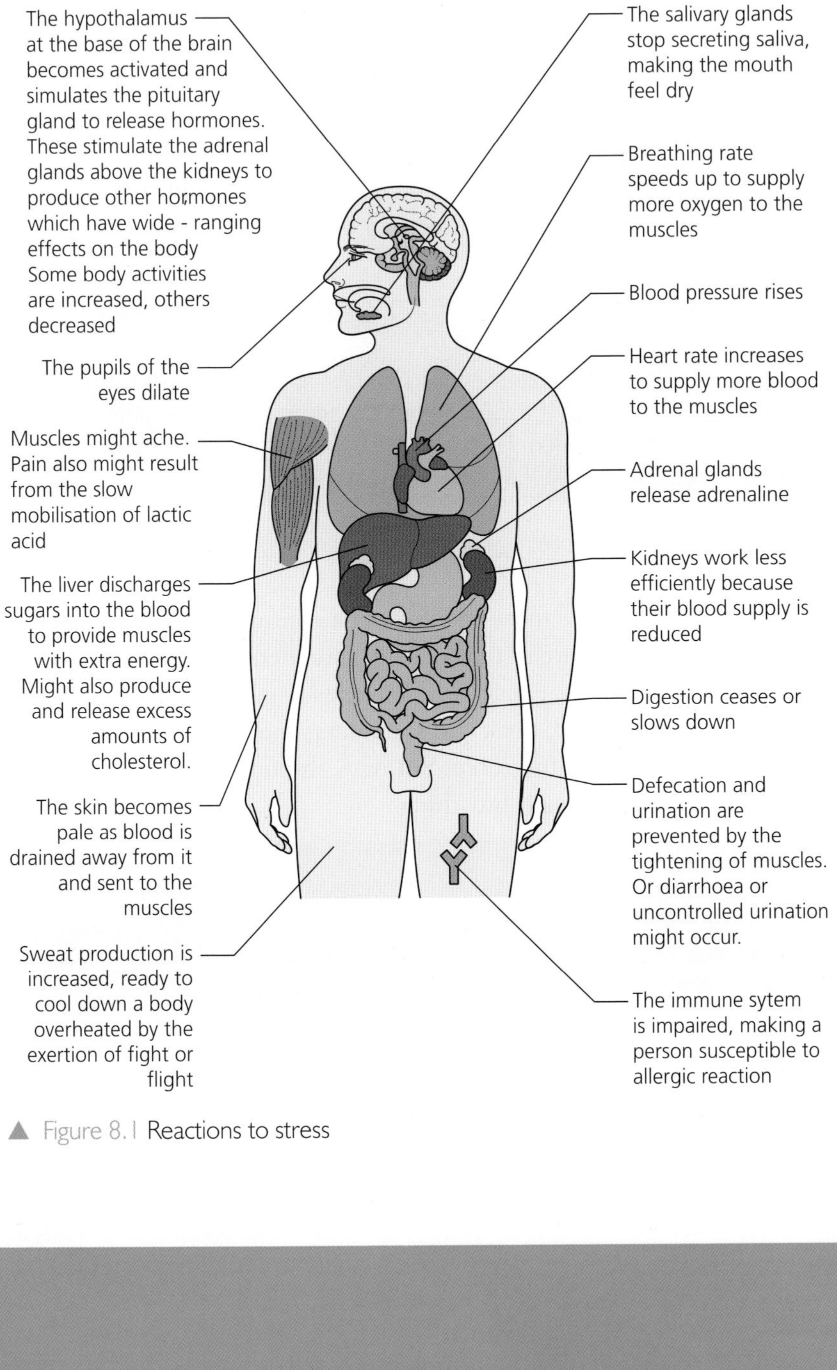
The hypothalamus at the base of the brain becomes activated and simulates the pituitary gland to release hormones. These stimulate the adrenal glands above the kidneys to produce other hormones which have wide - ranging effects on the body Some body activities are increased, others decreased
The pupils of the eyes dilate
Muscles might ache. Pain also might result from the slow mobilisation of lactic acid
The liver discharges sugars into the blood to provide muscles with extra energy. Might also produce and release excess amounts of cholesterol.
The skin becomes pale as blood is drained away from it and sent to the muscles
Sweat production is increased, ready to cool down a body overheated by the exertion of fight or flight
The salivary glands stop secreting saliva, making the mouth feel dry
Breathing rate speeds up to supply more oxygen to the muscles
Blood pressure rises
Heart rate increases to supply more blood to the muscles
Adrenal glands release adrenaline
Kidneys work less efficiently because their blood supply is reduced
Digestion ceases or slows down
Defecation and urination are prevented by the tightening of muscles. Or diarrhoea or uncontrolled urination might occur.
The immune sytem is impaired, making a person susceptible to allergic reaction

▲ Figure 8.1 Reactions to stress

> **Key fact**
>
> Increased cortisol secretion in stressful situations reduces the body's immune response, and the anti-inflammatory effect of cortisol can slow down healing too.

Areas of the body most vulnerable to stress

When the body is moving or stationary, a combination of muscle tension and relaxation exists in order to maintain posture. If a good balance is not achieved, the body suffers excessive muscle tension, which can cause pain and fatigue. If muscles are held tightly in a state of contraction, circulation is impeded, which results in a build-up of the products of fatigue. This can then result in muscular spasms, aches and pains.

When under stress, the entire body becomes tense and posture changes. Hours spent sitting and working at a desk can cause tension to accumulate in the upper body, particularly around the neck and shoulders. Large amounts of time spent in front of the computer screen can result in eye strain, where the eyes and surrounding muscles become tired.

Being tense and in a permanent state of alert can be uncomfortable and has the ability to throw the body out of balance. Tension uses up energy, but the energy is unproductive. Muscle tension can also affect our ability to function well, as it makes our thought processes less efficient.

> **Key fact**
>
> Tension can also have a debilitating effect on the immune system, predisposing people to colds and other diseases, because when we are in a constant state of alert, healing and tissue repair are inhibited. The key to stress relief is therefore relaxation, as healing can only take place when the body is at rest.

Shoulders

The shoulders are the place where most people hold a considerable amount of tension. When the body is in a state of tension, the shoulders are lifted towards the ears and often remain this way, causing the muscles to go into spasm. This restricts the blood flow to the head, neck and shoulders, and causes the neck and shoulders to become stiff and inflexible. Sitting with hunched shoulders can reduce chest capacity and thus impair breathing.

> **Key fact**
>
> Indian head massage can help to counterbalance the effects of stress by relaxing the shoulders; they will then drop and allow the energy to flow more freely to the area, encouraging deeper and easier breathing and improved joint flexibility

Upper arms

The upper arms are important for upper body movement; when the shoulders are tense, they tighten and restrict movement. When in a state of tension, the upper arms tend to hug the chest either at the sides or in front, while the elbows bend up.

Key fact

Indian head massage can help reduce tension and tightness in the upper arm muscles to help improve flexibility of the arms and shoulders.

Neck

When the body is balanced, the neck is designed to allow the head to move in a variety of directions. When the body is out of balance and under stress, the head tends to come forwards and the chin juts out. This then throws the body out of alignment, as the neck muscles tense and take the weight of the head. The neck muscles are then in a permanent state of contraction and can cause the neck to become stiff and tight. This tension then reduces mobility of the neck and shoulders.

Key fact

Working on the neck with Indian head massage helps to open up the energy flow from the spine to the whole head and can help to reduce tension and improve posture by realigning the muscles, thereby increasing mobility and allowing the head to move more freely.

Head

The face is an area of the body that cannot help but show tension; the jaw clamps tight, teeth grind together and the lips tighten. The scalp and temporal muscles tighten when under stress, restricting the blood flow and leading to headaches, eye strain, and neck and shoulder tension.

When the body is in balance it facilitates relaxation and a positive mental outlook, which are critical to successful stress management. If the shoulders and chest are free of tension, the ribs are free to allow deep, relaxed breathing; if the head and neck are well balanced they can support the shoulders and take pressure from the neck muscles.

The body is ideally equipped to deal with many different types of stressors; however, the ability to deal with stress can be inhibited by a heavy load of unresolved stress, which contributes to the development of disease and pain.

Key fact

Indian head massage helps to counterbalance stress in the head by improving the circulation and relaxing the muscles and nerve fibres, thereby relieving tension.

Stress-related disorders

Stress is considered to be a contributory factor in many conditions. Listed below are areas susceptible to stress-related diseases:

- skin: as the skin is often a manifestation of what is felt inside, skin disorders such as eczema and psoriasis are often exacerbated by stress; allergies may also be triggered by stress
- hair: some forms of hair loss are linked to stress

- heart: high blood pressure and conditions such as angina may be exacerbated by stress; if the blood supply to the heart is restricted by arteriosclerosis and the person's life is very stressful, a heart attack can result
- lungs: symptoms of asthma often worsen when the body is subjected to high levels of emotional stress
- muscles: muscle tension is often the result of stress
- brain: anxiety and depression may be triggered by stress
- reproductive: the reproductive hormones are reduced at times of stress; this is evidenced by stress-related problems such as infertility and menstrual disorders
- digestion: conditions that may be aggravated by stress include ulcers and irritable bowel syndrome.

Adaptation to stress

Fortunately, the body has the capacity to cope with stress, as the purpose of all the body's systems is to maintain a constant internal environment through homeostasis.

However, there are several factors that may affect the body's ability to deal with stress, including:

- genetics: the effects of stress on the body can be determined by genetic make-up and can dictate how well different organs respond and adapt to stressful situations
- physiological reserve: the body's response to stress depends on the ability to increase or decrease function according to its needs. If the ability of an organ to respond is diminished, it is difficult for the body to maintain homeostasis; even with small demands, imbalance and disease may ensue
- age: with age, the ability to adapt is diminished, and while a young, healthy individual may respond and adapt to stress easily, an elderly client may find the situation considerably more stressful
- health status: clients who are mentally and physically fit are able to adapt to stress placed on them more easily than those who are not fit
- nutrition: deficiencies or excesses of nutrition can impair one's ability to adapt to stressful situations
- sleep: irregular sleep patterns and wakefulness can reduce immunity as well as physical and psychological functions; sleep is important for restoring energy, and if sleep is inadequate, it can impair the body's ability to deal with stress
- psychological factors: psychological conditions such as anxiety and depression can make a person more susceptible to stress.

Knowledge check

1. What is the definition of stress?
2. What is the difference between survival stress signals and internally generated stress signals?
3. List six potential sources of stress.
4. List four short-term stress signals.
5. List four long-term stress signals.
6. List four factors that may affect a person's ability to cope with stress.

To see the answers to this knowledge check, scan the QR code below or visit www.hodderplus.co.uk/indianhead/chapter-8.

Managing stress

In order to be able to work towards preventing stress, it is important to be able to identify its causes. Part of the problem with stress is its familiarity; as people become used to living with stress, they may be unaware of how it is affecting them or those around them.

Mental attitude is a critical factor in dealing with stress, along with finding ways of reducing the effects of stress. Focusing on the ownership of the sources of the stress and not on the feelings they generate is the first step to counterbalancing it. Stress management can be approached in several different ways, and a client's stress management programme may typically consist of experiencing a range of holistic therapies, the use of relaxation and stress reduction techniques, as well as implementing lifestyle changes.

Holistic therapists can help clients to recognise their own stress by advising on ways in which they can combat it and start to manage their own stress positively. Stress management has to take into account the recognition of an individual's vulnerability to stress and their ability to be aware of possible sources of stress and to identify signs and symptoms of stress. What is most important is helping clients to learn how to manage stress and be able to identify the factors that contribute to it and so be able to control it.

Optimum stress levels

Stress levels vary, like any other human characteristic, and what may seem challenging and exciting to one person may seem stressful and threatening to another. The most positive approach to successful stress management is finding an optimum stress level in which the body can be sufficiently stimulated to perform well, while not becoming overstressed and unhappy.

The most effective way of finding an optimum level of stress is to keep a stress diary for a short period of time in order to identify what is causing the stress and whether it is being controlled effectively. The type of information that could be recorded in a stress diary is the stressful event and time, how stressful the event was (on a scale of one to ten), what made the event stressful and how the situation was handled. This can be the key to identifying whether it was the cause that was tackled or the symptom.

When analysing a stress diary, it should be possible to extract the following information:

- the level of stress that is optimum for an individual
- the main sources of unpleasant or negative stress, and whether the strategies for managing them are effective or not.

Key fact

It is important that each individual is able to monitor their own stress levels. Some people may operate most effectively at a low level of stress, while this may leave another person feeling bored or unmotivated. Alternatively, someone who performs only moderately at low level may find they excel at a high level when they are under more pressure.

Managing stress effectively

Once there is an understanding or recognition of what is causing the stress and the level of stress under which an individual can work effectively, the next stage is to work out how to manage the stress. An action plan for managing stress might include:

- controlling or eliminating the problems that are causing the stress
- using stress reduction techniques
- making lifestyle changes
- taking a holiday or break more often
- social and family support
- time management

- hobbies and leisure time
- being prepared to ask for help
- looking back at action taken and evaluating the effects.

Stress reduction techniques

When choosing methods for stress reduction, different strategies may be required for different people and different circumstances.

The main objective in managing stress is to help the client to improve the quality of their life and their resistance to stress by employing certain techniques, as well as making certain lifestyle changes. It is important to realise that as people react differently to stress, different techniques or combinations of techniques may be required for each individual. Stress can only be eliminated if the root causes are recognised and resolved. However, there are ways in which the unpleasant effects of stress may be reduced.

Relaxation techniques

Physical relaxation is something that often appears easy, but in reality it is a skill that needs to be learned and practised. By teaching clients physical relaxation techniques, you can help them to take responsibility for their stress reactions and reduce the distress of many conditions.

Tensing muscles and holding breath when tense becomes habitual; the key to relaxation is training the body to feel tension and recognise when breathing reflects tension. The body's reaction to stress involves breathing and muscle tension – the parts over which a person can gain control. The aim of relaxation is to control breathing and muscle tension in order to calm the mind and body.

Through learning physical relaxation, a person can learn to slow down their breathing, breathe deeply and relax their muscles. As the relaxation response starts to happen, other responses change automatically; and as the breathing calms down and the muscles relax, the heart rate simultaneously slows down. With relaxation, the key is in gaining control over breathing and muscles: the rest will happen automatically as the body responds positively to being in a state of relaxation.

Relaxation can help to:

- maintain emotional and physical health
- aid restful sleep
- reduce the harmful effects of stress
- relieve muscular tension
- promote optimum oxygen levels for the body
- aid the body to recover and repair.

Breathing

Deep breathing is a very effective method of relaxation and works well combined with other relaxation techniques such as relaxation imagery, meditation and progressive muscular relaxation.

On inhaling, the intercostal muscles, abdominal muscles and the diaphragm contract in order to increase the volume of the thoracic cavity, which causes air to pass into the lungs. While the breath is held, all these muscles remain tensed.

When they relax, the volume of the thoracic cavity decreases as the muscles return to their original relaxed position. Comfortable, healthy breathing brings air down into the depth of the lungs and the body is able to relax as the breath is let out. When the body is still tense, breathing becomes fast and the muscles in the upper part of the chest take over, to cause panting.

The experience of any physical or emotional stress will affect breathing. At times of stress, breathing becomes shallow and irregular, resulting in the brain being deprived of sufficient oxygen. This leads to a feeling of dizziness, inability to concentrate, and agitation. Learning how to breathe deeply helps to fill the body with positive energy and clears the mind. It can also help to prevent a person from getting stressed, or can help them gain control more quickly when they are feeling stressed.

Most people use only half of their lung capacity and breathe with their chest and not their diaphragm. Below are two breathing exercises that may be taught to clients for self-help. It is important for clients to practise breathing exercises regularly, in order that they may be prepared to use them the next time they feel anxious and stressed.

Health and safety note

After completing breathing exercises, clients should be advised to wait a few moments before getting up, in order to avoid dizziness.

Breathing exercises for successful stress control

Breathing exercise 1

1. Sit in a comfortable position and loosen tight clothing.
2. Place one hand on the chest and the other across the stomach.
3. Inhale deeply through the nose to fill the upper chest cavity and down to the lower part of the lungs, as if breathing into the stomach for a count of six.
4. Exhale slowly to a count of 12, allowing the air to escape from the top of your lungs before the lower part deflates.
5. Repeat this exercise six to eight times.

Breathing exercise 2

1. Apply the first two fingers of the right hand to the side of the right nostril and press gently to close it.
2. Breathe in slowly through the left nostril and hold for a count of three.
3. Transfer the first two fingers to the left nostril to close it.
4. Breathe out slowly through the right nostril on a count of three. Breathe in through the right nostril and hold for a count of three; while holding, transfer the fingers to the right nostril and breathe out.
5. Repeat the exercise six times.

Correct breathing is something that really needs to be practised often, until it feels natural; it may then be utilised as a counterbalance to stress. Breathing properly enables the body to relax and regain its natural balance, while calming the mind. If a client has difficulty breathing correctly, it may be advisable for them to attend classes that involve structured breathing, such as yoga.

The effects of poor breathing on the body can be damaging in that it:

- weakens the nervous system
- encourages muscle tension

- starves the body of nutrients
- blocks the circulation
- weakens the immune system
- disturbs digestion.

Progressive muscular relaxation

This is a physical technique designed to relax the body when it is tense. It may be applied to any group of muscles in the body, depending on whether one area is tense or whether it is the whole body.

Progressive muscular relaxation is achieved by tensing a group of muscles so that they are as tightly contracted as possible. The muscles are held in a state of tension for a few seconds and then relaxed. This should result in a feeling of deep relaxation in the muscles.

For maximum effect, this exercise should be combined with breathing exercises and imagery (such as the image of stress leaving the body).

Relaxation exercise

1. Find a place where you can feel comfortable.
2. Close your eyes and pull your feet towards you as far as you can; hold them for a count of five and then let them relax – let them drop as if you are a puppet on a string and the string had broken.
3. Curl your toes as if you were holding a pencil, hold them for a count of five and then relax.
4. Tighten and tense the calf muscles, count to five and then relax.
5. Tighten and tense the thighs, press them tightly together, count to five and then relax, allowing them to fall apart.
6. Tighten the abdominal muscles, pulling in the muscles, count to five and then relax.
7. Tighten the muscles in the hips and the buttocks, count to five and then relax.
8. Arch the back and tense the back muscles, count to five and then relax.
9. Tense the shoulders by raising them to the ears, count to five and then drop them.
10. Lift your arms up with the hands outstretched, as if you were reaching for something. Hold for a slow count of five and then let the arms drop down.
11. Tense the muscles in the forehead, count to five and then relax.
12. Tense the muscles around the eyes tightly, count to five and then relax.
13. Tense the muscles in the jaw and cheeks (as if gritting your teeth), hold for five and then relax.
14. By now you should feel relaxed and heavy, as if you are sinking into the floor or chair.
15. Check that all body parts are free from tension; if there are any areas left with tension, hold that part tense again before relaxing.
16. When you are ready, get up gradually, taking your time.

Note: this exercise will be easier to do if the instructions are on CD or downloaded to an iPod, preferably spoken by a person with a slow, calm and relaxing voice.

Imagery and visualisation

Imagery techniques can be useful in recreating a retreat from stress and pressure, by imagining a place or event that was happy and restful, and calling on it to help manage a stressful period.

Imagery and visualisation are often more effective and real if combined with sounds, smell, taste and warmth. It is important to realise that visualisation is a very individual skill. Clients should be encouraged to call on a happy experience and to gear their visualisation towards that image. Imagery and visualisation can often be enhanced by a relaxation tape, which may be played while the client is receiving treatment and can be purchased for home use.

Meditation

This is a very effective way of relaxing. The idea is to focus your thoughts on relaxing for a period of time, leaving the mind and body to recover from the problems and worries that have caused the stress. Meditation can help to reduce stress by slowing down breathing, helping muscular relaxation, reducing blood pressure, and encouraging clear thinking by focusing and concentrating the mind. The key to meditation is to quieten the mind and focus completely on one thing. With meditation, it is important for the body to be relaxed and in a comfortable position.

Meditation is a very personal experience and can involve a person sitting or lying quietly and focusing the mind, or it can be taught in a class situation. Therapists may also facilitate meditation by using positive mental imagery and visualisation, in order to help clients focus their minds and lift themselves into a state of passive awareness in order to relax.

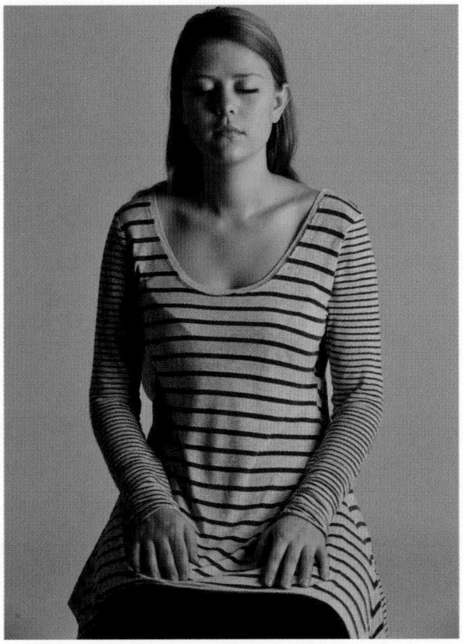

▲ Figure 8.2 Meditation

Relaxing at work

When a person spends hours sitting at a desk, driving or in meetings, tension can accumulate in the areas of the body most vulnerable to stress, such as the head, neck and shoulders. Using a simple relaxation routine while at work can help to release tension, reduce stress and renew the body's energy to carry on working effectively.

Start by loosening any tight clothing (collar, tie, scarf) and removing your shoes.

Five-minute stress reliever

Sit comfortably, with your back supported against the back of the chair, your feet firmly on the ground and your hands and arms open and relaxed and supported by armrests.

1. With a deep breath in, raise the shoulders towards the ears and hold them raised for a few seconds (be aware of the tension that may be accumulating in the shoulders); now take a long slow breath out and drop the shoulders down. Repeat this exercise several times.
2. Now lift your right shoulder and slowly pop it backwards several times, ensuring that the arms are kept loose and relaxed. Repeat the exercise with the left shoulder. Now pop both shoulders together. Repeat several times.
3. Place your left hand on your right shoulder, squeeze gently and then release. Repeat the exercise down the right arm to the elbow. Repeat several times. Now place your right hand on your left shoulder and repeat the exercise.
4. Place your hands over your shoulders. As you exhale, let your head fall backwards and slowly draw your fingers over the clavicles (collar bones). Repeat several times.
5. Place your hands over the top of your head and pull your head gently downwards, feeling the slight stretch in the back of the neck. Hold this position for several seconds and then repeat.
6. Place the fingers of both hands at the base of your skull; apply slow circular pressure from the base of the skull and behind the ears, gradually working down the neck. Repeat several times.
7. Exhale and turn the head to the right side. Hold there for a few seconds and use the right hand to massage the left side of the neck from behind the ear down to the clavicle (collar bone). Repeat the exercise on the other side of the neck.
8. Now close your eyes and relax the muscles in your face. Be aware of your eye muscles, your jaw and your forehead. Place the fingers of both hands on each side of the temples and slowly massage in a circular motion, repeating several times.
9. Place the fingertips of both hands in the centre of the forehead and perform slow, circular movements with both hands, working out towards the temples. Repeat several times.
10. Finish by cupping your hands over your eyes and holding for several seconds. This helps to release tension and tightness left in the face.

Clients can be encouraged to practise these exercises at least once a day during a break, and they may use individual exercises whenever they start to feel tense, to avoid stress building up.

Stress management is something that needs to be assessed in a holistic way, and will undoubtedly involve many other factors; these are outlined below.

Welcoming change

It is important to realise that in implementing a stress management programme, there will be an element of change, and success will often depend on adaptation to change. Changes in circumstances and lifestyle can be stressful; however, it is often the anticipation of the change that is more stressful than the change itself.

Attitude to stress

Attitude is a fundamental factor in stress management. A negative attitude can cause stress by alienating and irritating other people, whereas a positive attitude can help to draw the positive elements out of a situation and can make life more pleasurable and stress more manageable.

When the body is under stress, it is very easy to lose perspective; relatively minor problems can be perceived as threatening and intimidating. When faced with a seemingly overwhelming problem, it may help to view the problem in a different way – for instance, as a challenge or seeing what may be learned from it, whatever the outcome.

Study tip

It is important to be able to view mistakes as learning experiences, and realise that if something has been learned from an experience, then it has a positive value. Learning how to change the response to stress can help to transform it from a negative to a positive experience.

It may help to talk to someone who has had similar problems, or write the problem down in order to help put it into perspective. It is often helpful to break the problem down in order that it may be reduced to a smaller, more manageable size.

Positive thinking/cognitive therapy

Negative thoughts can cause stress, as they can damage confidence and harm effective performance by stifling rational thoughts. Common negative thoughts are feelings of inadequacy, self-criticism, dwelling on past mistakes and worrying about how you appear to others.

Awareness of negative thoughts can be the first step to counterbalancing stress. It is important to write negative thoughts down and review them rationally, deciding whether they are based on reality. It is useful to counter negative thoughts with positive affirmations in order to change a negative thought into a positive one, such as 'I can do this'.

Stress from the environment

Disorganised living and working conditions can be a major source of stress. A well-organised and pleasant environment can usually make a large contribution to reducing stress and increasing productivity. Stress may be reduced in the environment by improving air quality, lighting, decoration, untidiness and noise levels. Natural light can lift mood and help to prevent eye strain. Creating order out of disorder can help to clear a space mentally and physically in order to regain a state of calm.

When working in an office, it is advisable to consider the ergonomics of furniture as a potential source of stress. If you are working at a computer station, your chair should be checked for comfort and height, and the keyboard and monitor comfortably positioned and at the right height. Taking a short break from computer/desk work every hour or so can help to prevent tension and eye strain from building up.

Health and nutrition

Eating an unbalanced diet can cause stress to the body by depriving it of essential nutrients. Eating a well-balanced diet can help to eliminate chemical stress that may be caused by consumption of too much caffeine, too much alcohol, smoking, and food with high levels of sugar and salt.

Drinking more water may help to increase energy levels and the resistance to stress, by clearing toxins from the bloodstream. Eating sensible, well-balanced meals can help to calm or energise the mind and body and counteract the effects of stress. The best defence against negative stress is a healthy and nutritious diet.

Implementing the following guidelines with diet and nutrition can help towards successful stress control:

- take time out to eat properly (avoid working lunches)
- eat slowly and chew food well to aid digestion
- rest for a few minutes after eating
- eat fresh food to provide the body with essential vitamins and minerals
- avoid eating late at night to allow the body time to digest food properly
- avoid overeating, as it will decrease energy levels
- avoid eating if you are feeling angry, agitated or upset (practise relaxation techniques before eating).

A healthy diet to help beat stress will consist of:

- eating foods rich in vitamins, such as citrus fruits and dark green, leafy vegetables
- eating foods rich in vitamin A and folic acid
- cutting back on alcohol, caffeine, refined sugars, salt and saturated fats
- eating iron-rich foods, such as dried beans, peas and leafy green vegetables
- eating foods high in zinc and magnesium (seafood, wholegrains and dried beans)
- eating balanced amounts of protein, fat and carbohydrates to help provide the body with energy to be able to cope with stress
- eating plenty of whole, unprocessed foods (wholegrain bread and cereals, dried beans and peas, fresh fruit and vegetables, low-fat milk)
- drinking at least two pints of water a day.

Exercise

Taking frequent exercise is one way of reducing stress, as it helps to improve your health, relaxes tense muscles, relaxes the mind and helps induce sleep. Exercise can help to accelerate the flow of blood through the brain, helping the brain to function more clearly, and will remove waste products that have built up as a result of intensive mental energy. Exercise also releases chemicals called endorphins into the bloodstream that give a feeling of well-being.

When considering incorporating exercise into a stress management programme, thought should be given to the type of exercise and its suitability to the individual; if it is difficult or unenjoyable, it may cause stress and may not be continued long enough to produce long-term benefits.

Taking time out

A successful way of reducing long-term stress is to take up a hobby where there is little or no pressure for performance. Long-term stress can also be reduced by taking time out for undirected activities, such as reading a book, taking a walk, having a long bath or listening to music. It is important to take regular holidays or breaks in order to refresh mind and body and recharge energy levels. Taking a break can also help put problems into perspective.

Managing relationships (home and work)

Stress can be caused by relationships with other people, and although it is not possible to change a person's personality, a change of attitude will often determine the amount of stress experienced from the situation.

A useful technique to employ when dealing with other people is to try to understand the way they think and why they feel the way they do. Unfortunately, it is human nature that people will often attempt to exploit a relationship at the expense of another person. In this case, it is important to project the right approach – by being positive and pleasant, but assertive.

When dealing with a difficult, annoying or frustrating person, it is always a good policy to stay calm and neutral (take deep breaths) in order to be able to think more clearly and react more rationally. It is also important to be able to respect other people's opinions and to accept that some people or situations may not change.

Indian head massage as an antidote to stress

Holistic therapies such as Indian head massage can help clients to manage their stress, as they provide a period of time away from everyday stresses in order to relax and regain a sense of physical and emotional balance. A combination of relaxation and a holistic therapy programme can relieve tension and stress and allow the body energies to flow more freely. When the body reaches a state of relaxation, tense muscles start to unknot, blood pressure starts to lower, breathing becomes more regular and deeper, and the mind drifts into a state of passive awareness.

Indian head massage is particularly effective as an antidote to stress, as it relaxes and revitalises the mind and body, and can help with anxiety, tension and many stress-related conditions.

Key fact

It is unhealthy for a client to become reliant on a holistic therapist for their problems and see the therapist as the one to provide a solution to their stress. The key to successful stress management is for clients to be able to recognise their own stress and for the therapist to help guide them in managing it.

Other professional help

Although holistic therapies can provide a positive counterbalance to the negative effects of stress, it is important that a client does not become dependent on a therapist for any advice or service, other than that which is associated with the chosen treatment. Clients may need to consult another professional – for instance, if the client is deeply depressed, they may need to be referred to their GP or to a counsellor.

Study tip

Therapists should always take care to ensure that they remain objective with clients at all times, and realise that by not taking responsibility for the client's problems they are in fact helping the client to help themselves.

Time management

By employing time management skills effectively, time can be utilised in the most productive and effective way. Time management can help to reduce stress by increasing productivity, therefore allowing more time to relax outside work activities.

The important factor in time management is to concentrate on results and not on activity. This can be achieved by:

- assessing the value of your time and how it may be used most effectively
- focusing on priorities, while deciding which tasks can be delegated and which may be dropped
- managing and avoiding distractions
- finishing work that has been started and working systematically
- learning when to say no and avoiding feeling guilty for doing so
- avoiding being someone else's time problem and reducing commitments
- having a planner for the weeks of the year, including a plan for holidays and leisure.

This can help to reduce the effects of long-term stress by helping to put things back into perspective, giving a feeling of control and direction, and freeing up more quality time for relaxation and enjoyment of life outside work.

Evaluating stress from experience

In a stress management programme, it is important to look back and reassess in order to plan for the future. Planning ahead can help you to manage stress more effectively, rather than waiting for the distress signals. It is always useful to look back on a stressful situation, in order to assess whether it was dealt with successfully and decide what could be repeated or what needs to be changed.

Stress management in the workplace

Stress is a significant factor, costing billions of pounds a year, as it is thought that 60 per cent of absenteeism in the workplace is caused by stress-related disorders.

Over the last century, ever-increasing technological changes led to a faster pace of life and to an individual being required to perform the job descriptions that might previously have been assigned to several people.

Stress occurs when the body is required to perform beyond its normal range of capabilities; the net results of this can be harmful to both individuals and organisations. It is also important to realise that stress can be a motivator and that people need a certain amount of pressure in order to stimulate them into action. Positive stress is the type of stress that gives the body a kick-start when needed. It is a known fact that people with too much time on their hands and not enough stimulus suffer from symptoms of stress, just as those do who have too much work and too little time.

Companies are starting to realise that their staff members are more productive when they are able to deal with stress creatively, and any factors that can help to reduce the damaging effects of stress can make the workforce happier and increase productivity.

An action plan for stress management at work might include the following:

- learn to recognise the warning signals of stress and act on them in order to start taking control of stress responses
- enlist the support of colleagues and do not be afraid to talk about stressful situations in order to relieve some of the feeling of pressure
- take regular breaks away from the desk or workspace and get some fresh air (even if it means opening a window or door)
- pay attention to the ergonomics of office furniture and try to keep your workspace uncluttered
- eat healthily and regularly
- eat slowly and digest food properly
- learn to delegate and use time management skills – making lists and prioritising
- keep a stress diary, noting the days when high stress levels are experienced, and learn from this to help counterbalance the negative effects in the future
- set realistic goals to avoid the stress of failing to meet an unrealistic deadline
- concentrate on one task at a time
- pause after completing one task before starting another
- plan activities for days off
- try to view problems as challenges and opportunities
- think positively – negative thought processes can be disabling and very destructive
- learn to see the funny side of stressful situations
- look after yourself
- use relaxation techniques regularly.

Indian head massage as a counterbalance to stress in the workplace

Many companies and individuals are now aware of the costs that negative stress can have on their company and their staff. Staff illness can lead to reduced productivity and increased pressure being placed on other individuals, leading to low morale and high staff turnover. Frequent complaints of work-related stress include the following:

'My neck and shoulders ache constantly from using the phone all day.'

'I frequently suffer from headaches at work and feel under pressure all the time to meet tight deadlines.'

'I never have time for a lunch hour as there is always too much work and not enough time to complete it in.'

'I feel stressed out and tired before I even start work and am too exhausted to enjoy a social life.'

Comments like those above sound all too familiar to those suffering from the negative effects of stress at work, who could benefit from stress reduction techniques.

Some organisations have occupational health advisors, who look after the welfare of their staff and are interested in ways in which staff stress levels may be managed effectively. Indian head massage is well suited to the work environment due to its portable nature. An area of the workplace (preferably private) can be assigned for the treatment, which is performed in an ordinary chair and is short enough in duration to be slotted into a break or lunch hour. It is also advantageous in that the client does not have to undress.

The benefits of Indian head massage to organisations and individuals are that it helps to:

- increase staff morale by alleviating depression and anxiety
- relieve stress and muscular tension
- relieve headaches, neck and backache
- relieve eye strain
- relieve mental and physical strain
- improve concentration levels, memory and mental alertness
- increase energy levels to improve productivity.

Multiple-choice self-assessment questions

1. **Which of the following statements is *false*?**
   - a Stress is the imbalance between the demands of everyday life and the ability to cope.
   - b Too much stress can affect a person's ability to function effectively.
   - c Stress is caused by external pressures, such as work.
   - d Stress can involve any interference that disturbs a person's emotional and physical well-being.
2. **Which of the following is a symptom of short-term stress?**
   - a Rapid breathing
   - b Digestive problems
   - c Excessive tiredness
   - d Mood changes
3. **Which hormone increases in production when the body is under stress?**
   - a Thyroxine
   - b Adrenaline
   - c Oestrogen
   - d Oxytocin
4. **Which of the following factors may affect the body's capacity to deal with stress effectively?**
   - a Age
   - b Psychological factors
   - c Physiological reserve
   - d All of the above
5. **Which of the following effects on the body are associated with the alarm stage of stress, as defined by Dr Hans Selye?**
   - a Increased heart and ventilation rate
   - b Colds and flu
   - c High blood pressure
   - d Anxiety and depression
6. **Which of the following is a symptom of long-term stress?**
   - a Dry mouth
   - b Headaches
   - c Nausea
   - d Increased sweating
7. **The best way to protect the body from the harmful effects of stress is to**
   - a learn how to avoid it
   - b learn how to manage it
   - c take your anger out on inanimate objects
   - d take a long walk and bottle up your frustration.
8. **Extreme fatigue, exhaustion and burnout are all signs of**
   - a short-term stress
   - b long-term stress
   - c behavioural stress
   - d emotional stress.
9. **The type of stress when the body reacts to meet the demands of a physically or emotionally threatening situation is known as**
   - a survival stress
   - b negative stress
   - c work-related stress
   - d internally generated stress.
10. **Which of the following statements is *false* in relation to stress?**
    - a When under stress, the entire body becomes tense and posture changes.
    - b Large amounts of time spent in front of a computer can result in eye-strain headaches.
    - c Tension uses up energy, but the energy is largely productive.
    - d Muscle tension affects our ability to function well.

To see the answers, visit www.hodderplus.co.uk/indianhead/chapter-8. To access an interactive version of these multiple-choice self-assessment questions visit www.hodderplus.co.uk/indianhead/chapter-8.

To access an interactive crossword for this chapter visit www.hodderplus.co.uk/indianhead/chapter-8.

9 Health, safety, security and employment standards

Introduction

In order to be fully competent in their working role, a therapist is required to support and maintain workplace standards and codes of practice. This role covers following health, safety and security procedures when providing services to the general public, and safeguarding their own safety and that of their colleagues and clients.

The success of a therapist lies not only in their ability to perform their own job roles effectively, but also to be able to contribute to the overall efficiency and operation of a business, on which their livelihood ultimately depends.

Learning objectives

By the end of this chapter you will be able to understand and apply the following knowledge to your workplace practice:

- workplace standards and industry codes of practice
- hygienic precautions required for the professional practice of Indian head massage
- health, safety and security procedures in the workplace
- professional codes of practice in the workplace
- supporting and maintaining efficient workplace services and operations
- the implications of relevant legislation in relation to Indian head massage.

Workplace standards and industry code of practice

A therapist carrying out the professional practice of Indian head massage needs to understand that their work activities and responsibilities must comply with the individual establishment rules in which they are working.

Establishment rules lay down a benchmark of standards required by the workplace and are set according to the requirements of the individual business. They will include codes of professional dress, conduct and specific responsibilities. Below is an example of an establishment's rules.

Establishment rules

It is each therapist's responsibility to ensure that the following procedures and regulations are observed and adhered to during salon operational periods. These duties are required in line with establishment rules, health and safety policies, local by-laws and awarding body guidelines.

Professional appearance

Workwear

All therapists must wear professional workwear for ALL practical sessions in the salon, in order to present a professional image of the establishment and to maintain hygiene.

Footwear

Footwear should be low-heeled, comfortable, clean, enclosed at the toes and of smart and professional appearance. This is for health, safety and hygienic reasons.

Hair

Hair should be clean, neatly styled and secured away from the face. It is important to tie back long hair for hygienic and practical reasons.

Jewellery and accessories

Hands and arms should be bare of jewellery, other than a wedding band. All other jewellery must be unobtrusive.

Jewellery has the potential to harbour germs and is not considered to be hygienic.

Hands

These should be kept as soft as possible and protected from harsh chemicals. Nails must be kept short and without nail enamel.

Personal hygiene

Due to the close nature of therapy treatments, close attention should be paid to maintaining personal hygiene to avoid offending a client by having bad breath or body odour. Attention is also drawn to the need to avoid strong-smelling foods, smoking and the wearing of highly scented products when in close contact with clients.

Professional conduct

Therapists should adopt a professional attitude to clients, colleagues and staff at all times. This will include adherence to establishment rules and workplace policies, including being punctual and ready for work, in order to promote a continuity of professional service within the workplace.

All therapists need to observe the salon's code of ethics at all times.

Damages, breakages and accidents

All incidents, including damages, breakages or accidents, must be reported to the salon manager. All accidents must be recorded in the accident book.

Health and safety note

Nail enamel must be removed as a client may be allergic to it and nails may be harbouring germs underneath it.

Hands must be cleansed immediately before and after physical contact with the client.

Health and safety note

All therapists are reminded of the importance of health and safety and hygiene precautions, and these must be observed at all times in accordance with the specific treatment/s provided.

Liaising with colleagues

All therapists are to contribute to the efficiency of the salon's operation by assisting colleagues and informing them of any changes in procedures (client running late/client arriving early/client cancelled, and so on).

Security

Windows and doors

Please ensure that all windows and doors are secured at the end of each session.

Personal belongings

The salon is unable to accept liability for loss or damage to personal possessions while on the premises. Therapists must therefore be vigilant over their own property, as well as that of clients, and keep handbags and other items of value in a safe place.

Records

In order to maintain confidentiality, it is essential that client records and other confidential papers are secured and locked away when unattended. In the event of any problems or breaches of security, these should be reported to the salon manager.

Dealing with clients

Greeting clients

Clients visiting the salon are to be attended to promptly and efficiently in a professional manner at all times. Therapists are responsible for greeting their own clients promptly at reception, carrying out the treatment in a professional manner and booking the client's next appointment.

Processing client payments

It is each therapist's responsibility to ensure that the correct fee is taken for the treatment provided. The treatment and payment made must be recorded on the record of payments sheet, so that a reconciliation may be made at the end of the session.

Record-keeping

It is essential that a central record is kept of all salon treatments and that client confidentiality is observed at all times. It is each therapist's responsibility to ensure that all records are completed fully at the conclusion of the treatment and are updated accordingly.

Cost-effectiveness

It is each therapist's responsibility to ensure that cost-effective use of all resources is maintained. Due to the volume of products used in the clinic, please ensure that you split couch roll and only use the designated amount of products/towels, and so on for each treatment, in order to avoid wastage.

Note: attention is also drawn to the requirement of carrying out treatments in a commercially acceptable time.

Maintaining salon resources

Work areas

All therapists are responsible for the preparation of their work area prior to the client's arrival, and for tidying up and leaving the work area ready for re-use.

Equipment/resource cupboards

All items that are designated for storage in specific cupboards should be placed in the relevant cupboard on the shelves clearly marked for that item. The cupboard should always be kept clean and tidy, as should the items placed within it.

Shortages of stock

All breakages, spillages, damages or shortages in salon stock are to be reported immediately to the salon manager for action.

Laundry

All dirty linen should be folded neatly into a dirty linen bag, ready for laundering.

Bins

All bins and waste must be emptied at the end of each session.

Final check

At the end of your working day please ensure that:

- all waste has been removed and disposed of
- client records have been updated and filed away
- your work area is tidy and ready for re-use
- all electrical appliances have been switched off
- the salon has been left secure (windows and doors locked)

Maintaining a hygienic working environment

A therapist is responsible for applying the appropriate hygiene procedures at all times, to:

- ensure compliance with legislative and workplace requirements
- prevent cross-infection and contamination
- promote client confidence.

Hygiene precautions

- A smart and hygienic appearance should be presented at all times (including attention to personal hygiene).

- Cover any cuts and abrasions on your hands with a clean plaster or dressing to avoid the risk of secondary infection.
- Avoid treatment if you or the client is harbouring an infectious condition.
- All equipment should be disinfected and sterilised regularly.
- Rubbish should be disposed of regularly, in a sealed bin.
- All jewellery should be removed from the client and the therapist before treatment (with the exception of a wedding band).
- All materials and consumables used should be clean and hygienic, ensuring all tops are secured tightly after use.
- Therapist's hands should be washed with an antibacterial soap/hand cleanser before and after each client.

Methods of sterilisation and disinfection

Sterilisation and disinfection procedures are used in a salon in order to minimise or destroy the harmful micro-organisms that could cause infection, such as bacteria, viruses and fungi.

- Sterilisation is the total destruction of all living micro-organisms.
- Disinfection is the destruction of some, but not all, micro-organisms.

Sterilisation methods commonly used in a salon involve the use of physical agents such as radiation (for example, a UV steriliser), heat (for example, an autoclave) or chemical solutions (for example, Cidex or other manufacturer-specific brands such as Sterilsafe).

Disinfection will involve chemical agents such as antiseptic and disinfectants.

Health and safety note

It is important always to follow manufacturer's instructions and relevant COSHH guidelines (see pages 234–5) when carrying our sterilisation and disinfection procedures.

Health and safety

Health and safety procedures are of paramount importance in the workplace. The law demands that every place of employment is a healthy and, above all, safe place to work, not only for employees, but also for their clients and other visitors who may enter the workplace.

Failure to comply with legislation may have serious consequences, such as:

- claims from injured staff or clients
- loss of trade through bad publicity
- closure of the business.

Study tip

While the acts and legislation described here are deemed current at the time of writing, legislation is constantly changing and being amended regularly. Good sources of information on the most current legislation and act amendments can be found at www.legislation.gov.uk

Health and safety legislation

Health and Safety at Work Act 1974

The basis of British health and safety law is the Health and Safety at Work Act 1974.

It is a piece of legislation that is continually being reviewed and it lays down the minimum standards of health, safety and welfare in the workplace.

The Act sets out the general duties that employers have towards employees and members of the public, and that employees have to themselves and to each other.

It provides a comprehensive legal framework to promote and encourage high standards of health and safety in the workplace.

Both the employer and the employee have responsibilities under the Act.

The responsibilities of the employer are to:

- safeguard as far as possible the health, safety and welfare of themselves, their employees, contractors' employees and members of the public
- keep all equipment up to health and safety standards
- provide appropriate safety equipment and clothing and have it checked regularly
- ensure the environment is free from toxic fumes
- ensure that all staff are aware of safety procedures, by providing safety information and training
- ensure safe systems of working practices and operations
- provide toilets, washing facilities and drinking water, and adequate first aid facilities
- maintain relevant insurances.

The responsibilities of the employee are to:

- adhere to the workplace rules and regulations concerning safety
- follow safe working practices and attend training as required
- take reasonable care to avoid injury to themselves and others
- cooperate with others in all matters relating to health and safety
- not interfere or wilfully misuse anything provided to protect their health and safety.

Note: the Health and Safety Executive (HSE) has produced a guide to the laws on health and safety and it is a requirement that an employer displays a copy of this poster in the workplace (see below).

Health and safety note

The Health and Safety Executive is the body appointed to support health and safety law. The HSE appoints inspectors called environmental health officers, whose role is to enforce health and safety law by visiting workplaces to check compliance with all relevant health and safety legislation.

Health and Safety (Information for Employees) Regulations 1989

This legislation requires an employer to provide health and safety information in the form of leaflets, posters and notices.

An employer with five or more employees must formulate a written health and safety policy, which must be issued and discussed with each employee.

A written health and safety policy, as a minimum, should include information such as:

- the responsibilities of both the employee and the employer
- risk assessment guidance and records (including storage and handling of hazardous substances and details of checks made on electrical equipment)
- escape routes and emergency evacuation procedures
- who to report to in an emergency
- who to report significant risks to
- first aid equipment and appointed first-aider in the workplace.

Health and safety policies must be reviewed regularly to ensure that they meet all relevant guidelines and updates.

Health and safety regulations required to be displayed in the workplace include:

- fire evacuation procedures
- Health and Safety (Information for Employees) Regulations updated 2009 poster (copied may be obtained from the HSE)
- public liability insurance certificate
- health and safety policy (if five or more employees)
- risk assessment records and guidance.

Study tip

The HSE has produced a number of publications relating to the laws on health and safety, including a poster, which employers are required to display, telling employees what they need to know about health and safety.

The Management of Health and Safety at Work (Amendment) Regulations 2006 (the Management Regulations)

These generally make more explicit what employers are required to do to manage health and safety under the Health and Safety at Work Act. Like the Act, they apply to every work activity.

The main requirement of employers is to carry out a risk assessment. Employers with five or more employees need to record the significant findings of the risk assessment.

What is a risk assessment?

A risk assessment is simply a careful examination of what in the workplace could cause harm to people, so that it can be weighed up whether enough precautions have been taken to prevent harm. Workers and others have a right to be protected from harm caused by a failure to take reasonable control measures.

> **Study tip**
>
> Risk assessment should be straightforward in a simple workplace such as a small salon. It should only be complicated if it deals with serious hazards, such as those in a laboratory.

Undertaking risk assessments on a regular basis can help to identify areas where staff training is needed, in line with their work or new equipment/products that might be introduced into the business. Regular risk assessment is good business practice, as it promotes continued review of safe working operations and helps to maintain and update records.

The law does not expect employers to eliminate all risk, but they are required to protect people as far as 'reasonably practicable'.

How to undertake a risk assessment

1. Identify the hazards.
2. Decide who might be harmed and how.
3. Evaluate the risks and decide on precautions.
4. Record your findings and implement them.
5. Review your assessment and update if necessary.

The process does not need to be overcomplicated.

> **Study tip**
>
> Few workplaces stay the same. Sooner or later, there will be new equipment, substances and procedures that could lead to new hazards. It makes sense, therefore, to review what you are doing on an ongoing basis. Every year or so, formally review where you are, to make sure that you are still improving.

If you run a small salon and you are confident that you understand what is involved, you can do the assessment yourself. You do not have to be a health and safety expert.

If you work in a larger salon or spa, you could ask a health and safety adviser to help you. If you are not confident, get help from someone who is competent. In all cases, you should make sure that you involve your staff or their representatives in the process. They will have useful information about how the work is done that will make your assessment of the risk more thorough and effective.

When thinking about risk assessment, remember:

- a hazard is anything that may cause harm, such as chemicals, electricity, working from ladders, an open drawer

- the risk is the chance, high or low, that somebody could be harmed by these and other hazards, together with an indication of how serious the harm could be.

Types of risk assessment

Types of risk assessment that need to be considered individually as part of the overall assessment include the following.

Risk assessment of space

Check that the work area is suitable. Consideration should be given to heating, lighting, ventilation, layout and design.

Risk assessment of chemicals

This involves safe use and disposal procedures, storage, handling and access to data sheets.

Risk assessment of equipment

This is the type of equipment, the safe operation/use of the equipment, the training required, handling, lifting, maintenance and repairs.

Risk assessment associated with security

This involves control systems, procedures, ordering, handling and storage of stock, as well as the handling of cash, point of sale, when in transit and implications to staff, and also security relating to people, including staff, clients, visitors, personal belongings, systems, emergency evacuation, storage of data, records and business information.

Risk assessment associated with buildings

This is the maintenance of internal and external security, and commercially available systems.

Risk assessment associated with emergency procedures

This involves accidents, first aid, fire evacuation, incidents, personnel and records.

While the above list covers most aspects relating to risk assessments associated with the workplace, it is not exhaustive, and each business should undertake a risk assessment at a level appropriate to its operations.

While it is a legal requirement that all employers must conduct a risk assessment, it is only necessary that employers with five or more employees record the significant findings of their risk assessment, although it is sensible and good practice to document things in all cases where appropriate.

Table 9.1 is an example of a risk assessment form that an employer could use when undertaking a full risk assessment of the workplace. A simple risk assessment form could then be used on a daily, weekly or monthly basis, as deemed necessary, in relation to the level of risk associated with the workplace.

What are the hazards?	Who might be harmed and how?	What are you already doing?	Control action required	Action by whom?	Action by when?	Done
Slips and trips	Staff and visitors may be injured if they trip over objects or slip on spillages.	General good housekeeping. All areas well lit, including stairs. No trailing leads or cables. Staff keep work areas clear (e.g. no boxes left in walkways, deliveries stored immediately, offices cleaned each evening).	Better housekeeping in staff kitchen needed (e.g. on spills). Arrange for loose carpet tile on second floor to be repaired/replaced.	All staff; supervisor to monitor manager.	From now on 01/10/11	01/10/11
Electrical equipment	Staff using equipment	Checked before use by staff for visible damage and correct operation Annual PAT testing undertaken by electric company	Ongoing monitoring and PAT testing. Report to manager any items considered faulty or dangerous. Arrange to replace/ repair items if necessary.	All staff; supervisor to monitor manager	From now on 01/10/11	01/10/11

▲ Table 9.1 Example of a risk assessment form

Besides carrying out a risk assessment, employers also need to:

- make arrangements for implementing the health and safety measures identified as necessary by the risk assessment
- appoint competent people (often themselves or company colleagues) to help them to implement the arrangements
- set up emergency procedures
- provide clear information and training to employees
- work together with other employers sharing the same workplace.

Other regulations require action in response to particular hazards, or in industries where hazards are particularly high.

To see the answers to this knowledge check, scan the QR code below or visit www.hodderplus.co.uk/indianhead/chapter-9.

Knowledge check 1

1. Who is the body appointed to support health and safety law?
2. What is the main requirement of employers under the Management of Health and Safety at Work Regulations?
3. Outline the steps necessary in undertaking a risk assessment.
4. What is the difference between a hazard and a risk?
5. List three items that may be assessed as part of a risk assessment.

Other health and safety legislation

Reporting of Injuries, Diseases and Dangerous Occurrences Regulations (RIDDOR) 1995

This legislation requires that all accidents that occur in the workplace, however minor, MUST be entered into an accident register. This is a requirement of the Health and Safety at Work Act.

The legislation relates to employees, the self-employed, trainees or visitors in the workplace.

An accident report form should detail the following information:

- details of the injured person (age, sex, occupation and contact details)
- date and time of the accident
- place where the accident occurred
- a brief description of the accident
- the nature of the injury
- the action taken
- signatures of all parties concerned (preferable).

Cases where employees or trainees suffer personal injury at work resulting in three consecutive days' absence must be notified to the HSE Incident Contact Centre (local authority) with ten days of the initial incident. In the event that the incident results in major injury or more than 24 hours in hospital, or death, the incident must be reported by telephone immediately, followed by a written report (HSE Form F2508) within ten days.

Manual Handling Operations Regulations 1992

This legislation covers musculoskeletal disorders primarily caused by manual handling and lifting, repetitive strain disorders and unsuitable posture causing back pain.

The regulations under this legislation cover minimising risks from lifting and handling large or heavy objects and require certain measures to be taken, such as correct lifting techniques to avoid musculoskeletal disorders.

An employer is required to undertake a risk assessment of all activities involving manual lifting and should keep records of this being carried out, including the risk of injury and action taken to minimise potential risks.

Health and safety note

When lifting, take care to ensure that you lift from the knees and not from the back (keep back straight) in order to avoid injury. If an item is heavy, assess the risk and ask for help.

Cash handling

Under the Health and Safety at Work Act, failure to provide a safe system of cash handling could lead to prosecution of the employer. Employers must therefore ensure compliance with this legislation and avoid sending an individual to the bank in a way that exposes the employee to risk.

Provision and Use of Work Regulations (PUWER) 1998

This legislation lays down the important health and safety controls on the provision of work equipment to prevent risk. The provisions relate to both old and new equipment and include duties for both employers and users, including the self-employed.

Health and Safety (Display Screen Equipment) Regulations 1992

This legislation relates to the use of visual display units and computer screens, and includes the specifications for the acceptable levels of radiation emissions from the screen, correct posture and seating positions, permitted working heights and rest periods.

Health and safety note

Employers have a duty to comply with this legislation in order to avoid the potential risks associated with VDUs, such as muscle fatigue, musculoskeletal problems, headaches and eye strain.

Health and safety note

First-aiders must undertake training and obtain qualifications approved by the HSE. At present, first aid certificates are valid for three years. Refresher courses should be started before a certificate expires, otherwise a full course will need to be taken.

Health and safety note

The HSE has produced a handy first aid booklet called Basic Advice on First Aid at Work INDG347 (Rev 1), which may be kept in the first aid box as a handy reference guide.

Health and safety note

Personal protective equipment (PPE) should be 'CE' marked, which indicates that it complies with basic safety requirements.

Health and Safety (First Aid) Regulation 1981

Under these regulations, workplaces must have adequate first aid provision in the event of injury or illness.

The form it should take will depend on various factors, including the nature and degree of hazards at work, what medical services are available and the number of employees.

It is recommended that at least one person holds an HSE-approved basic first aid qualification in the workplace.

All employees should be informed of the first aid procedures in the workplace, including:

- where the first aid box is located
- who is responsible for the maintenance of the first aid box
- who to report to in the event of an accident or illness
- who to report to in the event of an accident or emergency.

First aid kits

Health and Safety (First Aid) Regulation 1981 states that workplaces must have adequate first aid provision. An adequately stocked first aid kit should be available that complies with health and safety first aid regulations, and is suitable for the number of employees.

First-aiders should record all cases they treat. Each record should include at least the name of the patient, date, place, time and circumstances of the accident and details of the injury and treatment given.

Personal Protective Equipment (PPE) Regulations 2002

This legislation requires an employer to identify through a risk assessment those activities requiring special protective equipment or clothing. The employer has an obligation to:

- provide suitable protective clothing and equipment for all employees, to ensure safety in the workplace
- ensure that staff are adequately trained in the use of chemicals and equipment
- ensure that equipment is suitable for its purpose and is kept in a good state of repair.

Potentially hazardous substances may include aerosols or disinfectants, which may cause harm or chemical irritation to the skin.

Control of Substances Hazardous to Health (Amendment) Regulations (COSHH) 2004

These regulations require employers to regulate employees' exposure to hazardous substances, which may cause ill health or injury in the workplace and involve risk assessment.

Risk assessment involves making an itemised list of all the substances used in the workplace or sold to clients that may be hazardous to health. Attention is drawn to any substances that may cause irritation, cause allergic reactions, burn the skin or give off fumes.

Instructions for handling and disposing of all hazardous substances must be made available to all staff, and training provided if required.

Hazardous substances are usually identified by the symbols shown in Figure 9.1.

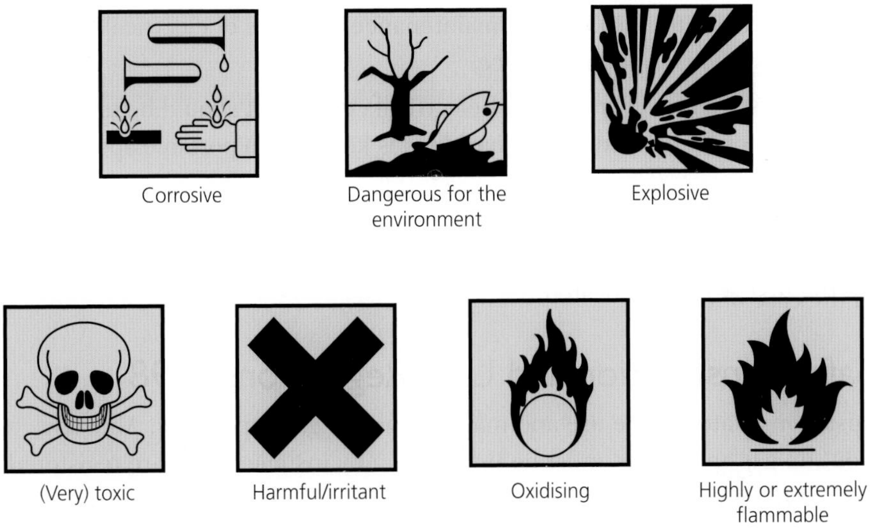

▲ Figure 9.1 Hazard symbols

Cosmetic Products (Safety) (Amendment No. 2) Regulations 2010

This legislation implements EEC regulations regarding the description of cosmetic products, their labelling, composition and marketing.

It is concerned with the supply of any cosmetic product that is liable to cause damage to human health when it is applied under:

- normal conditions of use or
- conditions of use that are reasonably foreseeable, taking into account all the circumstances, including the cosmetic product's presentation, labelling, any instructions for its use and disposal, and any other information or indication provided by the manufacturer, the manufacturer's agent or the person who supplies the cosmetic product on the first occasion that it is supplied in the Community.

Labelling and marking of cosmetic products

Cosmetic products must be supplied in packaging that includes (in lettering that is visible, indelible and easily legible):

- a list of its cosmetic ingredients (preceded by the word 'ingredients')
- the weight or volume
- the name or trade name of the product
- the address or registered office of the manufacturer of the product
- a 'best before' date if there is an expiry date
- any particular precautions to be observed during use and any special precautionary information on a cosmetic product for professional use, in particular in hairdressing

Health and safety note

Every supplier is legally required to make guidelines available on how materials should be stored and used. All products should be stored as guided by the material safety data sheets (MSDS), which may be supplied on request to suppliers/manufacturers), in order to comply with COSHH regulations.

Study tip

Essential information on COSHH regulations is available on the HSE website, in a section called COSHH and your industry.

Health and safety note

Remember that hazardous substances may enter the body via the skin, eyes, nose, mouth or by piercing the skin.

Health and safety note

In addition to the annual PAT test, it is important for staff to regularly check electrical items and to report and remove any potential hazards, such as exposed wires, cracked plugs, broken or overloaded sockets.

Any pieces of equipment that are faulty should be labelled as such to ensure they are not used by accident.

- a means of identifying the batch in which the product was manufactured
- the function of the product, unless this is clear from its presentation.

Electricity at Work Regulations 1989

This legislation covers the installation, maintenance and uses of electrical equipment and systems in the workplace.

The regulations state that every piece of electrical equipment should be tested every 12 months by a qualified electrician. This is known as a portable appliance test (PAT).

All checks should be listed in a record book, which must be retained for inspection, stating the results of the tests and the recommendations and action taken in the case of defects.

Gas Safety (Installation and Use) Regulations 1998

This legislation relates to the use and maintenance of gas appliances. All work carried out on gas appliances must be undertaken by installers who are registered under the CORGI scheme. The Rights of Entry Regulations 1996 gives gas and HSE inspectors rights to enter premises and order the disconnection of dangerous appliances. (HSE inspectors will not normally be CORGI registered and cannot personally undertake any work on a gas appliance, including disconnection.)

To see the answers to this knowledge check, scan the QR code below or visit www.hodderplus.co.uk/indianhead/chapter-9.

Knowledge check 2

1. Which legislative act requires all incidents, however minor, to be recorded in an accident book?
2. Which legislative act deals with minimising risks from lifting and repetitive strain disorders?
3. Which hazardous symbol indicates a substance that is very toxic?
4. How often should electrical equipment be tested under the Electricity at Work Regulations 1989?

Fire health and safety

Regulatory Reform (Fire Safety) Order 2005

This legislation replaces all previous legislation relating to fire, including fire certificates that are no longer valid.

The legislation places responsibility for fire safety onto a 'responsible person', usually the employer. A 'responsible person' is someone who has some level of control in a premises and who must take reasonable steps to reduce risk from fire, making sure people can safely escape in the event of a fire.

The Regulatory Reform (Fire Safety) Order 2005 applies to virtually all premises and covers nearly every type of building, structure and open space. Anyone who has control of premises or who has a degree of control over certain areas is responsible for complying with the order. This could be the employer, the occupier of the premises or any person who has some control over a part of the premises.

The main rules under the order mean that it is necessary to:

- carry out a fire risk assessment
- consider who may be especially at risk
- remove or reduce the risk of fire where reasonably possible
- implement control measures if flammable or explosive materials are used or stored
- have an emergency plan in place
- record findings
- review findings.

Undertaking a fire risk assessment

1. Identify fire hazards
   - sources of ignition
   - sources of fuel
   - sources of oxygen.
2. Identify people at risk
   - people in and around the premises
   - people especially at risk.
3. Evaluate, remove or reduce and protect from risk
   - evaluate the risk of fire starting
   - evaluate the risk to people from a fire
   - remove or reduce fire hazards
   - remove or reduce the risks to people from a fire
   - protect people by providing fire precaution.
4. Record, plan, inform, instruct and train
   - record any major findings and action you have taken
   - discuss and work with other responsible people
   - prepare an emergency plan
   - inform and instruct relevant people
   - provide training.
5. Review
   - review your fire risk assessment regularly
   - make changes when necessary.

General fire precautions

There are a number of things you need to consider; these include but are not limited to:

- a fire detection system
- a way of fighting a small fire
- safe routes for people to leave the premises
- suitable fire exit doors (which must be clearly marked, free from obstruction and remain unlocked during working hours)
- the possible need for emergency lighting
- suitable fire safety signs
- training for staff and other relevant people
- a system of management to maintain your fire safety systems.

Health and safety note

All staff must be trained in fire and emergency evacuation procedures for their workplace.

Fire extinguishers

There are different fire extinguishers designed to deal with different types of fire.

Fire extinguisher colour	Contents	Type of fire
Red	Water	Paper, wood, fabrics and textiles (NOT on burning liquids, electrical or flammable metal fires)
Black	Carbon dioxide (CO_2)	Electrical fires, fats, grease, oils, paint, flammable liquids (NOT on flammable metal fires)
Blue	Dry powder	Electrical fires, oils, alcohols, solvents, paint, flammable liquids and gases (NOT on flammable metal fires)
Cream	Foam	Flammable liquids (NOT on electrical or flammable metal fires)

▲ Table 9.2 The main types of fire extinguishers

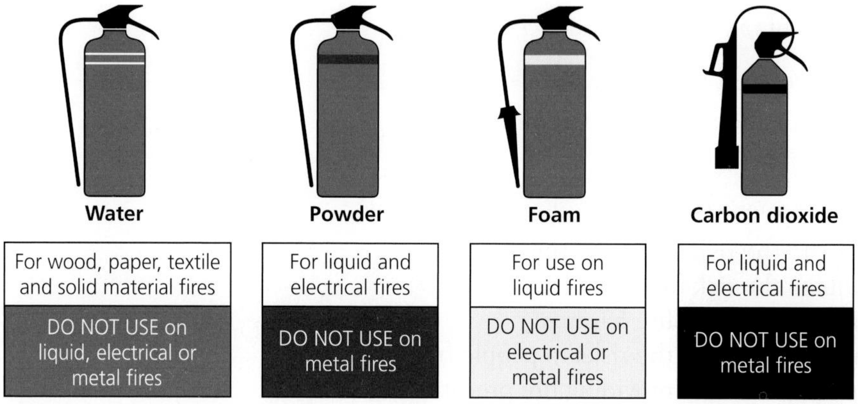

▲ Figure 9.2 Fire extinguishers

The fire extinguishers set out above are coded in order to allow quick and easy identification and to avoid using the wrong type and putting yourself and others in danger.

If you are in any doubt about the type of fire extinguisher to use in the workplace, it is advisable to contact your local fire safety department for advice.

Health and safety note

Further information on fire safety can be found at www.hse.gov.uk

Waste disposal

When disposing of waste, therapists have a responsibility to protect the environment, and also to ensure they are working within the hygienic practices of their workplace.

All waste should be disposed of in an enclosed waste bin with a polythene bin liner durable enough to resist tearing. The bin should be regularly disinfected in a well-ventilated area, wearing protective gloves.

Any waste considered to be hazardous must be disposed of following COSHH guidelines and training by the employer.

Health and safety note

Clinical waste (contaminated waste from blood and tissue fluids) should be disposed of as recommended by the Controlled Waste Regulations 1992.

Contact your local environmental health office (EHO) for advice on disposal arrangements for clinical waste.

Environmental Protection Act 1990

This act defines the structure for waste management (collection and disposal of waste) and the control of emissions from the environment.

Waste Electronic and Electrical Equipment Regulations 2007

These regulations require the safe disposal of electrical products. If you wish to dispose of an unwanted electrical item, it should be taken to a registered site able to accept electrical waste.

? Knowledge check 3

1. Which legislation replaces all previous legislation relating to fire?
2. List three important considerations in relation to a fire exit door.
3. Which fire extinguishers would be suitable for use on a electrical fire?

To see the answers to this knowledge check, scan the QR code below or visit www.hodderplus.co.uk/indianhead/chapter-9.

Dealing with spillages, breakages and waste in the workplace

When handling a spillage:

- wipe up immediately and warn staff and clientele; if the area is still wet, display a sign indicating the potential hazard.

When handling breakages:

- clear up immediately
- wrap up sharp items such as glass before placing them into the waste refuse.

When handling waste:

- dispose of in a covered bin
- remove daily
- refer to organisational and local authority guidelines regarding disposal of waste.

Registration and inspection of premises

Local authority by-laws

Larger local authority areas in the UK may impose their own legislation under which therapy establishments are licensed, and a 'special treatments' license will be required for massage.

The position is not uniform from one authority to another; therefore, practising therapists should obtain advice from their local EHO.

Local Government (Miscellaneous Provisions) Act 1982

This Act provides local authorities with powers of registration of persons practising acupuncture, tattooing, electrical epilation and ear piercing, among other things. These treatments present additional risks as they may produce blood and tissue fluid. Inspection of the premises is therefore necessary before such services can be offered to the public.

An inspector from the local authority will visit the premises and ensure that all requirements of the Local Government (Miscellaneous Provisions) Act 1982 are being met, including complying with all relevant health and safety laws, before a certificate of registration is issued.

Employers' Liability (Compulsory Insurance) (Amendment) Regulations 2011

This legislation requires the employer to take out and maintain an approved insurance policy with authorised insurers, against liability for bodily injury or disease sustained by their employees in the course of their employment.

A certificate of employers' liability insurance must be displayed at each place of business for the information of the employees.

Safety and security in the workplace

Therapists also require knowledge of security issues and measures in connection with premises, people and their belongings. Business requirements for the security of stock, equipment, money and records should be known. The proprietor of a salon or clinic is required by law to ensure adequate security of their business premises. The following steps may be taken to ensure maximum security. This is important not only for peace of mind, but also for insurance requirements.

Security recommendations include:

- fitting locks and bolts on doors and windows
- installing a burglar alarm
- fitting security lights
- ensuring there is a minimum number of key holders
- leaving a light on at night, preferably at the front of the premises
- ensuring all windows and doors are checked before leaving the premises
- ensuring that staff communicate any security breaches with the employer, police and relevant authorities appropriately
- ensuring that staff are adequately trained to deal with the situation and what actions to take, as incorrect action or failure to observe correct procedures could result in loss of employment.

Money

- Have a safe for short-term storage of money and valuables.
- Always keep the till locked, with a minimum number of key holders.
- Never leave money in the till overnight.

Stock

A good stock control system is needed in the workplace in order to monitor the use of consumables and retail products; this should be documented in a stock control book.

Recommendations for safeguarding stock include:

- always keeping supplies in a locked cupboard
- issuing keys to a limited number of authorised staff only
- having a locked cabinet for display purposes, or using 'dummy stock' to avoid shoplifting.

Records

In order to maintain confidentiality, it is essential that client records and other confidential papers are secured and locked away when unattended. In the case of a security breach, the data protection register and clients should be advised accordingly.

Personal belongings

It is not possible for therapists to take responsibility for a client's personal belongings when they attend for treatments. It is important for clients to be aware of this by displaying a disclaimer sign in a reception area.

When clients are removing jewellery, it is important for valuable items to be placed in a safe place for the duration of the treatment. In order to minimise risks, it is advisable to recommend that clients keep a minimum amount of money and valuables on them.

Staff should be vigilant over their own property as well as that of clients, and keep handbags and other items of value in a safe place.

Health and safety of the client

Therapists need to have knowledge of health and safety in relation to the client, which includes risk assessment, contraindications and contra-actions.

A therapist needs to fully understand that a contraindication may mean a client being adversely affected by the treatment, or that treatment could be ineffective, and that an adapted or shortened treatment might be possible.

Note: therapists must understand that diagnosis of a medical condition is the role of the medical profession; therefore suggestions should never be made to a client about a condition. It is the responsibility of the client to ask for medical advice concerning a contraindication.

Any condition that does not appear to be normal should be brought to the attention of the client and medical consultation advised before treatment is given.

Contra-actions (adverse reactions) to treatment must be explained and avoided where possible. In the event of a contra-action, the corrective action to be taken must be understood, as well as how to advise the client. It is also important to ensure that contra-actions are recorded.

Consumer Protection Act 1987

This Act provides the consumer with protection when buying goods or services, to ensure that products are safe for use on the client during the treatment, or are safe to be sold as a retail product.

In the past, those injured had to prove a manufacturer negligent before they could successfully sue for damages. The Consumer Protection Act removed the need to prove negligence.

The Act provides the same rights to anyone injured by a defective product, whether the product was sold to them or not. The Act also covers giving misleading price indications about goods, services or facilities. The term 'price indication' also includes price comparisons. To be misleading includes any wrongful indications about conditions attached to a price, about what you expect to happen to a price in the future and what you say in price comparisons.

It is essential to understand the implications of this legislation, including the promotion of special offers, as an offence could result in legal proceedings.

Sale and Supply of Goods Act 1994

As consumers of products and services, clients do have rights under this legislation. This legislation identifies the contract of sale, which takes place between the retailer (the clinic/salon) and the consumer (the client).

This legislation amends the previous Act (Sale of Goods Act 1979), which was the first of the laws and covers rights including the goods being accurately described without misleading the consumer.

The Sale and Supply of Goods Act 1994 is associated with the Supply of Goods and Services Act 1982, the Unfair Contract Terms Act 1977 and the Supply of Goods (Implied Terms) Act 1973.

These Acts cover consumer rights, including goods being of satisfactory quality, the conditions under which goods may be returned after purchase and whether goods are fit for their intended purpose.

Trade Descriptions Act 1968 (amended 1988)

This Act prohibits the use of false descriptions or selling or offering for sale goods that have been described falsely. This Act covers advertisements such as oral descriptions and display cards, and applies to quality and quantity as well as fitness for purpose and price.

It is important to understand this legislation, especially where the description is given by another person and repeated. Thus, to repeat a manufacturer's claim is to be equally liable.

Copyright Designs and Patents Act 1988 (Amendment) Regulations 2010

If a therapist is using relaxation music when carrying out treatments in the workplace, it may be necessary to obtain a licence from Phonographic Performance Ltd (PPL) or the Performing Rights Society (PRS), which is a organisation that collects licence payments as royalties on behalf of performers and record companies, whose music is protected under the Copyright Designs and Patent Act 1998.

Any use of music in treatment premises or waiting rooms, or music played on a switchboard holding system, is termed a public performance. The PPL and PRS have the backing of the Copyright Designs and Patents Act 1988 and can take legal action against those who seek to avoid paying its licence fees.

Helpful tip: it should be noted that a lot of music comes from composers who are not members of the above schemes. In such cases the music is 'copyright free', and no fee is due to PPL or PRS. Therapists are advised to check the position with the supplier of the music.

Data Protection Act 1998

This legislation protects clients' personal information being stored on a computer.

If client records are stored on computer, the establishment must be registered under this Act.

The Data Protection Act operates to ensure that the information stored is only used for the purposes for which it was given. Therefore, none of the information may be given to any outsider, without the client's permission.

Clients can seek compensation through the courts for any infringement of their rights established by giving information in the first instance for a specific purpose.

Businesses should therefore ensure that they:

- only hold information that is relevant
- allow individuals access to the information held on them
- prevent unauthorised access to the information.

Professional codes of practice

The role of a professional representative therapy body is to define limitations on procedures and practices for public protection.

A professional therapist is bound by the rules of a professional representative therapy body (such as the Federation of Holistic Therapists or the British Association of Beauty Therapy and Cosmetology) and its code of ethics, which exists to ensure that social, ethical and moral standards exist in a professional's day-to-day work.

Codes of ethics are rules of conduct binding on those who join a professional body. Infringement of these codes is taken very seriously by professional bodies and can result in penalties, including expulsion from membership.

A code of ethics also exists to determine the demarcation lines that enable a non-medical therapist to exist harmoniously in the industry with medical and medical-auxiliary practitioners. Therapists must therefore not practise beyond the scope of their profession.

Code of ethics

Professional codes of ethics are standards of acceptable professional behaviour by which a person or business conducts their business. Each professional association has its own code of ethics, which they require their members to adhere to.

The following guidelines reflect, in general terms, a code of ethics expected from a professional therapist. Therapists must:

- not treat any person who is suffering from a medical condition; in the event of a client presenting a medical condition, they should be referred to their GP
- conduct themselves in a professional manner and be courteous and respectful to a client at all times

- always bear in mind that their primary concern should be for the client and that they should practise their skills to the best of their ability at all times
- have respect for the religious, spiritual, social or political views of their clients, irrespective of creed, race, colour or sex
- never abuse the relationship between themselves and a client
- act in a cooperative manner with other health care professionals, and refer cases that are out of the sphere of the therapy field in which they practise
- explain the treatment and discuss any fees involved with the client before any treatment commences
- keep accurate, up-to-date records of treatments carried out on a client and the results, which should include client's confidential details, medical history, dates and details of treatment and any advice given
- never disclose client information without the prior written permission of the client, except when required to do so by law
- never claim to cure
- never diagnose a medical condition
- never give unqualified advice
- keep their personal and professional life separate
- ensure that any advertising represents their business in the most professional manner
- ensure that their working premises comply with all current health, safety and hygiene legislation
- be adequately insured to practise the therapy in which they are qualified
- become a member of a professional association that sets high standards for the industry
- continue their own professional development.

Antidiscrimination practices

Antidiscrimination practices involve therapists ensuring equal treatment of all those with whom they come into contact.

It is each therapist's responsibility to examine their procedures and practices to ensure that they are non-discriminatory, and that cultural differences are fully respected when dealing with clients and colleagues.

A therapist needs to understand the nature and diversity of communities, and that there are subgroups of different economic, cultural or other divisions that coexist within a geographical location.

Knowledge is therefore necessary of the existence of different communities within the larger community as a whole, in order to ensure that the provision of services encompasses the needs of the diversity of different groups within the local community. This may involve communication with other professionals (medical and non-medical) within the community, to forge relationships that foster mutual respect and raise awareness, to encourage integration of their chosen therapy within the community.

Therapists should understand that in the process of making professional contact with all parts of the community, they could improve knowledge and raise awareness of the benefits of the therapy to different groups within the area.

Antidiscrimination legislation

Discrimination occurs if one individual is treated less favourably than another.

Equality Act 2010

The Act was designed to simplify the law and make it easier to understand by replacing previous antidiscrimination Acts with one single Act.

The Act encompasses certain characteristics that cannot be used to treat an individual unfairly. The Act affords protection to all individuals, as one or more of the characteristics can be applied to every person. The characteristics covered under the Act are:

- age
- disability
- gender reassignment
- marriage and civil partnership
- pregnancy and maternity
- race
- religion or belief
- sex
- sexual orientation.

The Act explains the ways in which it is unlawful to treat someone, and details what is prohibited.

Health and safety note

It is always important to take note of any modifications a client or member of staff may require to a service provided, without discriminating against them for their individual characteristics – for instance, in the case of a client or therapist being pregnant.

Protection for the therapist and the client

When in professional practice, therapists may be in contact with various members of the community, including the elderly, infirm, those unable to give consent, clients with special needs and clients of the opposite gender to the therapist.

Specific attention is drawn to the law regarding the protection of minors (a person below the legal age of consent). Therapists need to be aware that a minor should not be examined or treated unless a parent or guardian is present, or has given written permission for examination and a chaperone is present.

Specific precautions also exist in relation to those individuals in specific categories (elderly, infirm, those unable to give consent, those with special needs). In the treatments of these client groups, attention is drawn to the need for a companion or appropriate adult (such as a carer) to be present, to offer protection for the individual and the therapist. Any special precautions should be considered and requested before any treatment is undertaken.

Providing a safe working environment

Therapists need to be aware of special precautions to ensure that clients do not feel vulnerable or at risk at any time.

The working environment in which the therapist practises must allow clients to feel comfortable and at ease at all times. Treatment processes should be not be invasive and all procedures must be explained to the client beforehand to ensure their consent is given for treatment to proceed.

Special precautions that therapists need to be aware of include having someone else nearby, working in an easily accessible working area and checking clients' details before offering treatment. As far as therapists are concerned, for personal protection, they may refuse to treat anyone they have concerns about.

Legislation for the protection of minors

Relevant legislation includes the following.

Children Act 2004

The Act is an amendment of the Children Act 1989 and is designed to make the UK a better and safer place for all children. It also specifically encompasses provision for disabled children.

Protection of Children Act 1999

This Act requires a list to be kept of persons considered unsuitable to work with children. It also makes provisions to extend the power of the regulations of the Education Reform Act 1988. It is designed to enable the protection afforded to children to be extended to those with any mental impairment.

Note: the Criminal Records Bureau may be consulted by employers of people with access to minors.

Sex Offenders Act 1997

This Act primarily requires persons who have committed certain sexual offences to notify the police and provide information in relation to the offences.

Any person convicted of a sexual crime will be placed on the Sex Offenders Register.

Knowledge check 4

1. Which local authority department deals with the regulation and inspection of premises?
2. Which legislative Act requires employers to take compulsory insurance against liability for bodily injury or disease sustained by their employees in the course of their employment?
3. State the legislative Act that protects the storage of client information held.
4. Which Act replaces all previous antidiscrimination legislation?
5. What legislation exists to assist in the protection of minors?
6. What is a code of ethics?

To see the answers to this knowledge check, scan the QR code below or visit www.hodderplus.co.uk/indianhead/chapter-9.

Maintaining operations and services

The role of a therapist in the context of the workplace is not merely in the provision of treatments, but in monitoring and maintaining operations to meet the requirements of both the establishment and the client. They are concerned with matters that help to make a business run smoothly and efficiently, with the ultimate aim of clients who are satisfied with the service provided, and the result of repeat business.

Therapists are expected to understand what is required to support workplace efficiency, within their given area of responsibility.

There are several important factors to be taken into account when working as a therapist, in order to monitor and maintain the standard of service offered to clients.

It is important not only to be able to perform a skill competently, but to be able to apply it in a way that is commercially acceptable.

In the workplace, therapists have a responsibility to their manager or supervisor, to their clients and to their colleagues.

Responsibilities of a therapist to a supervisor

These are to ensure that the therapist:

- adheres to the establishment's rules
- understands and adheres to legislation in relation to the provision of services
- reports any hazard or potential danger observed in the workplace
- has a sincere commitment to provide a high standard of work, to enhance the reputation and image of the establishment
- carries out work practices with honesty and integrity
- completes records fully and accurately
- uses their initiative to make the best use of time at work
- provides a high standard of work, to ensure client satisfaction and repeat business
- creates a good working relationship with other colleagues, to enhance a good working environment
- avoids wastage of resources
- makes recommendations for improvement in workplace practices, where appropriate
- understands how their job role contributes to the success of the business.

Responsibilities of a therapist to a client

These are to:

- treat clients with dignity and respect
- respond to clients' requests politely and efficiently
- accurately inform clients of the services provided by the establishment
- provide treatment only when there is a reasonable expectation that it will be advantageous to the client
- take appropriate measures to protect clients' rights to privacy and confidentiality
- provide a high standard of service, to ensure client satisfaction and the fostering of repeat business
- make recommendations for future treatments that would benefit the clients
- make recommendations for home care products that may enhance the clients' condition.

Responsibilities of a therapist to their colleagues

These are to:

- create a good working environment, by being friendly, helpful and approachable
- share responsibilities fairly, to enhance a good team spirit
- ensure good communication channels, pass on messages promptly and record messages accurately
- inform others of any changes in establishment procedure.

Maintaining effective relationships with colleagues

A successful business depends on a good image and reputation, but also on the way in which staff work together as a team to maintain the image and professionalism of the establishment.

Working with colleagues as a team helps to enhance smooth operations and promotes a pleasant working environment and a friendly atmosphere.

Working as a team involves:

- building a good rapport with each other
- understanding each other's responsibilities
- working efficiently within your own job responsibilities
- responding to each other's requests politely and cooperatively
- providing support and assistance, when required
- working together for the needs of the business.

Communication is essential when working with others in a team; regular meetings can help to maintain effective working relationships.

Meetings provide an opportunity to:

- identify and resolve problems in the workplace
- avoid breakdown in communication and misunderstandings
- contribute and exchange ideas on how workplace practices may be enhanced
- identify training needs
- maintain good working relationships.

Investing in staff

An employer should also remember that one of their most valuable assets is their staff. By maintaining the level of staff competency and staff feelings of fulfilment in their employment, an employer will reap the benefits. It is therefore good practice for an employer to keep staff up to date with matters affecting the business, by informing them verbally or with written information and leaflets, and also to make sure that staff skills are maintained, with the necessary training being provided. It is also good practice to make staff feel valued and part of a team, and that they can have their own input into the business through methods such as an open-door policy or suggestion boxes. The better that staff function, the better the business will function and the more likely it is to succeed.

Communication skills

Whether a business is small or large, a successful business relies on good communication in order to promote good understanding and efficient working relationships. Communication skills are extremely important when there are several colleagues working together; if communication breaks down, it can have a dramatic effect on the service given and the overall efficiency and image of the establishment. It is therefore important for a therapist to be able to communicate effectively with clients, colleagues and other visitors who may visit or telephone the establishment.

Communication skills may be used to:

- identify clients' needs
- inform clients about a service
- inform clients and colleagues of changes in procedures and problems arising
- maintain workplace records
- pass on recommendations for improving employment standards.

Communication skills involve verbal communication, listening, non-verbal communication and written communication.

Verbal communication

This involves sending and receiving information and is a cooperative effort between two parties. In order to facilitate effective verbal communication, it is important to pause periodically in order to verify that the message received was the message intended. In this way, corrections to the conversation may be made.

The objective of verbal communication is to be heard and understood.

For clarity, it is important to choose words that convey intent clearly, concisely and tactfully.

Listening

Although it is important to facilitate effective verbal communication, it is equally important to have good listening skills in order to develop optimal client–therapist relationships and relationships between colleagues. Effective listening involves understanding and evaluating the person's needs, including the tone and emotion in which the message is delivered. The objective of listening is focusing on understanding the message heard.

Good communication may be enhanced by maintaining eye contact, nodding and using verbal phrases or facial expression in order to encourage the speaker to continue.

When listening, it is important for therapists to clarify information received from clients or colleagues in order to ensure that the message has been understood correctly.

Non-verbal communication

This involves messages transmitted other than by the spoken word and may be exhibited by posture, gestures and facial expressions.

Non-verbal communication often projects more information about how a person is feeling and their emotions.

As a therapist's role is in dealing with people, it is helpful to be aware of body language, as this may have more meaning than the spoken word.

Written communication

An efficient working environment providing services to clients relies on accurate, legible record keeping, which is kept up to date.

Records may either be computer-based or handwritten.

Written communication may involve the recording of messages to colleagues to ensure continuity of service, or the completion of client records in the workplace to ensure therapeutic continuity.

In the workplace, it is very important that all messages are recorded accurately, to ensure continuity of operation and services.

Written communication should be clear, dated and timed, along with the action required. It should be placed somewhere that the person it is intended for will notice it.

Client records should be completed fully, accurately and legibly at the time of the treatment and stored securely and confidentially.

Responding to clients' requests

As clients are at the centre of every business, it is essential for therapists to respond to their requests promptly, accurately and enthusiastically.

Requests for information may come from a telephone enquiry or a personal visit to the workplace, or may be in the form of a written request.

It is important to assume a friendly and approachable manner when dealing with clients' requests, and use phrases such as 'How may I help you?'

It is also important to provide accurate information on treatments, such as:

- the benefits of the services
- the cost (of individual treatment and courses of treatment)
- the treatment duration
- any pre-treatment advice
- how often the client should attend for maximum benefit.

Providing as much useful information as possible at the time of request will increase the chances of the client booking an appointment. Even if the client does not book immediately, it will certainly give them a good impression of the professionalism of the establishment.

The best source of information should be from the professional themselves (the therapist); however, when this is not possible it is important to consider that leaflets and brochures may also help to sell treatments to clients. The information contained within leaflets and brochures should therefore be educational and informative, to increase client awareness of the treatment, as well as being attractive enough to stimulate interest.

Quality assurance

Every business, however small, should have a quality assurance policy in order to ensure that their services and operations are conducted in a systematic way.

Quality assurance policies help to monitor the quality and standard of the service provided, and are useful in analysing whether the clients' needs are met efficiently, effectively and consistently.

Effective ways of monitoring quality assurance include:

- examining your own workplace practice and how it relates to client needs and the needs of the business
- ensuring that you do not become complacent and that you continue updating your skills and knowledge
- distributing client satisfaction questionnaires
- introducing a client suggestions box
- implementing changes based on recommendations from clients and staff
- encouraging communication with clients on a regular basis.

Efficient work practices and cost-effectiveness

Efficient work practice requires a therapist to perform a skill to the required standard of the establishment and the industry, and in a time that is considered to be commercially acceptable.

Cost-effectiveness in terms of the workplace means maintaining treatment times and minimising waste, in order to avoid loss of revenue for the establishment.

Therapists need to be aware that by adhering to their appointment times and avoiding wastage, they are in fact helping to preserve the business's precious resources and thereby helping to maintain the security of their own employment.

Multiple-choice self-assessment questions

1. **Why is it important to understand national and local legislation?**
   - a Because it is part of the Health and Safety Act.
   - b So that you do not inadvertently break the law.
   - c To make sure that you are offering the correct treatments.
   - d It will help the business to operate more efficiently.
2. **Why is it important to understand cultural differences when dealing with colleagues, customers and other visitors to the workplace?**
   - a In order to ensure equal treatment of all those with whom you come into contact.
   - b Because it is part of the Care Standards Act.
   - c Because it will be helpful when visiting other countries.
   - d To make sure that you use the correct products when providing treatments.
3. **Why must practices and procedures be non-discriminatory at all times?**
   - a To ensure that all treatments keep to the same timings.
   - b Because it will increase business.
   - c Because it is the law and good business practice.
   - d In order to protect the client.
4. **COSHH stands for**
   - a Control of Special Health Hazards
   - b Control of Substances Hazardous to Health.
   - c Control of Severe Hazards to Health
   - d Control of Substances and Health Hazards.
5. **RIDDOR stands for**
   - a Reporting of Incidents, Diseases and Dangerous Occurrences
   - b Reporting of Injuries, Damages and Dangerous Occurrences
   - c Reporting of Injuries, Diseases and Dangerous Occupations
   - d Reporting of Injuries, Diseases and Dangerous Occurrences.
6. **The Health and Safety at Work Act provides a comprehensive legal framework to**
   - a promote and encourage high standards of health and safety in the workplace
   - b promote standards of responsibility in the workplace
   - c encourage employers to be more responsible
   - d encourage employees to be more responsible.
7. **Why is it important to wear professional workwear when carrying out therapy treatments?**
   - a Because it is a requirement of the Workplace (Health, Safety and Welfare) Regulations Act.
   - b In order to maintain a professional image and maintain hygiene.
   - c So that clients think you are a professional.
   - d In order to maintain personal hygiene.
8. **Good communication skills are essential in order to develop optimal relationships within the workplace. Effective communication involves which important skill?**
   - a Talking loudly so that the client can hear you
   - b Maintaining eye contact at all times
   - c Listening
   - d Verbal communication
9. **What are the legislative regulations that require employers to carry out a risk assessment in the workplace?**
   - a Employers' Liability Act
   - b Consumer Protection Act
   - c Children's Act
   - d Management of Health and Safety at Work Regulations
10. **What is a workplace risk assessment?**
    - a Checking if the workplace is at risk.
    - b An examination of what could cause harm to people within the workplace.
    - c A procedure to check risks associated with staff.
    - d A procedure to check risks associated with clients.
11. **What is involved when carrying out a risk assessment?**
    - a Making sure you are wearing the correct protective clothing when undertaking the assessment.
    - b Identifying potential hazards, the level of risk associated with a hazard and implementing appropriate precautions.
    - c Ensuring that all staff are aware of each assessment that takes place.
    - d Recording your findings in detail if there are fewer than five employees.

12. What actions would you take following a risk assessment?
- a Formulate a written health and safety policy.
- b Report your findings to your local business licensing council.
- c Implement steps to reduce the level of risk associated with a hazard, so that harm is unlikely.
- d Remove all hazardous items from the business.

13. State the legislative Act that is concerned with all electrical equipment being checked regularly.
- a COSHH
- b RIDDOR
- c Electricity at Work Regulations
- d Employers' Liability Act

14. State the legislative Act that is concerned with the reporting of accidents.
- a COSHH
- b RIDDOR
- c Electricity at Work Regulations
- d Employers' Liability Act

15. State the legislative Act that is concerned with regulating exposure to hazardous substances.
- a COSHH
- b RIDDOR
- c Electricity at Work Regulations
- d Employers' Liability Act

16. In the event of a problem in the workplace, who would you report to?
- a Health and Safety Executive
- b A colleague
- c A friend
- d Your manager

17. State the correct way to lift heavy items in order to avoid injury.
- a Keep knees bent and back bent forwards
- b Keep knees bent and back straight
- c Lock knees and bend back forwards
- d Lean backwards and keep knees bent

18. State which symbol represents a harmful hazard.
- a A cross
- b A flame
- c A hand
- d A skull

19. Which of the following fire extinguishers should NOT be used to extinguish a liquid fire?
- a Water
- b Powder
- c Carbon dioxide
- d Foam

20. What must you do under the Regulatory Reform (Fire Safety) Order 2005?
- a Keep all doors closed to prevent fire spreading.
- b Carry out a fire risk assessment.
- c Have colour-coded smoke alarms.
- d Register with the local authority.

21. What is the first consideration in the event of a fire in the workplace?
- a Collect your client's belongings and make sure your client is safe.
- b Try to put the fire out with a fire axe.
- c Check that no one is trapped.
- d Raise the alarm and exit the premises.

22. Who is responsible for the client's personal belongings in the workplace?
- a The salon
- b The owner
- c The therapist
- d The client

23. What consideration must be observed if providing a treatment to a minor?
- a Treatments need to be shorter in duration.
- b They should not receive treatment unless a parent, guardian or chaperone is present.
- c You may need to help them fill in their consultation form.
- d You need to take care if you are using oils in the treatment.

24. Why is confidentiality important?
- a To protect the client and comply with the Data Protection Act.
- b To protect the client and comply with the Consumer Protection Act.
- c To protect the client and comply with the Children's Protection Act.
- d In case information is needed by other professionals.

25. What should an employer do as part of their health and safety support for their staff?

a Issue staff with a written contract of employment.

b Undertake regular customer surveys to ascertain levels of satisfaction with services provided.

c Ensure that all staff are aware of safety procedures, by providing safety information and training.

d Make sure that there is a one-to-three staff-to-supervisor ratio.

26. Which of the following statements is *false*?

a In all cases of personal injury, an entry must be made in the workplace accident book.

b Every beauty supplier is legally required to make guidelines available on how materials should be stored and used.

c The Data Protection Act (1998) only applies to a business that uses computers.

d The display of a public liability insurance certificate is an example of compliance with health and safety in the workplace.

To see the answers, scan the QR code opposite or visit www.hodderplus.co.uk/indianhead/chapter-9. To access an interactive version of these multiple-choice self-assessment questions visit www.hodderplus.co.uk/indianhead/chapter-9.

To access an interactive crossword for this chapter visit www.hodderplus.co.uk/indianhead/chapter-9.

10 Promotion and marketing

Introduction

Marketing is the means by which you tell potential clients what you have to offer and how it will benefit them. In order to be successful in business, it is not enough for therapists to have excellent skills in the therapy they practise; they also need to get to grips with the important skill of marketing. It is important to consider the marketing of services such as Indian head massage carefully, as it is a specialist market and the marketing must therefore be selective.

Learning objectives

By the end of this chapter, you will be able to:

- understand the fundamental issues of marketing and promotion
- design a marketing plan for business success in Indian head massage.

Raising awareness with marketing

Marketing in the holistic therapy industry is educational and is about raising awareness of who you are and what you do. It is important for therapists to consider that marketing is about matching their service to clients' needs; therefore the focus is not so much on selling, but on identifying needs.

Marketing involves finding out:

- who your potential clients are
- what their needs are
- how much they would be prepared to pay for the service
- where they are and how to reach them
- how often they would visit.

Study tip

The key to successful marketing is to view every aspect of your marketing through the clients' eyes, and match their needs and desires to your products and services.

Researching clients

It is essential to use market research to assess the needs of the market. Knowing and understanding who your potential clients are is crucial to devising a marketing plan and deciding who to target in advertising and promotion. Market research enables you to identify potential clients, discover what influences them and find out how to reach them. Knowing the market then enables you to refine the message you wish to send to potential clients. There are very few services that will appeal to everyone; there is always a sector of the market that is going to be more inclined to buy. Therefore, you need to find out who makes up this sector and focus the attention of your marketing on them.

When building client profiles, it is helpful to consider the following factors:

- age
- gender
- income
- interests
- location.

Gathering client information

As clients are at the centre of every business, it is vital to find out about them and what they want. Carrying out marketing surveys using questionnaires is an effective way of gathering information. A great deal of thought needs to be given to the design of a marketing questionnaire, in order to give both quantitative and qualitative results.

When designing marketing questionnaires, it is important to keep questions short, simple and to the point, in order to get an exact answer. If questions are structured, it is simpler and quicker for the respondent to reply. Another important consideration is the type of questions to ask. Closed questions require only yes/no/don't know responses, while open questions allow the respondent to answer in their own way.

When designing questionnaires, it is also important to remember to avoid prejudging the participant's response – in other words, do not assume that you know what they are going to say. Neither should you leave them with no alternative but to agree with you.

In order to get the best results from your marketing questionnaire, bear in mind the following:

- keep it simple, attractive, interesting and relevant
- include a short introduction to the questionnaire in order to stimulate the respondent's enthusiasm and motivation to complete it
- offer an incentive to complete the questionnaire (such as a free prize or entry into a free prize draw)
- make it known to the respondents that there is a deadline to reply to the questionnaire.

You may wish to carry out a pilot survey on a group of individuals (friends, family, colleagues); however, check that the individuals concerned are within the same category as potential clients, otherwise this may prove to be a fruitless exercise.

(There is an example of a market research questionnaire for Indian head massage on page 272.)

Client surveys are useful tools in market research in that by gaining the client's input they:

- demonstrate your desire to offer the best possible service
- help you to fulfil the client's needs
- direct you towards potential sales triggers
- guide you towards potential strengths and weaknesses.

If sending out market research questionnaires, always make the response easy for the client by providing a stamped addressed envelope. As Indian head massage involves a personal and specialised service, it tends to appeal to certain segments of the market. Selecting a target market enables you to modify your advertising and promotional activities to appeal to a specific group.

Helpful tip: with the advantages of social media as a strong marketing tool, it is considered much more efficient in terms of time and money to conduct online marketing surveys. See page 263.

Consider the type of clientele you want to attract or, if you have an existing clientele, examine who is already using your services and what they have in common.

When targeting client markets, it is wise to target more than one sector, the number being dependent on your preference and expertise and the size of your practice.

In order to make marketing more effective, it is helpful to create a niche market by addressing the needs of a specific group of people. Your name then becomes linked with providing a particular service for a particular target group.

Assessing marketing needs

Marketing needs will be dependent on the following factors:

- your target market
- the size of your practice
- the amount of money you can afford
- the amount of time you can devote to marketing.

If you are a therapist starting out in business and do not have a large clientele, more time and energy can be devoted to making contacts and giving talks and presentations to help get your name and what you do known. The activities involving client education and awareness will be low-cost but time-consuming.

If you are an established business, you may have the financial budget to concentrate on other marketing methods, such as targeted advertising or mailshots to announce the introduction of a new service such as Indian head massage into the business.

> **Study tip**
> An important factor to consider in marketing is that it takes time and money to become known in business.

Compiling a marketing plan

Once you have established where the market for Indian head massage is and how extensive it is, the next stage is to put all the findings together in the form of objectives – this will form a marketing plan. A marketing plan will form the basis of how you intend to promote the service to generate clients. Before compiling a marketing plan, it is essential to carry out a SWOT analysis in order to self-assess your strengths, weaknesses, opportunities and threats, so that you can be realistic in your plan.

Strengths

These may include:

- specialism
- location of the business

- pricing
- opening hours
- personality
- customer service
- flexibility.

Weaknesses

Possible weaknesses may be:

- lack of experience
- opening hours
- location
- range of skills offered.

Opportunities

These could include:

- expansion into other sectors of the market – for example, the workplace.

Threats

Potential threats may include:

- local competition.

Getting the balance right in marketing

Successful marketing usually involves a mix of different methods, and the chemistry or 'mix' has to be right for the individual business.

Marketing can be divided into four factors and each of these will influence how you develop your marketing plan. Marketing can be seen as a balancing act; if adjustments are made to one or more of the four factors, a compensating adjustment has to be made among the other factors in order for the approach to be balanced.

Product/service

This includes the features and benefits of the product/service being offered, including the quality of service. For marketing to be effective, it is important to create demand. With products and services, it is also important to consider the image of the business being projected by the service itself, the marketing material and the staff.

Price

This is the cost of the service to the client. When setting prices for services it is vital that you charge:

- enough to cover your overheads, meet your expenses and make a profit
- what clients are prepared to pay
- a price in line with your competitors.

Place

This is where you are located in relation to your clients. Careful consideration needs to be given to the location and opening hours of the business to ensure that the service is available to potential clients.

Location is an important factor in business; it affects the distribution of services. Because of the portable nature of Indian head massage, therapists should consider the many locations or settings in which the therapy may be practised – for example, in the workplace, in hairdressing salons and hospitals, and in beauty spas and clinics.

> **Key fact**
> A marketing plan should also include your unique selling point (USP), which is what makes your business and service different to others.

Promotion

The objective of promotion is to become known and to create a desire in potential clients to use your services. The promotion of services such as Indian head massage is largely educational in nature and is the means by which potential clients learn who you are, what you do and how your services will benefit them.

In any form of promotion it is important for therapists to realise that they are marketing themselves as well as their treatments. Marketing is the art of promoting yourself and the services you offer in order to attract clients. There are many marketing strategies that can be used to sell the services you intend to offer. However, one of the most important attributes for holistic therapists is to have self-confidence, a positive attitude and belief in themselves and their abilities. As the holistic therapy business is a personal service, it is essential that therapists feel confident enough to sell their services and products to potential clients.

In order to be able to sell a service or product effectively, it is important for a therapist to:

- know the services well enough and have enough experience to be able to sell their benefits to potential clients
- be aware of the services of competitors and have identified their strengths and weaknesses
- be able to sell solutions
- identify with the potential client's needs and personalise the sale.

Personality selling

The concept of personality selling is very important in business. Some clients may decide whether to have a treatment based on factual information. In this case, the benefits of the treatment need to be stressed in a very factual and analytical way. Other clients may need to have a picture created for them, enhanced by imaginative therapeutic words to stimulate their interest.

No amount of advertising can make up for the personal touch, and with Indian head massage it is best to consider the direct and more personal approach first and turn personal skills to your advantage. By creating a positive environment for treatment provision, therapists can sell through one of the most powerful senses – the therapeutic touch. When planning advertising and promotion, it is essential to use a mix of methods in order to reach different target markets and help to evaluate the overall effectiveness of the activities.

> **Key fact**
> Some therapists may feel uncomfortable with the idea of selling and may need to attend sales training in order to enhance this very important skill.

The direct approach to marketing and promotion

Personal recommendation/word of mouth

This is the most valuable form of advertising for personal treatments like Indian head massage. Once a therapist has established a reputation for excellent customer service and quality skills, a satisfied client will automatically recommend the service to another potential client. It is important for therapists to tell as many people as possible about Indian head massage and communicate their enthusiasm. Positive enthusiasm is infectious, and even if the person you are speaking to does not need the information, they may pass it on to someone who does. The power of the spoken word is very effective in the marketing of services.

Talks and demonstrations

Talks and demonstrations are an effective way of presenting the service to a targeted group and they usually work best when presented together.

Talks should be informative and educational in nature (they should tell potential clients how Indian head massage will benefit them) and the demonstration should show the target audience the effects and help to break down barriers or preconceptions they may hold about the therapy.

It is useful to identify the needs of the target audience prior to the presentation, as this gives the therapist the advantage of being able to personalise the session. Talks and demonstrations are best limited to a maximum of 30 to 40 minutes, with time left to answer questions and to distribute business cards and literature.

The focus of the talk should be about identifying with and providing solutions to the client's needs.

A useful checklist when preparing for talks is to:

- find out as much as possible about the target group before the talk
- confirm the number of people who will be attending
- check out the venue and its suitability
- plan out the talk with a basic outline format
- have a plentiful supply of literature to hand out
- prepare a list of possible questions you might be asked
- take some relaxation music to help create a relaxing ambience
- aim to involve the audience in the session (encourage questions or volunteer models for demonstrations)
- take your appointment book with you, along with forms for clients to complete with their email addresses to allow you to send out follow-up marketing newsletters.

Exhibitions

Exhibitions are an effective way to communicate with lots of potential clients in one place. They are a useful way of distributing brochures and leaflets and persuading new clients to watch a demonstration of a new service and sample it. When exhibiting at a show it is important to ensure that it is the right type of show for the image of the business. It is also important to speak to people who have attended the show to gain feedback from them.

In order to project the right image at an exhibition it is important to ensure that:

- the stand looks attractive, neat and tidy
- the stand is accessible and situated to your best advantage
- staff manning the stand look warm and welcoming, and are approachable and easy to talk to
- there is space for people to browse without feeling intimidated.

It is also important, if possible, to take the names and contact details (including email addresses) of those who visit the stand, so that you can contact them after the exhibition.

Building a referral network

This is one of the most successful and inexpensive ways of creating new business. Current satisfied clients are one of the most effective means of advertising.

Referrals can be encouraged by:

- offering existing clients incentives to introduce new clients to use your service
- establishing links with other professionals by making yourself and what you do known to them.

Public relations

This is a way for therapists to get their name in the public eye without actually paying for advertising.

There are a variety of ways in which it can be done.

1. Offering a free talk and demonstration to a particular client group in the community is an ideal way of marketing Indian head massage and helping to get your name and reputation established.

   Public interest in holistic therapies is increasing all the time and there are many groups that meet regularly that might be keen to hear from you (a list of contact names, addresses and phone numbers may be obtained from your local library). (See talks and demonstrations on page 260.)
2. Send information or news concerning your business to editors of newspapers or magazines in the form of a news article. Every day, editors and journalists are looking for stories and information to fill their newspapers or magazines.

   An important consideration when sending information to journalists is to send only information that is truly of interest to the community and their readers.
3. Donate your time, money or products to a local worthwhile charity. There are many charitable organisations that rely on donations each year in order to survive. An event linked to funding or sponsoring a charity would be a newsworthy article, as well as helping to meet the needs of the community.
4. Try to get a regular or one-off slot on local radio (see radio on page 268).
5. Compile a press release that may be sent to local and national newspapers and magazines.

When compiling a press release, the following guidelines may help to increase your chances of publication:

- think of an original, interesting, thought-provoking or even humorous headline
- avoid trying to sell your service
- it should be newsworthy and of interest to the journalists and their readers
- address the information directly to a named editor or journalist, preferably one with whom you have already established contact
- ensure that it is laid out clearly (preferably with double-line spacing) and is no longer than two pages
- always include a contact name, address and telephone number.

The indirect approach to marketing and promotion

Study tip

Advertising strategies usually involve a mix of different media and should be scheduled over a period of time for maximum effect. Isolated advertisements rarely sustain enough interest.

There are several other methods of advertising or marketing that may be used in order to reach the potential clients you cannot reach in person. These include:

- online marketing
- newspaper advertising
- specialist magazines
- national directories
- mailshots
- leaflets and promotional material
- the internet
- local radio
- cross-merchandising promotional literature.

Online marketing

With the continuing development of the internet, social media and electronic communications, there are many more marketing opportunities and avenues available to a therapist, at a fraction of the financial cost, than those available only five years ago. However, while many of the marketing media available today are in fact free from financial cost, time and effort is still a crucial ingredient to generate success, and the clever marketer will always look to attain the best mix of both online and offline marketing, as there will always be times when one method will be more fruitful than the other.

The beauty with online marketing is that it can be integrated to afford a much wider range for penetration into the client market. However, it should be noted that while there are many marketing avenues available, it is best to find out which ones are best suited to your needs, as they will not always all be productive.

Websites

With the continued growth in the number of people using the internet, it is fairly essential to have a website in order to market yourself and have an online presence. Your website should function as your virtual shop front, and present you and your services in an appealing manner, not just to your prospective clients, but also to your existing clients in order to maintain their custom.

Websites come in all shapes, sizes and costs, from practically free to thousands of pounds. While you can now have a website for next to nothing, it is essential to make an investment in the optimisation of the website in order that you will appear reasonably high up on search engine results, so that you are visible to your potential clients.

Email

Email has been around for some years now, but is often overlooked as part of a marketing strategy. It is therefore a good idea to collect email addresses from your clients so that you can keep them informed of special offers and other news you may have.

It is easy to obtain a free email address, such as Gmail (Google) or Hotmail (Microsoft). However, if you have a website that is being hosted by an Internet Service Provider (ISP), you will normally get quite a few email accounts with this service, so that you can have yourname@yourcompany.co.uk. This is the best option as it gives a more professional look to your email address.

Online surveys

Once you have a good-sized database of your clients' email addresses, you can use free services (paid if it goes over a certain number), such as SurveyMonkey, to obtain quality information to help you with your marketing, by asking your clients to take part in an online survey that you send them by email. You can also offer a free incentive to encourage them to complete the survey, as the results can provide you with information that will help you decide what your customers want and what areas to put your marketing efforts into.

Social media

Since the last edition of this book, social media platforms have seen phenomenal growth and present a fantastic marketing opportunity for your business. The main social media platforms at the time of writing are:

- Facebook
- Twitter
- YouTube
- LinkedIn.

It is possible to set up accounts with all of the above at no cost apart from your time. But you can also have paid options, where you can advertise and target specific target markets.

Facebook (www.facebook.com)

With Facebook it is possible to have a business page that people can subscribe to by 'liking' your page. You can upload static information about your services, business and opening hours for people to see. The most important thing with Facebook is to post regularly to keep your subscribers interested. But remember, you do not want to keep pushing sales talk on them, as they will soon get fed up and go elsewhere.

> **Health and safety note**
>
> When seeking to send out a newsletter to a potential client via email, it is essential to obtain their permission to send them marketing emails, as there are antispamming laws that can incur heavy fines.

Twitter (www.twitter.com)

Twitter is similar to Facebook in that you can post regular updates to your subscribers (or followers, as they are called), but it was originally designed as a micro-blog that was limited to 140 characters, in order to tell people what you were doing at the time of writing. It has since expanded, as many businesses have found it to be a great marketing tool to keep their followers up to date with short sharp posts known as tweets.

YouTube (www.youtube.com)

YouTube was founded in 2005, but has become a great media for businesses to advertise themselves using video. You can set up your own channel on YouTube to upload videos, and for a relatively low cost you can create your own short promotional videos to market to your potential clients.

LinkedIn (www.linkedin.com)

LinkedIn is useful as a networking medium and can help you to develop business contacts or form links through your business connections.

With all social media, much of the marketing activity will require continued and regular input from you, so it is important to allocate the time and effort required to make these avenues work for you.

In-depth details on the above media can be found at each individual website. There are also other good sources and information on online marketing to be found through Business Link (www.businesslink.gov.uk).

Newspaper advertising

Advertising is about getting your message across. Important considerations when considering an advertisement are:

- what do you want to say to potential clients?
- who is your target audience?
- how will you communicate with them what you want to say?

It is essential to follow the tried and tested AIDA formula when considering your publicity:

- A (attracting *attention*): this can be created by an appropriate heading that attracts attention.
- I (generating *interest*): this can be created by stating what is on offer.
- D (creating *desire*): this can be created by stating why what you have to offer is needed and getting potential clients to believe in the benefits.
- A (motivating *action*): this can be created by offering the reader an incentive (special offer).

Good advertisements are usually targeted to the right audience, are accurate, not misleading, and are catchy, concise and memorable.

Effective adverts must have a good headline to have immediate impact. A good headline will:

- attract the reader's attention
- compel the person to read further

- improve response
- express the most important benefits.

A good advert should be easy to read and should be written to:

- touch people's emotions
- be informative
- promote the service
- raise awareness
- motivate the reader to act.

When designing adverts, ask yourself what adverts you responded to and why.

Local papers

There are two types of advertisements in newspapers: display advertisements and business classified. Display advertising is more expensive and could appear anywhere in the paper, unless you have paid to have a particular space, such as the front or back page or the television page (any of which could prove very expensive).

It is always a gamble when relying on display advertising, as it may be largely dependent on the following:

- the day of the week the paper is printed
- the time of the year
- the page the advert appears on
- the layout of the advert in relation to the other advertisers.

An important point to consider with display advertising is that people buy papers for many reasons other than to read adverts (reading news, announcements and events, crosswords, horoscopes). It is therefore important to consider how your advert is going to grab their attention, bearing in mind that newspapers have a short lifespan, and also bearing in mind the AIDA principle.

It is also useful to consider that the person reading the news and features may come across your display advert and may not be thinking about a massage until he or she sees your advert, or they may not be ready to have a massage for some while. In fact, it may take many exposures to your advert before this person feels you are sufficiently familiar to give you a try. It is therefore important that adverts are repeated regularly in the same way, in order to create familiarity. It can also help to have a picture of yourself in the advert, as it will be more eye-catching and will help the potential client to feel that they know you.

It is important to remember when writing adverts that you are speaking directly to your potential clients and the reader will be initially attracted by your headline message, rather than the name of your business. It is often helpful to give the reader a reason to reply immediately, such as a deadline on a special offer, as this motivates action.

When you have designed an advert, it is often helpful to ask friends and colleagues to cast an eye over the design and the wording for critical review; often, by looking with a fresh pair of eyes, they can add constructive comments.

Display advertising is usually more effective when it is combined with some editorial. Often papers run special features on health-related matters, and it may

Study tip

Words that tend to sell in adverts include:

you, new, results, health, free, complimentary, benefits, now, yes.

> **Key fact**
> Editorials in newspapers and magazines are seen to be credible and true, as readers place a considerable amount of trust in the objectivity of journalists. It is therefore worth getting to know editors and journalists and being persistent, as the articles they write tend to hold a lot of weight with readers.

be more appropriate to consider a display advert within a feature, as it draws the reader's attention to a more focused subject. Classified advertising is more cost-effective than display advertising, as it is more targeted to the service to be provided. The disadvantage with classified advertising is that there may not always be an appropriate section for holistic therapists and advertisements will need to be placed frequently in order to make it effective.

Specialist magazines

These are usually targeted to a specific audience, and those related to health are normally of interest to a holistic therapist. The main drawback with them is that they are not local, but national, and whether the advertising will be effective will depend on the readership and the location of the therapist.

Promotional material

> **Key fact**
> Check the readership profile before committing to advertising in magazines, and check circulation radius and readership numbers.

When writing and designing promotional material, the key to success is to write it as if you know the client personally. Choose words carefully so that they strike a chord with the client. Remember that many clients reading promotional material may not know they are looking for your service until they see it.

It is also important when developing marketing material to ensure that it reflects the image you wish to portray and that it appeals to the target market.

Promotional materials such as leaflets, brochures and posters are the means by which clients will decide whether to contact you for an appointment. Promotional material must be attractive enough to make clients read it, and wording should be positive, direct and, above all, personal. Brochures and posters with a question-and-answer format can help clients to overcome their reservations, and visual aids can help to attract attention.

It is also important to use positive language and turn a negative statement (such as a client's problem) into a positive one (how your treatment is going to help them). Including testimonials from satisfied clients (with their permission) can also help to build credibility and break down barriers.

Mailshots

> **Key fact**
> When writing to companies it is worth offering the incentive of corporate membership as a promotion, to motivate more clients to use your service. Each employee may be issued with a corporate membership card, which entitles them to a certain percentage discount.

Mailshots can be a worthwhile exercise, but require a degree of planning and forethought. It is far more effective to target a specific group when designing a mailshot, as the main theme has to address the needs of all the recipients.

You may choose to target self-help groups with a common need of relaxation, or to write to the occupational health adviser at local companies, offering to give free talks and demonstrations as part of their stress management programme.

The letter should be sent on headed notepaper and should be brief and concise. The focus should be on the recipient's needs, although it is helpful to send background information on yourself, as well as information on Indian head massage.

Mailshots usually have a success or response rate of around 2 per cent, although this may be enhanced to 5 per cent by follow-up phone calls.

When sending a mailshot it is important to consider the day it is mailed out, as this could have a significant effect on the result. If sending a mailshot to clients' homes, aim to send it to arrive on a Friday or Saturday, ready for the weekend, when they may have more time to consider what you are offering. If sending mailshots to companies, aim to send the information to arrive on a Tuesday or Wednesday, and preferably not on a Friday or Monday.

Acquiring corporate clients

Indian head massage is ideally suited to the workplace because of its unique selling points:

- it is portable in nature
- it is quick
- it provides a solution to the client's problems
- it is a personal service
- there is no need for the client to undress
- no special resources are required.

If your objective is to secure contracts with corporate clients, first consider which companies (both large and small) are within your catchment area and the profile of the staff members.

When approaching corporate clients, it is important to create a corporate image for yourself, even if you are not part of a large organisation. The first point of contact should be by letter or email, directly to the person within the organisation who is responsible for the health and welfare of staff (this may be an occupational health adviser, staff nurse, health and safety officer or managing director). The letter, if sent in the traditional way, should be sent on quality headed notepaper. The main theme of the letter should focus on the workplace benefits of Indian head massage and how it can benefit the staff and the organisation (see Chapter 8 on stress management). When approaching corporate clients it is advisable to avoid 'flowery' therapy language, and be specific and accurate in terms of the outcome (the benefits). Offer to go in and give a free talk and demonstration, with no obligation. Once the letter or email has been sent, keep a record of it and follow it up with a phone call approximately seven to ten days afterwards.

Remember that businesses, whether large or small, receive a lot of paperwork through the post. Do not assume that the reason you have not heard from them is that they are not interested. They may simply not have had time to read your letter or email.

Publications and directories

Advertising in national publications and directories such as Yellow Pages can be an effective way of advertising, as entries are classified by therapy type. It is also a long-term form of advertising and can prove to be cost-effective, as many are annual publications.

Therapists should also consider their geographical location; if they are situated between two counties, it may be advisable to take an advert in more than one directory.

If there are several therapists advertising under the same category, it is important to consider your USP and stress this in order to make your entry stand out from your competitors.

Radio

Radio is an excellent form of media in raising awareness of treatments such as Indian head massage. Consider contacting your local radio station, with a view to having either a regular or a one-off spot on the radio to promote Indian head massage. It is important when approaching the station to make the proposal interesting and one that will interest their listeners. It is important to respond to local trends or issues (for instance, lifestyle or reducing stress) when presenting information on the radio, as it has to be topical and of value to listeners. Assessing growth trends within the industry will help you to assess the opportunities on offer to you.

When preparing to talk on the radio it is important to find out as much as possible about the programme you will be appearing on, the profile of the listeners and, most importantly, the style of the radio presenter. Some presenters prefer to work to a script and will run through a list of questions before the programme; others prefer to work unscripted and make the presentation more spontaneous.

> **Key fact**
>
> Local radio stations often look for gifts that can be given to listeners in exchange for on-air promotions. Donating your services is an easy and effective way of getting your name out on the airwaves without buying advertising time.

Cross-merchandising promotional literature

Consider other local businesses that cater for clientele similar to yours – for example, hairdressers, osteopaths – and who may be in a position to influence clients to try Indian head massage. Exchange promotional literature and brochures with them; this will allow each party additional exposure to the type of clients they wish to attract. When approaching other local businesses with a view to cross-merchandising, it is important to establish a friendly, approachable and cooperative working relationship, as this will enhance the success of the promotion on both sides.

Encouraging client retention

The first goal of marketing is to encourage potential clients to try out your services; the next goal is to encourage them to come back again. There are several ways of fostering repeat business:

- Create an understanding of the benefits of the treatments you provide to clients by encouraging them to book regular treatments.
- Award loyalty bonuses and reward schemes (such as ones offered by major supermarket chains).
- Stay in touch with your clients and inform them of special offers and any new treatments you may have added to your treatment menu (and how these can benefit them).
- Invite clients to attend talks and events you may be holding.

Helpful tip: remember that you can keep in touch with your clients very easily through social media network marketing, through Facebook, Twitter and LinkedIn.

Maximising marketing opportunities

Because of the widespread appeal of Indian head massage, it is well suited to clinics, salons and spas, as well as other associated trades, such as hairdressers, osteopaths, chiropractors and health clinics. Consider all the places where people attend regularly for reasons of health, beauty and relaxation.

A local hairdresser may be interested in adding Indian head massage to their treatment menu, to give a different marketing angle to their customer service. Osteopaths and chiropractors may be interested in Indian head massage for clients with soft-tissue problems of the head, neck and shoulders. A GP surgery may be interested in helping patients with stress, anxiety and depression, or with musculoskeletal problems.

If you have a local regional airport nearby, there may be interest in a business proposal to offer treatments to tired business executives in need of stress relief. A local school may benefit from a regular visit to help teachers and students to manage their stress levels.

If you use your imagination, there are a multitude of different opportunities for marketing Indian head massage.

Selling of associated products

As providing treatments is a labour-intensive service, consider selling complementary products for clients' home use. Clients are more likely to buy products such as scalp oils and relaxation tapes at the time of their treatment. It is therefore advisable to have a display of items available for purchase at reception or wherever the client is likely to pay. Clients are also more likely to buy from their therapist, with whom they have a trusting relationship.

Creative marketing opportunities

Other creative marketing opportunities could be to offer gift certificates linked to promotions at specific times of the year, such as Christmas, Valentine's Day, birthdays, Mother's Day or Father's Day. Specially packaged courses of treatment often attract interest, as they are designed specifically to address the needs of the recipient.

Male clients

An area that is often left unexploited is the male market. Marketing treatments such as Indian head massage to men can require a different strategy from selling to female clients. Men often respond more to factual and benefit-related words rather than the more aesthetic language women tend to respond to. Think of male-dominated markets and how that target market may be reached. Local sports clubs and associations might be a good place to start, as well as men's barbers and health clubs.

An important consideration when marketing to male clients is whether the environment you are practising in is male-friendly (it may be difficult to attract male clients into a salon that looks too pretty and feminine). Some men are also conscious of their body image; it may therefore be more prudent to schedule specific times for male clients to attend.

Defining marketing objectives

Once you have put together the right mix of marketing methods, the next stage is to define your marketing objectives. Marketing objectives are closely linked to overall business objectives and will define what you want to achieve from your marketing and how you intend to meet the objectives. Below is an example of marketing objectives for a therapist practising Indian head massage.

Objectives

Short-term

To introduce Indian head massage to existing clientele

Medium-term

To expand the existing client base to secure new clients

Long-term

To introduce Indian head massage into the workplace

Strategy

1. Send a newsletter to all existing clients, advising them of the benefits of Indian head massage and how it can help them. Include a voucher with a special introductory offer.
2. Contact the editor of a local newspaper to offer an article on Indian head massage that is going to be of interest to readers, plus a free demonstration.
3. Write to 20 local companies with a short but informative introductory letter. Offer a corporate discount. Follow up with a phone call in seven to ten days, with a view to securing a meeting to offer a free talk and demonstration.

Monitoring marketing methods

It is important to regularly monitor the response to marketing methods, so you can assess which methods are helping you to meet your business objectives. It is essential to constantly monitor, review and adapt your strategies in order to ensure continued business success. Marketing methods may change, with a difference in trend, or may simply become outdated.

A simple and effective way of monitoring the response to your marketing methods is to ask each new client how they heard of you and keep a record of this, in order to review it in line with your business objectives. Provided you know how much each method cost and how many clients were generated from it, you will then be in a position to analyse which methods are cost-effective. Once you establish a clientele, you can build up information such as how often they attend for treatments, how much they spend and what marketing methods they respond to.

For marketing to have the desired effects it should be:

- sufficient – it has to be done regularly, even when you are busy
- efficient – it has to be cost-effective to be worthwhile
- effective – it has to work and get results.

How to encourage repeat business

Maintaining excellent customer service is the key to encouraging repeat business.

It is important to make it easy for clients to come to you by:

- making client needs a priority
- concentrating all your actions and efforts for the business with the client in mind
- treating every client like a new client and avoiding complacency
- delivering an excellent service
- building an open relationship with clients by encouraging feedback.

Keeping ahead of business

Many businesses fail to realise their potential because they do not continually market themselves. An important factor to consider is that many clients may have to see your advert or marketing material many times before responding.

Many therapists fail to be consistent in marketing methods, believing that they already have enough clients. Even if the appointment book is full, it is important to keep on marketing, to raise client awareness and to maintain your professional image, as you never know when you are going to lose current clients because of various circumstances – for example, client's personal or financial circumstances, or clients moving out of the area.

Indian Head Massage Questionnaire

Indian head massage is a traditional massage treatment originating in India. It involves the application of massage techniques to the upper back and shoulders, upper arms, neck, face and scalp. The treatment is applied through the clothes, with the recipient remaining seated in a chair.

Indian head massage has many benefits, including helping to relieve muscular tension, relieving headaches and reducing stress levels.

This questionnaire is designed to establish current levels of awareness and interest in Indian head massage.

1. Have you heard of Indian head massage before? (Delete as applicable.) Yes/No

2. If yes, when did you hear about it?

___

___

3. Do you experience any of the following on a regular basis? (Please circle any that apply.)

High stress levels Muscular tension in the back, neck or shoulders Headaches

Eyestrain Anxiety Depression Poor concentration levels

4. What measures do you take (if any) to help with any of the above?

___

___

5. Would you be interested in trying a treatment? Yes/No

6. Would you like further information on Indian head massage and its benefits? Yes/No

Thank you for your time and cooperation in completing this form. If you would like further information or would like to book a complimentary introductory treatment, please give your details below.

Name ___

Address ___

___

Email address ___

Telephone number(s) ___

▲ Figure 10.1 Indian head massage questionnaire

To access editable and printable versions of this form scan the QR code opposite or visit www.hodderplus.co.uk/indianhead/chapter-10.

Activity

Design a marketing plan for Indian head massage based on the following outline:

1. Description of the service to be offered – that is, Indian head massage

   Include your unique selling points and a full description of the service and how it can benefit clients.
2. Objectives of the marketing campaign

   This could be to increase your client market or to raise awareness of Indian head massage.
3. A profile of your intended client market

   This is who you want to target and why you think they will pay for the service. Include as much information as possible, based on what you have discovered about your potential clients (market questionnaires, interviews, etc.). Also include information on competitors, if applicable, as this will help you to identify how much your potential clients are currently spending on a similar service.
4. Where you intend to offer the service (location)

   Because of its portability, consider the different locations where Indian head massage treatment may be offered.
5. Details of your SWOT analysis (strengths, weaknesses, opportunities, threats)
6. Intended marketing strategies

   Consider how you intend to advertise the service, what media you will use and how often you will advertise.

   Consider all the direct and indirect forms of marketing and promotion that will help your business to succeed.

   Design a promotional leaflet for Indian head massage.

   Remember to allocate a budget for marketing activities and to plan the activities over a period of time for maximum effect.

Frequently asked questions

Can Indian head massage be carried out daily as it is in India?

Indian head massage is generally carried out daily in Indian families as it is part of family life. Treatment is short and is generally restricted to the head only. Indian head massage has developed in the western world as a more comprehensive treatment, which, if carried out daily, may prove too stimulating and provoke adverse reactions. It is therefore best to leave 48 hours between treatments to allow the body to rest and respond to any reactions.

When massaging the scalp I find the oil application difficult. Do you have any advice?

First, it is best to use a bottle with a slow-drip cap to ensure that only a small amount of oil is released at a time. If you are massaging a client with thick or long hair, it is best to section the hair off with clips, by parting down the centre and then dividing the scalp into quarter sections to ensure even coverage of the oil to be absorbed into the scalp and hair follicles.

If a client has curly hair, what is the best way of carrying out the hair tugging without causing the client discomfort/getting your fingers stuck in the hair?

First, ensure the hair is free from hair products such as mousse, hairspray or gel. When carrying out the hair tugging on curly hair, ensure that you tug the hair from the root only, by clasping the hair between the fingers, but keeping them *fixed at the root* as you tug. If you attempt to draw the fingers upwards and through the hair (as is usual with this technique), your fingers will invariably get stuck and will be likely to cause discomfort.

With clients with little or no hair, do I simply miss out the scalp massage?

No, you can still carry out the scalp massage, omitting techniques such as the hair tugging; despite the fact that your client may have little or no hair, they will still benefit from the relaxation of the muscle fibres of the scalp.

Where is the best place to buy authentic Indian oils for Indian head massage?

The best place to buy authentic Indian oils is from a local Indian supermarket or from an Ayurvedic supplier (see Resources section on page 286).

What is the best way to promote Indian head massage?

The best way to promote Indian head massage is simply to demonstrate it in as many locations as possible – the more public the place, the better (such as exhibitions and shows). Take advantage of the fact that Indian head massage is portable and demonstrate an aspect of the treatment where clients will look their most relaxed (massaging the scalp).

When I was carrying out Indian head massage on one of my clients recently, she started to experience a feeling of faintness when I started to massage the head. Why is this, and what action should be taken in the event of this happening during a treatment?

This can be a common reaction to Indian head massage due to the increased blood supply to the head. Some clients may feel dizzy due to stress or tiredness, or their blood sugar levels or blood pressure may have dropped during the treatment. Always monitor and discuss your client's reactions during treatments, and if they start to feel faint it is best to stop the treatment and ensure their continued comfort by offering them a glass of water and advising that they get some fresh air, if appropriate.

I have a client who suffers from osteoarthritis in the neck who wants to try Indian head massage. Is it possible to carry out a treatment on this client?

It may be possible to carry out an adapted form of treatment, but this depends on the severity of the client's condition. In cases where pain and discomfort are severe, it is best for a client to seek medical advice.

Care would need to be taken to ensure there was no excessive movement of the neck joint during treatment, in order to avoid pain, discomfort and potential joint damage. In most cases, gentle massage can help to ease pain and gently increase mobility. Care should also be taken to position the client according to individual comfort and offer additional supports for the neck.

Remember that if the client's condition is acutely inflamed at the time of the treatment, it would be best to avoid massage, as the increased circulation arising from the massage may exacerbate the symptoms.

Glossary

abducens nerve a mixed nerve that innervates only the lateral rectus muscle of the eye

abduction movement of a limb away from the midline

accessory nerve innervates muscles in the neck and upper back, as well as muscles of the palate, pharynx and larynx

acne vulgaris a common inflammatory disorder of the sebaceous glands that leads to the overproduction of sebum

adduction movement of a limb towards the midline

adipose tissue type of tissue containing fat cells, found in the subcutaneous layer of skin

adrenaline hormone secreted by the medulla of the adrenal glands; prepares the body for 'fright, fight or flight' response

Ajna the brow chakra located in the middle of the forehead, over the 'third eye' area

albinism a condition in which there is an inherited absence of pigmentation in the skin, hair and eyes

allergic reaction a disorder in which the body becomes hypersensitive to a particular allergen and produces histamine in the skin as part of the body's defence

alopecia temporary baldness or severe hair loss, which may follow illness, shock or a period of extreme stress

Anahata the heart chakra, located in the centre of the chest

angina pain in the left side of the chest and usually radiating to the left arm, caused by insufficient blood reaching the heart muscle

ankylosing spondylitis a systemic joint disease

anxiety a psychological illness that can vary from a mild form to panic attacks and severe phobias

arthritis: osteoarthritis a joint disease involving varying degrees of joint pain, stiffness, limitation of movement, joint instability and deformity

arthritis: rheumatoid chronic inflammation of peripheral joints, resulting in pain, stiffness and potential damage to joints

asthma shortness of breath and difficulty breathing caused by spasm or swelling of the bronchial tubes

autonomic nervous system part of the nervous system that controls the automatic activities of smooth and cardiac muscle, and the activities of glands

Ayurveda world's oldest Indian healing system ('the science of life and longevity')

basal cell layer (stratum germinativum) deepest and innermost of the five layers of epidermis

Bell's palsy a disorder of the seventh cranial nerve (facial nerve) that results in paralysis on one side of the face

biceps a muscle on the anterior of the upper arm

boil an inflamed nodule forming a pocket of bacteria around the base of a hair follicle, or a break in the skin

brachialis a muscle attaching to the distal half of the anterior surface of the humerus at one end, and to the ulna at the other

brachioradialis an anterior muscle of the forearm, connecting the humerus to the radius

brainstem the enlarged extension upwards within the skull of the spinal cord, consisting of the medulla oblongata, the pons and the midbrain

bronchi two short tubes that carry air into each lung

bronchiole a subdivision of the bronchial tree

bronchitis a chronic or acute inflammation of the bronchial tubes

buccinator the main muscle of the cheek, attached to both the upper and the lower jaw

cardiac muscle special type of involuntary muscle found only in the heart

carotid artery either of the two main arteries of the neck whose branches supply the head and neck

carpals eight small bones forming the wrist

central nervous system (CNS) part of the nervous system consisting of the brain and spinal cord

cerebellum cauliflower-shaped structure located at the posterior of the cranium, below the cerebrum

cerebral palsy a condition caused by damage to a baby's central nervous system during pregnancy, delivery or soon after birth

cerebrum largest portion of the brain, making up the front and top part of the brain

cervical nodes lymph nodes located within the neck

cervical plexuses spinal nerves supplying the skin and muscles of the head, neck and upper region of the shoulders

cervical vertebrae seven vertebrae of the neck

chakras non-physical energy centres, located about 2.5 cm away from the physical body

chloasma a pigmentation disorder that presents with irregular areas of increased pigmentation, usually on the face

clavicle bone forming the anterior of the shoulder girdle

clear layer (stratum lucidum) epidermal layer below the most superficial layer

coccygeal plexus supplies the skin in the area of the coccyx and the muscles of the pelvic floor

coccygeal vertebrae (coccyx) four fused vertebrae at the base of spine, forming the tail bone

collagen protein in the dermis that gives the skin its strength and resilience

comedone a collection of sebum, keratinised cells and wastes that accumulate in the entrance of a hair follicle

compression a form of petrissage in which the muscles are gently pressed against a surface

conjunctivitis a bacterial infection following irritation of the conjunctiva of the eye

contact dermatitis red, dry and inflamed skin caused by a primary irritant

corrugator a muscle located on the inner edge of the eyebrow

cranial nerves set of 12 pairs of nerves originating from the brain

cuticle outer layer of hair

deltoid thick, triangular muscle that caps the top of the humerus and the shoulder

depression a psychological condition that combines symptoms of lowered mood, loss of appetite, poor sleep, lack of concentration and interest

dermal papilla elevation at the base of the hair bulb; contains a rich blood supply

dermis deeper layer of the skin found below the epidermis

desquamation the shedding of dead skin cells from the horny layer (stratum corneum)

diabetes a metabolic disorder, of which there are two types: diabetes mellitus, in which sugars are not oxidised to produce enough energy due to lack of the pancreatic hormone insulin, is the most common form; diabetes insipidus, in which a person produces large quantities of dilute urine and is constantly thirsty, is a less common form

diaphragm dome-shaped muscle of respiration that separates the thorax from the abdomen

dosha subtle life-giving force

eccrine gland simple, coiled, tubular sweat gland that opens directly on to the surface of the skin

effleurage a stroking or smoothing movement that signals the beginning and end of a massage

embolism obstruction or closure of a vessel by an embolus

embolus substance such as a blood clot that is carried by the blood and obstructs a blood vessel

epidermis outermost, superficial layer of the skin

epilepsy a neurological disorder that makes the individual susceptible to recurrent and temporary seizures

erector pili muscle small, smooth muscle attached at an angle to the base of a hair follicle

erector spinae a long, postural muscle in three bands either side of the spine, attaching to the spine, ribcage and head

erythema reddening of the skin due to the dilation of blood capillaries just below the epidermis

ethmoid skull bone forming part of the wall of the orbit, the roof of the nasal cavity and part of the nasal septum

extensor carpi radialis a muscle extending along the radial side of the posterior of the forearm

extensor carpi ulnaris a muscle extending along the ulnar side of the posterior of the forearm

extensor digitorum a muscle extending along the lateral side of the posterior of the forearm

facial nerve a mixed nerve that conducts impulses to and from several areas in the face and neck

fibromyalgia a chronic condition that produces musculoskeletal pain

flexor carpi digitorum an anterior muscle of the forearm extending from the medial end of the humerus, the anterior of the ulna and radius to the anterior surfaces of the second to fifth fingers

flexor carpi radialis a muscle of the forearm extending along the radial side of the anterior of forearm

flexor carpi ulnaris an anterior muscle of the forearm extending along the ulnar side of the anterior of the forearm

folliculitis a bacterial infection that occurs in the hair follicles of the skin

frictions deeper massage movements, causing the skin to rub against the underlying structures

frontal skull bone forming the forehead

frontalis muscle that extends over the front of the skull and the width of the forehead

frozen shoulder (adhesive capsulitis) a chronic condition in which there is pain and stiffness and reduced mobility, or locking, of the shoulder joint

glossopharyngeal nerve a mixed nerve that innervates structures in the mouth and throat

granular layer (stratum granulosum) layer of epidermis linking the living cells of the epidermis (basal and prickle cell layers) to the dead cells above

haemorrhage loss of blood from the circulatory system; bleeding

hair bulb the enlarged part at the base of the hair root

hair root part of the hair found below the surface of the skin

hair shaft part of the hair that lies above the surface of the skin

hair tugging a technique used in the scalp massage where the roots of the hair are lifted and pulled upwards in order to stimulate hair growth

herpes simplex (cold sore) a viral infection normally found on the face and around the lips

herpes zoster (shingles) painful infection along the sensory nerves caused by the virus that causes chicken pox

high blood pressure when the resting blood pressure is above normal (consistently exceeding 160 mmHg systolic and 95 mmHg diastolic)

homeostasis process by which the body maintains a stable internal environment for its cells and tissues

horny layer (stratum corneum) most superficial, outer layer of the skin, consisting of dead, flattened, keratinised cells

humerus long bone of the upper arm

hypothenar eminence a projection of soft tissue located on the ulnar side of the palm of the hand; consists of three muscles: abductor digiti minimi manus, flexor digiti minimi manus and opponens digiti minimi

impetigo a superficial, contagious, inflammatory disease caused by streptococcal and staphylococcal bacteria

infraspinatus a muscle that attaches to the middle two-thirds of the scapula, below the spine of the scapula at one end and the top of the humerus at the other

intercostal muscles muscles that occupy the spaces between the ribs and are responsible for controlling some of the movements of the ribs

jugular vein major vein draining blood from the head and neck (divides into internal and external branches)

kapha one of the three doshas; said to be responsible for growth

keratin tough fibrous protein found in the epidermis, the hair and the nails

keratinisation process that cells undergo when they change from living cells with a nucleus to dead, horny cells without a nucleus

kyphosis an abnormally increased outward curvature of the thoracic spine

lacrimal bones smallest of the facial bones, located close to the medial part of the orbital cavity

larynx (voice box) short passage connecting the pharynx to the trachea

levator labii superiorus a muscle located towards the inner cheek beside the nose, extending from the upper jaw to the skin of the corners of the mouth and the upper lip

levator scapula a strap-like muscle that runs almost vertically through the neck, connecting the cervical vertebrae to the scapula

low blood pressure when the blood pressure is below normal (consistently 99 mmHg or less systolic and less than 59 mmHg diastolic)

lymph transparent, colourless, watery liquid, derived from tissue fluid

lymphatic capillaries minute, blind-end tubes that commence in the tissue spaces of the body

lymphatic node oval or bean-shaped structure that filters lymph

lymphatic vessels tubes similar in structure to veins, with thin, collapsible walls and valves; responsible for transporting lymph

malignant melanoma a deeply pigmented mole that is life-threatening if it is not recognised and treated promptly

mandible only moveable bone of the skull, forming the lower jaw

Manipura the solar plexus chakra, located at approximately waist level

marma points subtle pressure points that stimulate the life force or pranic flow

masseter a thick muscle in the cheek, extending from the zygomatic arch to the outer corner of the mandible

mastication the process of chewing food

mastoid nodes lymph nodes located behind the ear; they drain lymph from the skin of the ear and the temporal region of the scalp

matrix (hair) area of mitotic activity of the hair cells, located at the lower part of the hair bulb

maxilla largest bone of the face, forming the upper jaw

mentalis a muscle radiating from the lower lip over the centre of the chin

metacarpals five long bones in the palm of the hand

migraine specific form of headache, usually unilateral (one side of the head), associated with nausea or vomiting

milia pearly, white, hard nodules under the skin

Muladhara the base or root chakra, located at the base of the spine, concerned with issues of a physical nature

multiple sclerosis disease of the central nervous system in which the myelin sheath is destroyed and various functions become impaired

muscle tone state of partial contraction of a muscle

nasal bone small facial bone forming the bridge of the nose

nasalis a muscle located at the sides of the nose

occipital bone skull bone forming the back of the skull

occipital nodes lymph nodes located at the base of the skull

occipitalis muscle found at the back of the head, attached to the occipital bone and the skin of the scalp

oculomotor nerve a mixed nerve that innervates the internal and external muscles of the eye and a muscle of the upper eyelid

oedema an abnormal swelling of body tissues due to an accumulation of fluid

orbicularis oculi a circular muscle that surrounds the eye

orbicularis oris a circular muscle that surrounds the mouth

osteoporosis brittle bones due to ageing and the lack of the hormone oestrogen, which affects the ability to deposit calcium in the matrix of bone

palatine L-shaped bones that form the anterior part of the roof of the mouth

papillary layer most superficial layer of the dermis, situated above the reticular layer

parasympathetic nervous system one of the two divisions of the autonomic nervous system; creates the conditions needed for rest and sleep

parietal bones bones forming the upper sides of the skull and the back of the roof of the skull

parotid nodes lymph nodes located at the angle of the jaw; they drain lymph from the nose, eyelids and ear

pectoralis major a thick, fan-shaped muscle covering the anterior surface of the upper chest

pectoralis minor a thin muscle that lies beneath the pectoralis major

pediculosis (lice) a contagious parasitic infection, commonly known as lice; the lice live off blood sucked from the skin

petrissage deeper massage movements using the whole hand, thumbs or fingers (picking up, squeezing and releasing, rolling, etc.)

pharynx (throat) serves as an air and food passage

pitta one of the three doshas, which is said to be responsible for the process of transformation or metabolism

pityriasis capitis (dandruff) a scaly, flaking scalp condition

platysma a superficial neck muscle that extends from the chest up either side of the neck to the chin

prana the vital force (*pra* = before, *ana* = breath)

pressure points vital energy points similar to acupressure used in Chinese medicine

prickle cell layer (stratum spinosum) binding and transitional layer between the stratum granulosum (granular layer) and the stratum germinativum (basal cell layer)

procerus a muscle located between the eyebrows

progressive muscular relaxation a physical technique designed to relax the body when it is tense

psoriasis chronic inflammatory skin condition

radius long bone of the forearm (on thumb side of forearm)

reticular fibres fibres found in the reticular layer of the dermis that help to maintain the skin's tone, strength and elasticity

reticular layer deepest layer of the dermis, situated below the papillary layer

rhomboids either of the two muscles situated in the upper part of the back, between the thoracic vertebrae and the scapula

ringworm a fungal infection of the skin

risorius a triangular-shaped muscle that lies horizontally on the cheek, joining at the corners of the mouth

rodent ulcer a malignant tumour; starts off as a slow-growing, pearly nodule, often at the site of a previous skin injury

rosacea a chronic inflammatory disease of the face, making the skin appear abnormally red

Sahasrara the crown chakra, located on top of the head, concerned with thinking and decision-making

scapula bone forming posterior of the shoulder girdle

scar a mark left on the skin after a wound has healed

sebaceous cyst a round, nodular lesion, with a smooth, shiny surface, which develops from a sebaceous gland

sebaceous gland small, sac-like pouches found all over the body (except for the soles of the feet and the palms of the hands), producing an oily substance called sebum

seborrhoea an excessive secretion of sebum by the sebaceous glands

seborrhoeic dermatitis a mild to chronic inflammatory disease of hairy areas that are well supplied with sebaceous glands; common sites are the scalp, face, axilla and groin

serratus anterior a broad, curved muscle located on the side of the chest/ribcage below the axilla

sinusitis a condition involving inflammation of the paranasal sinuses

skeletal/voluntary muscle attached to the skeleton, this type of muscle tissue is striped in appearance and is responsible for the movement of bones

smooth/involuntary muscle this type of muscle tissue is found in the walls of hollow organs such as the stomach, intestines, bladder and uterus, and in blood vessels

sphenoid skull bone located in front of the temporal bone

squamous cell carcinoma a malignant tumour that arises from the prickle cell layer of the epidermis

sternocleidomastoid long muscle that lies obliquely across each side of the neck

stress any factor that affects physical or emotional health

stroke the blocking of blood flow to the brain by an embolus in a cerebral blood vessel

stye acute inflammation of a gland at the base of an eyelash, caused by bacterial infection

subcutaneous layer thick layer of connective and adipose tissue found below the dermis

submandibular nodes lymph nodes located beneath the jaw; they drain lymph from the chin, lips, nose, cheeks and tongue

superficial cervical nodes lymph nodes located at the side of the neck; they drain lymph from the lower part of the ear and the cheek region

supraspinatus muscle located in the depression above the spine of the scapula

Swadhistana the sacral chakra, located at the level of the sacrum, between the navel and the base chakra

tapotement a series of light, brisk, springy movements applied with both hands in rapid succession (hacking, double hacking, tapping)

telangiecstasis dilated capillaries, where there is persistent vasodilation

temporal bone forms the sides of the skull, below the parietal bones and above and around the ears

temporalis a fan-shaped muscle situated on the side of the skull above and in front of the ear

temporomandibular joint tension (TMJ syndrome) a collection of symptoms and signs produced by disorders of the temporomandibular joint (the hinge joint between the mandible of the jaw and the temporal bone of the skull)

teres major a muscle that attaches to the bottom lateral edge of the scapula at one end and the back of the humerus (just below the shoulder joint) at the other

teres minor a muscle that attaches to the lateral edge of the scapula, above teres major at one end, and into the top of the posterior of the humerus at the other

thenar eminence a mound of soft tissue located on the radial side of the palm of the hand

thoracic cavity group of body parts (sternum, ribs and thoracic vertebrae) that protect the heart and lungs

thrombosis the formation of a thrombus in an unbroken blood vessel

thrombus a clot of coagulated blood that remains at its site of formation

tinea capitis a fungal infection of the scalp (a type of ringworm)

tinnitis condition where there is the sensation of sounds in the ears in the absence of an external sound source

trachea the windpipe that passes down into the thorax and connects the larynx with the bronchi

trapezius a large, triangular-shaped muscle in the upper back

triangularis a triangular-shaped muscle, located below the corners of the mouth

triceps a muscle on the posterior of the upper arm

trigeminal nerve a mixed nerve (containing motor and sensory nerves)

trigeminal neuralgia a painful condition caused by irritation of the fifth cranial nerve (the trigeminal nerve)

tumour an abnormal growth of tissue, which may be benign or malignant

turbinate bone layers of bone located either side of the outer walls of the nasal cavities

ulcer a slow-healing, open sore in the skin, extending to all its layers

ulna long bone of the forearm (on little finger side of forearm)

urticaria (hives) an itchy rash resulting from the release of histamine by mast cells

vacuole empty space within the cytoplasm containing waste materials or secretions formed by the cytoplasm

vagus nerve a cranial nerve with branches to numerous organs in the thorax and abdomen as well as the neck

vata one of the three doshas, which is said to govern the principle of movement and relates to the nervous system and the body's energy centre

vesicle small, sac-like blister

vibrations fine shaking, trembling or oscillating movements that are applied with one or both hands

Vishuddha the throat chakra, located at the base of the neck

vitiligo areas of the skin lacking pigmentation

vomer single bone at the back of the nasal septum

wart a benign growth on the skin caused by the human papilloma virus

weal a raised area of skin that contains fluid and is white in the centre, with a red edge

whiplash condition produced by damage to the muscles, ligaments, intervertebral discs or nerve tissues of the cervical region by sudden hyperextension and/or flexion of the neck

zygomatic bone facial bone forming the cheeks

zygomatic major and minor muscles lying in the cheek area, extending from the zygomatic bone to the angle of the mouth

Resources

For professional training courses, training DVDs and resources

Helen McGuinness Health and Beauty Training International
103 Bournemouth Rd
Chandlers Ford
Eastleigh
Hampshire SO53 3AZ
Tel: 02380 266448
www.helenmcguinness.com

For a selection of authentic Indian massage and hair oils

Ayurveda Limited
Beacon House
Willow Walk
Skelmersdale
Lancashire WN8 6UR
Tel: 01695 51015
Fax: 01695 50917
www.maharishi.co.uk/index.html

For an extensive range of therapy books and DVDs

Willen Limited
Three Crowns Yard
High Street
Market Harborough
Leicestershire LE16 7AF
Tel: 01858 410233
www.willenbooks.co.uk

DVDs

Indian Head Massage DVD
Helen McGuinness
A demonstration of a professional Indian head massage that covers the area around the upper back, neck, scalp, shoulders, arms and face. This DVD is suitable for those studying for a professional qualification and as a reference for qualified professionals.

Further reading

Aldred, Elaine Mary
A Guide to Starting your own Complementary Therapy Practice: A Manual for the Complementary Healthcare Profession
Churchill Livingstone (2006)
ISBN 978 0 443 10309 4

Brennan, Dr Donn
Live Better: Ayurveda Remedies and Inspirations for Well-being
Duncan Baird Publishers (2006)
ISBN 978 1 844 83291 0

Cash, Mel and Wadmore, Anne
The Pocket Atlas of the Moving Body
Ebury Press (1999)
ISBN 978 0 091 86512 2

Davis, Martha and Robbins Eshelman, Elizabeth
Relaxation and Stress Reduction Workbook
New Harbinger Publications, US, 6th rev. edn (2008)
ISBN 978 1 572 24549 5

Edwards, Paul, Edwards, Sarah and Clampitt Douglass, Laura
Getting Business to Come to You: Complete Do-it-yourself Guide to Attracting All the Business You Can Handle
T P Tarcher (1998)
ISBN 978 0 874 77845 8

Frawley, David, Ranade, Subhash and Lele, Avinash
Ayurveda and Marma Therapy: Energy Points in Yogic Healing
Lotus Press (2004)
ISBN 978 0 940 98559 9

Gardner, Joy
Vibrational Healing through the Chakras
Celestial Arts, Ten Speed Press (2005)
ISBN 978 1 580 91166 5

Gardner-Gordon, Joy
Pocket Guide to the Chakras
Pilgrims Publishing (2002)
ISBN 978 8 173 03221 9

Goodheart, Herbert P.
Goodheart's Photoguide to Common Skin Disorders: Diagnosis and Management
Lippincott Williams and Wilkins, 3rd rev. edn (2008)
ISBN 978 0 781 77143 6

Hayden, C.J.
Get Clients Now! A 28-Day Marketing Program for Professionals, Consultants, and Coaches
Amacom, 2nd edn (2006)
ISBN 978 0 814 47374 0

Heighway, Penny, Duncan, Mary and Chadder, Paul
Health and Safety at Work Essentials
Lawpack Publishing Ltd, 6th rev. edn (2010)
ISBN 978 1 906 97137 3

Jenkins, Gail, Kemnitz, Christopher and Tortora, Gerard J.
Anatomy and Physiology: From Science to Life
John Wiley & Sons, 3rd edn International Student Version (2012)
ISBN 978 1 118 09245 3

Johari, Harish
Ayurvedic Massage: Traditional Indian Techniques for Balancing Body and Mind
Healing Arts Press, Inner Traditions, Bear and Company (1996)
ISBN 978 0 892 81489 3

Johari, Harish
Chakras: Energy Centers of Transformation
Destiny Books, Inner Traditions, Bear and Company, rev. and enlarged edn (2000)
ISBN 978 0 892 81760 3

Kingsley, Philip
The Hair Bible
Aurum Press Ltd, new edn (2003)
ISBN 978 1 854 10906 4

McGuinness, Helen
Anatomy and Physiology: Therapy Basics
Hodder Education, 4th edn (2010)
ISBN 978 1 444 10923 8
www.hoddereducation.com

McGuinness, Helen
Facials and Skin Care in Essence (In Essence series)
Hodder Education (2007)
ISBN 978 0 340 92693 2
www.hoddereducation.com

Mehta, Narendra
Thorsons First Directions: Indian Head Massage
HarperCollins (2001)
ISBN 978 0 007 12356 8

Mehta, Narendra and Mehta, Kundan
The Face Lift Massage: Rejuvenate your Skin and Reduce Fine Lines and Wrinkles
HarperCollins (2004)
ISBN 978 0 007 15741 9

Mitchell, Tim and Kennedy, Cameron
Common Skin Disorders: Your Questions Answered
Churchill Livingstone (2005)
ISBN 978 0 443 07463 9

Premkumar, Kalyani
Pathology A to Z: A Handbook for Massage Therapists
Lippincott Williams and Wilkins, 2nd edn (2002)
ISBN 978 0 781 74098 2

Rickman, Cheryl D. and Roddick, Dame Anita
The Small Business Start-up Workbook: A Step-by-step Guide to Starting the Business you've Dreamed of
How To Books Ltd (2005)
ISBN 978 1 845 28038 3

Tortora, Gerard J.
Principles of Anatomy and Physiology
John Wiley & Sons, 13th international student edn, 2 vols (2011)
ISBN 978 0 470 92918 6

Turkington, Carol and Dover, Jeffrey S.
The Encyclopedia of Skin and Skin Disorders
Facts on File Inc., 3rd edn (2006)
ISBN 978 0 816 06403 8

Werner, Ruth
Massage Therapist's Guide to Pathology
Lippincott Williams & Wilkins, US, 4th rev, edn (2008)
ISBN 978 0 781 76919 8

Williams, Sara
The Financial Times Guide to Business Start-up 2012 (The FT Guides)
Financial Times/Prentice Hall, 7th edn (2011)
ISBN 978 0 273 76199 0

To access a list of useful weblinks scan the QR code opposite or visit www.hodderplus.co.uk/indianhead.

Index

Page numbers in *italics* represent illustrations. The abbreviation IHM refers to Indian head massage.